Mummies, magic and medicine in ancient Egypt

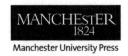

MANCHESTER
1824

Manchester University Press

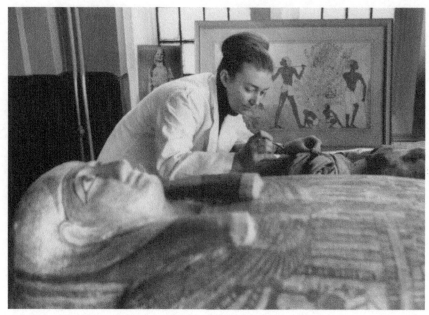

Rosalie David, c. 1974. (Courtesy of Manchester Museum,
University of Manchester.)

Mummies, magic and medicine in ancient Egypt

Multidisciplinary essays for Rosalie David

Edited by Campbell Price, Roger Forshaw,
Andrew Chamberlain and Paul T. Nicholson

with

Robert Morkot and Joyce Tyldesley

Manchester University Press

Published by Manchester University Press
Altrincham Street, Manchester M1 7JA, UK
www.manchesteruniversitypress.co.uk

British Library Cataloguing-in-Publication Data is available

ISBN 978 1 7849 9243 9 hardback

ISBN 978 1 7849 9244 6 paperback

First published by Manchester University Press in hardback 2016

This edition first published 2018

The publisher has no responsibility for the persistence or accuracy of URLs for any external or third-party internet websites referred to in this book, and does not guarantee that any content on such websites is, or will remain, accurate or appropriate.

Printed by TJ Books Limited, Padstow

To Rosalie and in memory of Antony

Contents

I: Pharaonic sacred landscapes

II: Magico-medical practices in ancient Egypt

III: Understanding Egyptian mummies

IV: Science and experimental approaches in Egyptology

Figures

Plates

following p. 226

Every effort has been made to obtain permission to reproduce copyright material, and the publisher will be pleased to be informed of any errors and omissions for correction in future editions.

Tables

Notes on contributors

Judith Adams qualified at University College Hospital London; after medical posts in Cambridge she began her radiology career in Manchester Royal Infirmary and the University of Manchester, where she is a consultant and professor of radiology. She is a musculo-skeletal radiologist with special interests in imaging of metabolic and endocrine diseases, in particular osteoporosis, and in quantitative methods of assessment of the skeleton, on which topics she has published widely. She has been involved in imaging of mummies, of both humans and animals, for over twenty years and has supervised students undertaking research projects in this field.

Carol Andrews was Assistant Keeper and Senior Research Assistant in the Department of Egyptian Antiquities at the British Museum from 1971 until 2000 and was closely involved with the Tutankhamun Exhibition. From 2000 until 2012 she tutored various Egyptology courses for Birkbeck College, University of London. She has written books on mummification and funerary artefacts, Egyptian jewellery, Egyptian amulets and the Rosetta Stone, provided catalogue entries on Egyptian glass, compiled a catalogue of demotic papyri for the Egyptian Exhibition which toured the Far East in 1999 and edited a translation of the Book of the Dead.

Stephanie Atherton-Woolham is a Research Associate at the KNH Centre for Biomedical Egyptology, University of Manchester. She has co-curated the Ancient Egyptian Animal Bio Bank project since its inception in 2011 and is Honorary Curator of Archaeozoology at the Manchester Museum. Her research focuses on bird mummification practices in ancient Egypt using imaging (radiographic and microscopic) techniques. She is particularly interested in the direct treatment of the bird body, especially the practical and ritual uses of resins and linen, alongside the chronological development of wrapping styles and techniques in animals and humans during the Late and Roman Periods.

Don Brothwell has been interested in the biology of the ancient Egyptians since he was a young graduate. He has published on various aspects, and co-edited with B. Chiarelli *Population Biology of the Ancient Egyptians* (1973). Mummy studies have taken him to various museums, as well as to the Valley of the Kings. He is currently Emeritus Professor of Archaeological Science in the University of York.

Andrew Chamberlain is Professor of Bioarchaeology and Director of the KNH Centre for Biomedical Egyptology at the University of Manchester. He has research interests in osteoarchaeology and biological anthropology, including the natural and artificial processes that influence the preservation of mummified organic materials, and he undertakes investigations in palaeodemography, the study of the composition and dynamics of past populations.

Jenefer Cockitt has studied ancient Egyptian mummies since 2001 and has completed a PhD in biomedical Egyptology at the University of Manchester, focusing on the radiocarbon dating of ancient Egyptian artefacts. She has undertaken research projects on experimental mummification and ancient Nubian human remains, and is currently reinvestigating the autopsy of Manchester mummy 1770.

Mark Collier was an undergraduate and doctoral student at University College London, and held postdoctoral positions at Corpus Christi College, Cambridge (concurrent with a British Academy postdoctoral fellowship), and then All Souls College, Oxford, before taking up a post at the University of Liverpool, where is he now Professor of Egyptology.

Robert Connolly joined the research staff of the University of Liverpool in 1961 initially at the School of Tropical Medicine, subsequently moving to Pathology and finally to Anatomy. Here, between teaching assignments, most of his research time was spent on Bronze Age, Anglo-Saxon, and medieval bone assemblages plus the Anne Mowbray–Princes in the Tower project, but then he became 'swept up' in Egyptology. Egyptology was interrupted in 1984 while he began excavating and working on Lindow Man, but now he is mainly involved with Egyptology once again.

David Counsell qualified in medicine at Leicester in 1982 and became a consultant cardiothoracic anaesthetist at Blackpool in 1991. From 2001 he was a consultant in Wrexham and from 2010 to 2015 Chief of Staff in Anaesthetics, Pain and Critical Care at Nuffield Health, The Grosvenor Hospital. He obtained the Certificate in Egyptology at the University of Manchester in 1996 and was awarded a PhD for his research into drug and intoxicant use in ancient Egypt. He became an Honorary Research Associate at the KNH Centre for Biomedical Egyptology at Manchester University and has lectured, published papers and made television appearances relating to opium, the blue lotus, cocaine, nicotine and the death of Tutankhamun.

Alan Curry obtained a BSc (zoology) in 1970 and a PhD (protozoology) in 1974 from the University of Manchester. He was appointed in 1973 to run the newly established electron microscopy unit at Withington Hospital, south Manchester. This unit was a joint Public Health Laboratory Service (later Health Protection Agency) and Department of Histopathology facility undertaking both diagnostic and research work. With the closure of Withington Hospital, the electron microscopy unit was relocated to Manchester Royal Infirmary in 2001. He was appointed an honorary university lecturer while at Manchester Royal Infirmary and retired in 2011 as a consultant clinical scientist.

John Denton's interest in biomedical Egyptology was kindled in 1974 after he met Rosalie David for the first time. Many years later he became a member of the newly opened KNH Centre for Biomedical Egyptology at the University of Manchester, where he was a supervisor for MSc and PhD students and contributed to the application of the field of modern histological techniques to that of ancient tissues. His Manchester University career started in 1967 when he was a technician in the Department of Rheumatology, and ended in 2011 when he retired as a senior pathology research fellow in the Department of Pathological Sciences.

Aidan Dodson is a Senior Research Fellow in the Department of Archaeology and Anthropology at the University of Bristol, and was Simpson Professor of Egyptology at the American University in Cairo for the spring semester of 2013. A graduate of Liverpool and Cambridge Universities, he was elected a Fellow of the Society of Antiquaries of London in 2003, and Chairman of Trustees of the Egypt Exploration Society in 2011.

Tosha L. Dupras is a Professor and Chair of Anthropology at the University of Central Florida. She received her PhD (1999) in anthropology from McMaster University (Ontario, Canada). She specialises in bioarchaeology, growth and development, dietary studies through isotopic analysis, palaeopathology, juvenile osteology and forensic archaeology. Dr Dupras conducts research at sites in the Sudan, Lithuania and south-east Asia, and has been a member of the Dakhleh Oasis Project (Egypt) since 1996 and a member of the expedition at Deir al Barsha (Egypt) since 2004.

Essam El Saeed is a Professor of Egyptology at Alexandria University, Director of the Writing and Scripts Center, Bibliotheca Alexandria, and the Director of the Coptic Institute at Alexandria University. Previously he was the cultural attaché in the Egyptian Embassy in Mauritania, and Director of the Egyptian Embassy in Nouakchott, Mauritania. From 2007 to 2014 he occupied the position of Honorary Scientific Visitor at the KNH Centre for Biomedical Egyptology at the University of Manchester.

Roger Forshaw, a retired dental surgeon, obtained an MSc in biomedical Egyptology and a PhD in Egyptology from the University of Manchester. He is a Research Associate at the KNH Centre for Biomedical Egyptology, where he has investigated the dental remains excavated by the first Archaeological Survey of Nubia and is currently examining mummy computed tomography scans for evidence of dental palaeopathology. He has published papers on healing practices as well as on dental disease and dental treatment in ancient Egypt. A recent published monograph is *The Role of the Lector in Ancient Egyptian Society* (2014).

Glenn Godenho took various Egyptological courses with Birkbeck College, London, in the mid- to late 1990s before studying for his BA, MA and PhD at the University of Liverpool. Following a one-year teaching post at Swansea University, he is now a Senior Lecturer in Egyptology at the University of Liverpool with additional responsibility for admissions and widening participation, and contributes to the online Egyptological initiatives run by Dr Joyce Tyldesley at the University of Manchester.

Mervyn Harris qualified as a dentist in 1971 and worked in that field for twenty-eight years. Following his retirement, he returned to university, where he obtained an MA in health care law and ethics in 1999, followed by an MSc and PhD in biomedical Egyptology from the University of Manchester in 2002 and 2006 respectively. His research interests include skeletal manifestations of systemic disease and interpretation of trauma in skeletal remains.

Rosalind Janssen is currently a Lecturer in education at the Institute of Education, University College London. She was previously a curator in the Petrie Museum, London, and then a lecturer in Egyptology at the Institute of Archaeology, London. She specialises in textiles and dress, ancient Egyptian social life and the recording of oral histories of Egyptology.

Diane Johnson is a Postdoctoral Research Associate based in the Department of Physical Sciences at the Open University. She has a special interest in the application of advanced analytical technology to ancient materials; her major areas of research are iron meteorites and iron in ancient Egypt. Diane completed the University of Manchester Certificate in Egyptology and is now studying for a Diploma in Egyptology.

Richard Johnston is a Senior Lecturer in the Materials Research Centre, Swansea University. Embracing a multidisciplinary approach, Richard's research has taken him from artificial intelligence in manufacturing, through gas turbine materials (abradables, nickel superalloys, ceramic matrix composites), and on to X-ray microtomography. He is Co-Director of the Advanced Imaging of Materials Centre at Swansea, collaborating with marine biologists, osteologists, bioengineers, Egyptologists, clinicians, glaciologists, and corrosion scientists among many others on broad research challenges in imaging.

Patricia Lambert-Zazulak qualified as a medical radiographer and has a degree in comparative religion. Combining research in ancient medicine and theology and focusing on Egyptian mummification, she was awarded a PhD in the Department of Religions and Theology at the University of Manchester. As a postdoctoral research associate, then fellow, she dedicated nine years' work to the creation and curation of the International Ancient Egyptian Mummy Tissue Bank and its archive, during which she collected and documented many samples from international depositors, and assisted researchers in various disciplines.

Conni Lord graduated in 2012 with a PhD in Egyptology from the University of Manchester. She has an MA degree in Egyptology from Macquarie University and a MSc in biomedical Egyptology from the University of Manchester. She is currently a member of the Amarna Cemetery Excavation Team and works at the Nicholson Museum, University of Sydney, Australia.

Robert D. Loynes was born in Manchester and qualified as a medical doctor at the University of Liverpool in 1966. He then trained as an orthopaedic surgeon, becoming a consultant in orthopaedics, trauma and hand surgery in Staffordshire in 1977. After retirement he was awarded a PhD in Egyptology in 2014 at the University of Manchester. His main sphere of research is in the use of computed tomography scans to explore the methods of mummification used by the ancient Egyptians.

Susan Martin trained as a textile designer and then worked in a number of museums and galleries in the UK, before taking up her current post at the Manchester Museum in 1999. In the museum she works with the Human Cultures collections, focusing mainly on collection care, conservation and collection management. In 2008 she completed a PhD project, supervised by Rosalie David, researching the textiles used to wrap the Manchester Museum mummy known as 1770.

Lidija McKnight holds a BSc in archaeology from the University of York and an MSc and PhD in biomedical Egyptology from the University of Manchester. Since 1999, Lidija has conducted research into animal mummification, particularly through the application of non-invasive radiographic imaging, and has presented and published widely on the subject. As founder of the Ancient Egyptian Animal Bio Bank, Lidija has studied numerous museum collections in the UK, Europe and the USA. Lidija holds the position of Honorary Curator of Archaeozoology at the Manchester Museum.

Ryan Metcalfe works at the University of Manchester and has lectured on and researched a variety of subjects related to biomedical Egyptology. His major research interests are in the preservation of soft tissues, the effects of mummification on biomolecular and chemical analysis and the roles played by grain products in ancient Egyptian medicine.

Robert G. Morkot is a Senior Lecturer in Archaeology at the University of Exeter. He studied ancient history and Egyptology at University College London (1977–80), followed by postgraduate studies at London including a year at the Humboldt University, Berlin. He is a leading authority on the relationship between Pharaonic Egypt and Nubia (Kush), and on the 25th Dynasty. His other main areas of interest are Egypt and Libya, the historiography of Egypt and the reception of antiquity in Western Europe.

Paul T. Nicholson is Professor of Archaeology at Cardiff University, where he teaches courses on Egyptian archaeology and early technology. He has worked in Egypt since 1983 and has directed excavations at Amarna, Memphis and Saqqara as well as working at Berenike, Hatnub, Thebes and elsewhere. His work has involved the investigation of the Sacred Animal Necropolis at Saqqara as well as early crafts and industries, particularly faïence and glass. He has published extensively on these subjects, including co-editing *Ancient Egyptian Material and Technology* (Cambridge University Press, 2000) with Ian Shaw.

J. Peter Phillips earned a degree in natural philosophy from the University of Glasgow and then worked in IT at the University of Manchester, where he developed his spare-time interest in Egyptology and gained the Certificate in Egyptology with distinction under Rosalie David. The subject of his dissertation, 'The columns of Egypt', became the basis for a book with the same title published in 2002. He is editor of *Ancient Egypt Magazine* and Chairman of the Manchester Ancient Egypt Society.

Campbell Price undertook his BA, MA and PhD in Egyptology at the University of Liverpool, where he is now an Honorary Research Fellow. Since 2011 he has been the Curator of Egypt and Sudan at the Manchester Museum,

University of Manchester, one of the UK's largest Egyptology collections. His research interests focus on elite culture of the first millennium BC, in particular the functions of non-royal sculpture.

Stephen Quirke is Edwards Professor of Egyptian Archaeology and Philology at the Institute of Archaeology, University College London. His research interests include Egyptian handwriting; state institutions; ethics and history of archaeology and museums; and Middle Kingdom history, with a focus on manual labour, social class and gender. His publications include *Exploring Religion in Ancient Egypt* (2014), *Going Out in Daylight: peret m heru – the Ancient Egyptian Book of the Dead* (2013), *Hidden Hands: Egyptian Workforces in Petrie Excavation Archives 1880–1924* (2010), *Egyptian Literature 1800BC: Questions and Readings* (2004) and, with Mark Collier, *The UCL Lahun Papyri* (2002–06).

Peter Robinson is a geography and archaeology graduate of Lancaster and Manchester Universities, and has studied Egyptology under Professor Rosalie David on her extra-mural Certificate in Egyptology course at Manchester. He has since become an independent scholar, joining a number of local Egyptology societies, and a freelance lecturer. He has a continuing interest in the religion and afterlives of the ancient Egyptians, and has presented and published papers on the geographical and sacred landscapes within a number of Egyptian after-life texts.

Patricia Rutherford completed an honours degree in biological sciences at the University of Lancaster in 1995. While teaching anatomy and physiology at the Blackpool and Fylde College she studied part-time at the University of Manchester and obtained an MSc and PhD in biomedical Egyptology, focusing on the study of schistosomiasis.

Peter G. Sheldrick, is a semi-retired family physician resident in Chatham (Ontario, Canada). He is a research associate at the Royal Ontario Museum and a trustee of the Society for the Study of Egyptian Antiquities in Toronto. He has been a permanent member of the Dakhleh Oasis Project since 1979, participating every year since. He assists with the excavation and analysis of human remains but has also worked with the prehistorians, palaeontologists and other aspects of the project.

Steven Snape is a graduate (BA, PhD) of the University of Liverpool, where he is currently Reader in Egyptian Archaeology. He is also Director of the Liverpool University Mission to Zawiyet Umm el-Rakham and Director of the Garstang Museum of Archaeology.

Denys Stocks completed a five-year technical apprenticeship in mechanical engineering. He was later awarded the University of Manchester Certificate in Egyptology (with distinction), which led to a research degree of MPhil and a Post-Graduate Certificate in Education from the Victoria University of Manchester. A post followed as a high-school teacher of design and technology and history. Stock has published *Experiments in Egyptian Archaeology: Stoneworking Technology in Ancient Egypt* (2003). He has also published a number of papers, had entries in several encyclopedias and appeared in television documentaries.

Kasia Szpakowska is Associate Professor of Egyptology at Swansea University, Fellow of the Society of Antiquaries and Director of the Ancient Egyptian Demonology Project, Second Millennium BC. She specialises in ancient Egyptian *Behind Closed Eyes* private religious practices, dreams, gender and the archaeology of magic. Her monographs include: *Dreams and Nightmares in Ancient Egypt* (2003) and *Daily Life in Ancient Egypt: Recreating Lahun* (2007). She is an avid proponent of interdisciplinary research and digital humanities, and her projects involve engineers, artists, glaciologists, computer scientists and developing an online database of liminal entities with 3D visualisation. Her current research interests include apotropaic devices and the iconography of "demonic" entities.

John H. Taylor is Assistant Keeper in the Department of Ancient Egypt and Sudan at the British Museum. Since joining the museum in 1988 he has published extensively on numerous aspects of ancient Egyptian funerary practices, particularly coffins, mummies and the Book of the Dead. He has curated several major exhibitions on these and other themes. His interests also include the Third Intermediate Period, the study of ancient bronze-working, the history of Egyptology and the formation of museum collections.

Angela Thomas studied Egyptology at the University of Liverpool and University College London. She spent her working life as a museum curator. From 2006 to 2012 she was a part-time honorary teaching fellow at the KNH Centre for Biomedical Egyptology, University of Manchester. She is the author of *Gurob: A New Kingdom Town*, two books in the Shire Egyptology Series and articles in a variety of journals.

Philip J. Turner was encouraged by Professor David on his retirement from clinical biology to pursue his interest in Egyptology, which culminated in the award by Manchester University of his PhD in 2013 for his studies on the god Seth. He and Professor David are now hoping to work together on the incidence of schistosomiasis in Ancient Egypt.

Joyce Tyldesley is a Senior Lecturer in Egyptology at the University of Manchester, where she teaches a suite of online courses to students around the world. She is the author of a number of Egyptology books written for both adults and children. Her most recent book, *Tutankhamen's Curse* (published in the USA as *Tutankhamen: The Search for an Egyptian King*) won the 2014 Felicia A. Holton Book Award, presented by the Archaeological Institute of America.

Sandra M. Wheeler is a Lecturer in Anthropology at the University of Central Florida, where she teaches courses in biological anthropology, archaeology and cultural anthropology. She received her PhD (2009) in anthropology from Western University (Ontario, Canada). She specialises in bioarchaeology, palaeopathology, juvenile osteology and mortuary archaeology. She has conducted fieldwork in Belize and Mexico, and continues to work with the Dakhleh Oasis Project in Egypt.

Lana J. Williams is a Lecturer in Anthropology at the University of Central Florida, where she teaches courses in biological anthropology, archaeology and cultural anthropology. She received her PhD (2008) in anthropology from Western University (Ontario, Canada). She specialises in stable isotope analysis, bioarchaeology, palaeopathology and mortuary archaeology. She conducts research in Turkey, and is a member of the bioarchaeology team of the Dakhleh Oasis Project, and also of the expedition at Deir al Barsha.

Penny Wilson is a Senior Lecturer in Egyptian Archaeology in the Department of Archaeology, Durham University. She is Field Director of the 'Royal City of Sais' Project and also part of the Egypt Exploration Society Delta Survey team currently in Kafr el Sheikh province and the site of Tell Mutubis. Her research interests include settlement archaeology in the Delta of all periods including the present day, cult practices in temples and shrines and ceramic assemblages and their stories.

Preface

Professor Rosalie David OBE has made a significant contribution to Egyptology both within Manchester University and far beyond. Presented on the occasion of her seventieth birthday in May 2016, this volume reflects the major Egyptological themes that have characterised Rosalie's academic career. 'Pharaonic sacred landscapes' addresses the ways in which the ancient inhabitants of the Nile valley conceptualised their landscape – funerary, ritual, mythic – and is a reminder that Rosalie's doctoral research involved a detailed study of the hieroglyphic inscriptions in the Sety I temple at Abydos; 'Magico-medical practices in ancient Egypt' includes contributions that represent her lifelong interest in Dynastic pharmacy and medicine; 'Understanding Egyptian mummies' reflects the pioneering work of the Manchester Museum Mummy Project, which Rosalie initiated, and the subsequent application of the 'Manchester method' to the study of mummified remains elsewhere; chapters presented under the heading 'Science and experimental approaches in Egyptology' stand testament to Rosalie's innovative approach to understanding ancient materials and technologies.

But these academic themes, and Rosalie's many books and articles, are not the whole story. Away from her laboratories and museum galleries, Rosalie has worked tirelessly to bring Egyptology – once perceived as the rather dull preserve of elderly gentlemen – to the widest possible audience. This has involved everything from formal teaching sessions through numerous television and radio appearances to advising awestruck schoolchildren on their future careers. By inspiring others to study the past she has brought great joy into many lives, and for this she is respected and admired throughout the world.

We hope that Rosalie will enjoy reading these articles written by colleagues who have benefited from her teaching, research and friendship. Many others would have liked to contribute, but were prevented from doing so by the constraints of time and space. They all send their best wishes to the 'Mummy Lady'. Happy birthday, Rosalie!

Campbell Price, Roger Forshaw, Andrew Chamberlain, Paul T. Nicholson, Robert G. Morkot and Joyce Tyldesley

Rosalie David: a biographical sketch

Joyce Tyldesley

Ann Rosalie David was born in Cardiff, Wales, in 1946, to parents Idris and Edna. Her father was a captain in the Merchant Navy, and it was perhaps from him that she inherited her fascination with travel and all things foreign. Her interest in Egyptology was first sparked at primary school, when a teacher talked about ancient Egypt and showed what Rosalie later realised was a reconstruction drawing of the three Abusir pyramids. This inspired the six-year-old Rosalie to tell her parents that she wanted to spend her life studying ancient Egypt. Clearly she already possessed the determination that would characterise her academic career, as she never changed her mind.

Aged eleven, Rosalie won a scholarship to Howell's School, Llandaff, Cardiff, which focused on the Classics. Still determined on a career as an Egyptologist, Rosalie selected subjects relevant to Egyptology. Avoiding games as much as possible, she studied Greek and Latin. Her holidays were spent working in the National Museum of Wales as a volunteer.

Rosalie first visited Egypt aged nineteen when, as an undergraduate student at University College London (UCL), she was awarded a travel grant donated by an anonymous American. She was able to see all the usual sites – and many unusual sites not normally visited by tourists – and this confirmed her impression that she was indeed studying the right subject. She found that she loved Egypt from the outset, both as a country and as a subject for academic study.

Rosalie had chosen to study at UCL because it offered a degree that included Egyptology as part of a wider study of the ancient world. One of just six students, and the only student to specialise in ancient Egypt, she had the valuable – but daunting – experience of individual tuition from the great philologist Raymond Faulkner. She graduated from UCL in 1967, and moved to the University of Liverpool to study for a PhD with Herbert Fairman. She took as her subject religious ritual within the Egyptian temple, focusing on inscriptions on the Abydos temple of Sety I. This required an extended stay at Abydos, where often she and the famous Omm Sety were the only temple visitors. On one occasion she overheard Omm Sety, in conversation with the son of King Farouk, describe her as the 'little lady Beatle from Liverpool' – this being the 1960s, and the height of Beatle-mania.

Back in Liverpool, Rosalie undertook some undergraduate teaching, following Fairman's good if somewhat brief advice to 'sit in front of the class, and if they begin to look bored, change tack'. At the same time she started to become involved in adult education, teaching evening classes around the north-west of England. She discovered this to be a very different form of teaching: challenging, exciting and, when done correctly, very rewarding. This experience – and her awareness of the great public interest in ancient Egypt – would eventually lead to the establishment of the internationally renowned Certificate in Egyptology at the University of Manchester. The certificate, which started life as a conventional taught course, then evolved via a postal course to be fully online, is today one of a suite of online courses taught from Egyptology Online in the University of Manchester. Many Egyptologists, amateur and professional alike, have gained their first glimpse of ancient Egypt through Rosalie's certificate course.

After nine months working at the Petrie Museum in London, Rosalie joined the Manchester Museum as Assistant Keeper of Archaeology in 1972. In so doing she became the latest in a line of women Egyptologists, starting with the formidable Margaret Murray, to take charge of the Manchester collection. She found the entire collection inspiring, but it was the mummies which really interested her. This was unusual. Egyptologists, in the 1970s, tended to avoid mummies, regarding them as rather tasteless objects of public fascination unsuitable for academic study. But Rosalie recognised that the mummies were essentially desiccated bundles of information, and realised that Manchester University, with its close links between the museum, the hospital and the medical teaching departments, was an ideal place to pursue a programme of serious academic mummy studies.

The Manchester Museum Mummy Project was established with the help of various experts throughout the university. Its two main aims were to look for evidence of disease and cause of death while gaining evidence of life and death in ancient Egypt, and to develop a standard method of examining ancient human remains that could be used worldwide. Work started with the re-examination of the 'Two Brothers', mummies originally autopsied by Margaret Murray seventy years previously. Then 1770, a mummy in a very poor state of preservation, was unwrapped and autopsied in June 1975. This, thanks to the involvement of television, brought mummy studies to the wider public. It even inspired a political cartoon in the *Daily Telegraph*, which showed Prime Minister Harold Wilson unwrapping a mummy labelled 'The Social Contract'.

Her groundbreaking mummy work led to the award of a personal chair in 2000 and her appointment as Officer of the Order of the British Empire (OBE) in 2003 for services to Egyptology. It also led to the establishment of a master's degree in biomedical Egyptology, which would allow the Mummy Project team to pass on their expertise to future generations of scientists. Out of this grew the KNH Centre for Biomedical Egyptology within the Faculty of Life Sciences at the University of Manchester. The centre was opened in 2003 with two ceremonies, attended by the Earl of Wessex and the Egyptian Consul General. Subsequently, it has published groundbreaking research on projects as diverse as Egyptian pharmacy (demonstrating that the remedies used by the ancient Egyptians were indeed effective), animal mummies and the work of Grafton Elliot Smith.

Rosalie's considerable achievements are, of course, all her own. But she has asked me to mention here two very special people whose support has been invaluable, and 'I can't imagine how everything would have developed without them!'

The first is Kay Hinckley, who was a passenger on a Swan Hellenic Nile cruise on which Rosalie was guest lecturer in the 1990s. From this initial meeting arose Kay's great interest in the biomedical mummy studies being carried out at Manchester. Kay was to provide considerable financial support for Egyptology at Manchester University over many years. At first, this was focussed on research into schistosomiasis in ancient Egypt, and then, in 2003, her patronage enabled the university to establish the KNH Centre for Biomedical Egyptology (an institution which carries her initials).

The second special person is Rosalie's late husband, Antony Edward David. Antony gained a degree in Egyptology from Cairo University and the Diploma in Archaeological Conservation from the Institute of Archaeology, University of London. He met Rosalie in Egypt 1969, and they were married in Alexandria and Cardiff in 1970. Antony then pursued a very successful career in archaeological conservation, retiring in 2004 from his position as Head of Conservation for Lancashire County Museums Service. His research interests included the conservation and preservation of mummies, and he shared joint publications with Rosalie on mummies and other Egyptological subjects.

In 2012 Rosalie retired as Director of the KNH Centre, assuming the title of Professor Emerita. She assures me that this is not so much a retirement as a freedom from university administration that will allow her the opportunity to catch up with her writing. I have no doubt that she will continue to enrich the field of Egyptology for many years to come.

My first meeting with Rosalie David

Kay Hinckley

When I think of the wonderful character and ability of Rosalie David, I cannot help but feel that it was no accident that our lives crossed. People are often sent at the right time in one's life to give a clear direction and help enhance the future.

Rosalie and I first met when I was a passenger on a Nile boat where she was a lecturer. I was amazed at the number of lectures she gave and, indeed, by the wonderful support given to Rosalie by her late husband Antony. Through a mutual friend we soon became very close. I was so interested in her lectures that I took notes and, having read them, Rosalie suggested that I join her Certificate of Egyptology course at the University of Manchester. It was wonderful to have a year of excellent teaching, which I thoroughly enjoyed. The present certificate course is delivered by Joyce Tyldesley, another clever Egyptologist and an example of Rosalie's fine judgement of people.

The KNH Centre for Biomedical Egyptology was born at a table in Christie's Bistro, Manchester University, where Rosalie told me the history of Egyptology at Manchester, and gave me her vision for the future. Afterwards I felt that here was another Jesse Haworth and Flinders Petrie partnership. I was attracted by the possibility of enabling young and clever people to achieve their interests and fulfil their talents. It was very pleasing to be able to endow a chair in a field that Manchester did not previously have: a chair in Egyptology had been an unfulfilled dream of Margaret Murray, and a reminder of the fact that many of Flinders Petrie's archaeological finds were donated to the museum by Jesse Howarth in the hope that they would form the basis of a teaching department.

We had an official opening of the KNH Centre by HRH Prince Edward, followed by an official dinner for the great and good of the university. Since then, my interest and financial support have been rewarded one thousand fold. The centre has gone from strength to strength and each member of the team has been totally admirable. We have even had a lovely romance among the centre staff! Rosalie and I wish her successor at the KNH Centre, Andrew Chamberlain, every success.

In the Valley of the Kings some years ago, Rosalie and I had just visited three tombs when a prominent Egyptian walked up to us and said, 'Ah Rosalie David; when you are in Egypt, she sings.' After thanking him sincerely, Rosalie turned to me and said, 'Come on Kay, we are going to a fourth tomb.' I think no finer tribute can be paid to a most remarkable career.

PART I

Pharaonic sacred landscapes

I

Go west: on the ancient means of approach to the Saqqara Necropolis

Aidan Dodson

I am delighted to offer this contribution in celebration of Rosalie David's career, particularly in my current role as Chairman of Trustees of the Egypt Exploration Society, in view of her role in founding the Northern Branch of the Society, and also for the way in which she has worked to bring Egyptology to the widest possible audience. The vitality of amateur Egyptology in the Greater Manchester area and beyond stands significantly to her credit.

The Egyptian ideal was that the physical and ritual journey to the next world would be a consistent one from east to west. However, this was sometimes complicated by the topography of the site chosen for a cemetery. Today, the tourist approach road to Saqqara (Figure 1.1) rises at a fairly gentle slope from close to the valley temple of Unas, to reach the plateau at a point above the southern end of the Bubastieion; from here, the road turns south-west, leading to the car park adjacent to the Step Pyramid. However, this route is bedded entirely on debris that has accumulated over the centuries against a steep escarpment, near the top of which 26th Dynasty rock-cut tomb chapels exist (LS23, LS24; Porter and Moss 1974–81: 588–91), with others doubtless buried below the level of the modern roadway. Accordingly, it is clear that while there may have been paths leading to and among tomb chapels in the area, this cannot have served anciently as a means of approaching the necropolis. This is further demonstrated by the location of the monuments on the Saqqara plateau itself: these were clearly located with reference to a number of ancient approach routes, the analysis of which is the subject of this chapter.

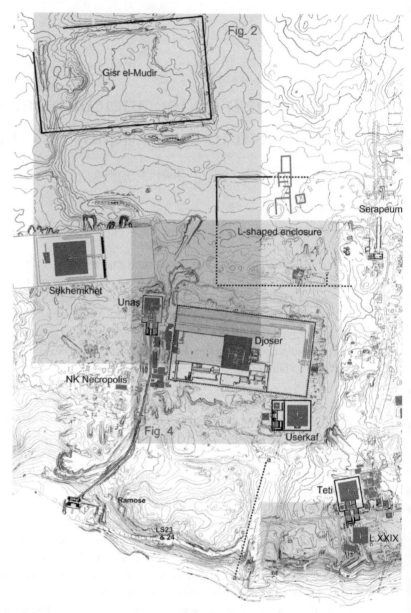

1.1 The North Saqqara necropolis. (Created by the author after Ministère de l'Habitat et de la Reconstruction, *Le Caire*, sheet H22.)

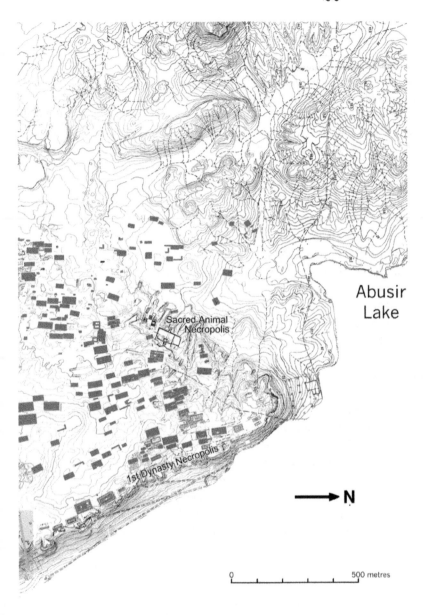

Abusir
Lake

Sacred Animal
Necropolis

1st Dynasty Necropolis

N

0   500 metres

The 2nd Dynasty royal tomb complexes

The earliest tombs at Saqqara stand on a high ridge that extends northward from the north-east corner of the plateau (Porter and Moss 1974–81: 435–47). Comprising the sepulchres of the highest non-kingly status of the 1st Dynasty, they were clearly intended to be visible from the new city of Memphis, directly below them to the east. To the west, the tombs overlooked a wide wadi that extended from what is now Abusir Lake (but in ancient times appears to have been low shelf of desert – Jeffreys 2001: 16) southward towards the site later occupied by the pyramid of Sekhemkhet. By – and probably long before – the Late Period this had become a formal processional way (cf. Davies and Smith 2005: 5), with the Sacred Animal Necropolis on its eastern flank.

As the ridge-top became increasingly full, tomb builders of the 2nd, 3rd and later dynasties of the Old Kingdom placed their own structures on the west-facing slope of wadi and, as this became congested, on its far western slope as well. Their willingness to do so, although wholly out of the view of the citizens of Memphis, further marks out the 'Abusir Wadi' as the principal direction of approach to the Saqqara necropolis (as already pointed out by Bárta and Vachala 2001, and Reader 2004: 63–7; cf. Martin 1989: 3; Awady 2009: 86–120).

This mode of approach explains much about the layout of the early 2nd Dynasty royal mortuary monuments at Saqqara (Figure 1.2). The subterranean parts of the tombs of Hetepsekhemwy and Ninetjer lie beyond the south-west corner of the Step Pyramid enclosure (Porter and Moss 1974–81: 613–14; Lacher 2008; Lacher-Raschdorff 2014), any superstructures having been obliterated by the building of the pyramid of Unas and its associated necropolis (but cf. Munro 1993; Lacher 2008: 431–3). Further into the desert lies a pair of huge rectangular enclosures (cf. Swelim 1991). Of these, the northern one (known as the 'L-Shaped Enclosure' from the prominence of its south-west corner in aerial photographs) possessed defining embankments that were composed of desert sand and gravel. Also incorporating brick and limestone traces, 140 m of the southern end of the west wall survive, together with probably 200 m of the south one (Mathieson and Tavares 1993: 27–8; cf. Spencer 1974: 3). Its full extent is unclear,[1] but the southern wall may have extended as far east as the southern end of the western arm of the so-called 'dry moat' of the Step Pyramid (discussed below).

The southern enclosure, known as the *Gisr el-Mudir* (Mathieson and Tavares 1993: 28–31; Mathieson *et al.* 1997; 1999: 36–41; Mathieson 2000), is of different

---

1   There are some indications on the ground that could suggest that it was actually square, but if these are unrelated to the enclosure, one would assume a rectangular form, with roughly the proportions of the Abydos enclosures, or the *Gisr el-Mudir*, discussed just below.

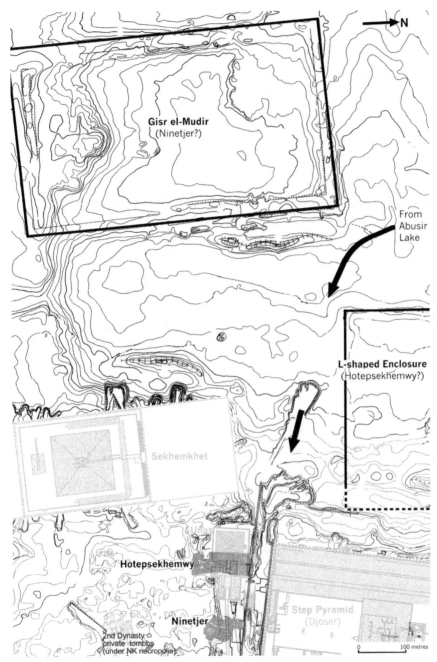

1.2 The area of the 2nd Dynasty royal tombs and enclosures. (Created by the author after Ministère de l'Habitat et de la Reconstruction, *Le Caire*, sheet H22.)

construction. Covering an area of some twenty-five hectares, it had fifteen-metre thick walls which comprised a mixed filling within pairs of walls of limestone blocks, still standing in places to a height of over three metres. The building technique of the latter is relatively primitive, supporting the 2nd–3rd Dynasty date suggested by pottery from the site. A prepared pavement extended at least 25 m from the wall inside the enclosure, but no trace of any structure at the centre has been identified. Given the lack of limestone walls in the construction of the perimeter of the L-Shaped Enclosure, this is likely to have been the earlier of the two monuments.

Given the aforementioned ceramic dating, and the presence of (brick) rectangular enclosures in association with the Early Dynastic royal tombs at Abydos, a correlation between the *two* enclosures and the *two* 2nd Dynasty royal tombs to their east is of course tempting, with the L-Shaped Enclosure potentially that of Hetepsekhemwy and the *Gisr el-Mudir* that of Ninetjer.[2] A problem has been, however, that while the Abydos enclosures lay adjacent to the processional route towards the tombs at Umm el-Qaab, those at Saqqara appear at first sight to reverse this relative positioning, thus undermining the parallelism and perhaps suggesting that another explanation might be needed for the Saqqara enclosures (e.g. the remarks of Awady 2009: 18). However, this 'problem' applies only if we view the tombs and enclosures from the 'modern' direction: if approached via the Abusir Wadi they are indeed interposed between the edge of the necropolis and the tombs with which they seem most likely to be associated.

It should be noted, however, that there has also been a tendency in recent years to date the *Gisr el-Mudir* to the end of the 2nd Dynasty, specifically to the time of Khasekhemwy (for references, see Regulski 2009: 226–7). It has been suggested that, rather than being associated with either of the known royal tombs at Saqqara, the *Gisr el-Mudir* may have been an arena for some kind of celebration linked with Khasekhemwy's reunification of Egypt, perhaps even a *sd*-festival (Regulski 2009: 227; Van Wetering 2004: 1071 attributes the L-Shaped Enclosure to Peribsen). However, this has been essentially based on a restrictive late 2nd–early 3rd Dynasty dating of the pottery found in the enclosure (complementing the presence of sealings of Khasekhemwy at the Step Pyramid complex), but one must question whether our understanding of pottery evolution during such an obscure period as the 2nd Dynasty is sufficiently

---

2   Although there is the complication of our lack of knowledge as to the location of the tomb of the king who seems to have ruled between them, Reneb, a stela of the type found outside royal tombs came onto the antiquities market in 1960, having allegedly been found at Mit Rahina (Metropolitan Museum of Art 60.144; Porter and Moss 1974–81: 870).

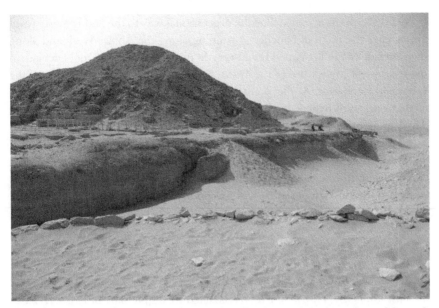

1.3 The western end of the rock-cutting forming the northern boundary of the 2nd
Dynasty royal burial precinct. (Photograph by the author.)

precise to rule out a date a decade or two earlier for the ceramics from the *Gisr*.[3]
It thus seems unwise to deny the distinctly suggestive dualism of the presence of
both a pair of enclosures and a pair of kings' tombs within a restricted area on
this subjective basis.

If our linking of the enclosures and the tombs is thus correct, their relative positions contribute to an explanation of the rock-cut trench that runs
parallel to, and just beyond, the southern edge of the Step Pyramid enclosure
(Figure 1.3). While this feature ultimately became part of the 'dry moat' around
the latter monument (see below), it seems clear that it actually predated the 3rd
Dynasty and was intimately connected with the tombs of Hetepsekhemwy and
Ninetjer, whose entrances were placed close to the rim of the southern wall of
the cutting and were orientated at right angles to it. Indeed, the cutting defines
the northern margin of a wide and deep graded area on which the 2nd Dynasty
royal tombs were constructed: a 2nd Dynasty royal burial precinct, raised up
above and separated from the area to the north.

3   It remains unclear how many years separate Ninetjer from Khasekhemwy, or even
    how the various royal names known from monuments (Sened; Sekhemib/Peribsen)
    and later sources relate to one another. It is clear that the latter half of the 2nd
    Dynasty was a time of civil war (cf. Gould 2003: 47–51), with the likelihood that some
    or all of the names represent contemporary rivals and the implication that the gap
    could perhaps be no more than a decade in real terms.

On this basis, one may define the processional way to the 2nd Dynasty royal tombs after the reign of Ninetjer as running along the Abusir Wadi and along the west side of the L-Shaped Enclosure. At this point, a visitor could deviate to the south-west to visit the *Gisr el-Mudir*, or turn left along the south side of the L-Shaped Enclosure. At this point, they would arrive at the south-east corner of that enclosure (where its principal entrance will have lain on the basis of Abydene parallels) and the beginning of the cutting, at which point steps or a ramp may have led up to the precinct occupied by the actual tombs. The approach route to the 2nd Dynasty private tombs that are now being revealed under the southern section of New Kingdom necropolis south of the Unas causeway (Regulski 2009, 2011) was presumably the same, but then along the west side of the tomb of Hetepsekhemwy.

The Step Pyramid and its 'moat'

As noted just above, what is seen here as a 2nd Dynasty confection had been (at least implicitly; cf. Swelim 1988) classified as simply part of a 3rd Dynasty work – the so-called 'dry moat' running around the Step Pyramid complex (Figure 1.4). The 'moat' separated the enclosure – and a wide area in front of the eastern wall – from the surrounding plateau by cuttings on all four sides, and thus should be seen as an extension of the concept of physical separation of the royal burial monument seen in the construction of the original 2nd Dynasty cutting. The 'moat' was not, however, complete; the south-eastern arm did not join the 2nd Dynasty cutting, but was placed a little further to the south, terminating to the east of the tomb of Ninetjer. This allowed for an access route from the 2nd Dynasty precinct into the new 3rd Dynasty one, the ancient approach to the Step Pyramid complex being thus an extension of the 2nd Dynasty route, ending on the wide terrace before the east front of the Step Pyramid enclosure, as defined by the eastern arm of the 'dry moat'.

This arrangement reinforced the status of the southern end of the Abusir Wadi as the place for a king to be seen dead in, something continued by Sekhemkhet, whose pyramid complex forms yet another part of the constellation of rectangular royal funerary enclosures apparently initiated by the L-Shaped Enclosure, the *Gisr el-Mudir* and the Step Pyramid. Interestingly, the complex of Sekhemkhet marks the last kingly tomb in the northern half of the Saqqara necropolis until the beginning of the 5th Dynasty: one wonders whether the fact that the end of the Abusir Wadi was now fully occupied by royal funerary monuments was a factor. Furthermore, the next pyramid after Sekhemkhet's, Khaba's Layer Pyramid at Zawiyet el-Aryan, moved not only to a new area, but also to a new kind of location, a raised site with a fairly easy slope down to the edge of the cultivation. Here there seems to have been no attempt to build

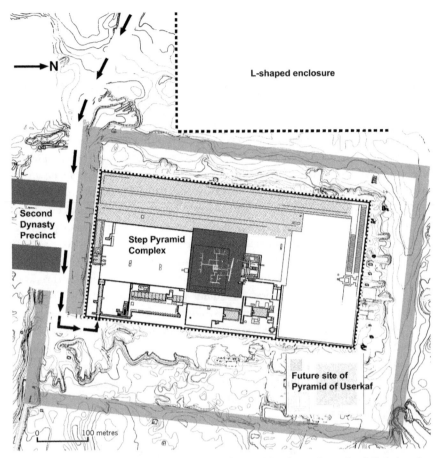

1.4 The 'dry moat' of the Step Pyramid. (Created by the author after Ministère de l'Habitat et de la Reconstruction, *Le Caire*, sheet H22.)

the kind of rectangular enclosure that had hitherto been standard in royal complexes, now-lost traces on the edge of the desert (Swelim 1983) suggesting that the Layer Pyramid may have been first to adopt the soon-standard pattern of an enclosure not much larger than the pyramid itself, now connected to the edge of the desert by an artificial causeway, rather than a natural wadi (cf. Reader 2004).

The aforementioned topography of the Saqqara escarpment was not well fitted to such an arrangement, and may thus have been a key reason why the kings of the later 3rd Dynasty, and then those of the 4th, put their tombs at the more suitable – that is, gentler-sloped – sites of Abu Rowash, Dahshur, Giza, Zawiyet el-Aryan and Saqqara-South. It was not until Userkaf came to build his pyramid that Saqqara-North once again hosted a king's tomb.

The pyramid complex of Userkaf

As has long been noted, the plan of the pyramid complex of Userkaf (Porter and Moss 1974–81: 397–8; Labrousse and Lauer 2000) is anomalous, with the majority of its mortuary temple placed south of the pyramid, and with only the offering-place itself located against the east face of the pyramid. The constraint involved is clear, as Userkaf built his monument on the wide terrace between the eastern enclosure wall of the Step Pyramid and the eastern arm of the latter's 'moat'. The arrangement adopted placed the entrance to the complex at the southern end of the eastern enclosure wall, the location employed in all royal rectangular funerary enclosures down to Sekhemkhet, and, at first sight, one might have considered that Userkaf might have employed the old 2nd and 3rd Dynasty approach route via the Abusir Wadi and the 2nd Dynasty precinct.

However, one of the blocks to the left of the entrance to the mortuary temple is cut in such a way as to indicate that an obliquely angled terminus for a causeway must have abutted it, while Perring mapped a 400-metre 'inclined road to [the Step and Userkaf] pyramids' – actually aligned towards that of Userkaf – which must have been the route of the middle section of Userkaf's causeway (Perring 1842: pl. VII). The 'road' is now partly lost under a section of a modern asphalt road, but its line has now been traced down as far as the twenty-metre contour (Labrousse and Lauer 2000: 40–1, fig. 39; see Figure 1.1 [a–a] above). Its lower end runs parallel to what Perring (followed by Maragioglio and Rinaldi 1970: 40–3) identified as an 'inclined causeway of crude bricks' – but what actually transpired to be the southern enclosure wall of the Late to Ptolemaic Bubastieion.[4] This parallelism of arrangement suggests that the orientation of the Bubastieion wall was purposely relative to that of Userkaf's causeway, and that the latter still formed an approach route in Late Period times. Its line represents one of the shallower descents from the plateau, although even here a 5 per cent slope is followed by one of 20 per cent to the edge of the cultivation. The access route provided by it may have influenced the development of the New Kingdom necropolis in the escarpment to the north, excavated by Zivie.

The upper part of the causeway, while almost flat, presents problems owing to the presence of the 'moat' between the temple and the upper end of the probable middle section, previously discussed. The two elements lie at the same level, leaving the question as to how the moat might have been bridged. Unfortunately, no remains have been recorded that might come from any structure that may have allowed the causeway to cross the approximately forty-metre gap (cf. Swelim 1988: 22; Labrousse and Lauer 2000: 41; Awady 2009: 106–7).

4 Jeffreys suggests that the Bubastieion wall was actually built over part of the Userkaf causeway (Jeffreys, Bourriau and Johnson 2000: 9).

As Swelim notes (1988: 22), the area within the moat to the north-west of Userkaf's pyramid was used extensively for the construction of tombs during the 5th Dynasty, and it would be interesting to know the mode of access to these structures – via the Userkaf causeway (however it bridged the moat), or via the old 3rd Dynasty route.

That the causeway remained usable until Saite times may be suggested by the use of the king's enclosure as a site for a series of large shaft tombs of that date (Porter and Moss 1974–81: 586–7). On the other hand, the attraction of an ancient monument in a time of archaism might have played a role, as it may also have done in the enclosure of Unas (see below).

The pyramid complexes of Menkauhor and Teti

The next attempt to access the Saqqara plateau from the east came towards the end of the 5th Dynasty, after the abandonment of the Abusir necropolis, presumably owing to a lack of remaining sites deemed suitable for another king's pyramid. At the beginning of the 6th Dynasty, Teti placed his pyramid 400 m north of the probable causeway route of Userkaf, but directly to the east lie the scanty remains of a pyramid (L.XXIX; Figure 1.5) whose dating has been a matter for debate for many years – yet whose date becomes clear when topographical and architectural data are combined.

The remains of L.XXIX were noted by Lepsius, and then examined on more than one occasion without adequate publication until fully excavated during 2005–08 (Hawass 2010). In the interim, the pyramid had been variously attributed to Menkauhor of the 5th Dynasty, to Merykare of the 10th Dynasty and to the Middle Kingdom, potentially for Amenemhat I (for references, see

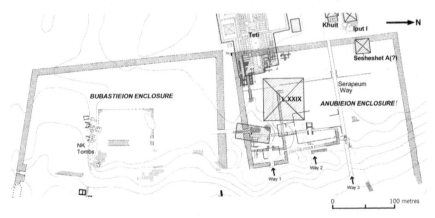

1.5 Plan of the Bubastieion/Anubieion area. (Adapted and augmented by the author from Jeffreys and Smith 1988, fig. 1.)

Hawass 2010: 159–61). However, it is now clear that the substructure possessed a distinctive oblique inner entrance passage, otherwise found only in the pyramids of Neferirkare, Neferefre and Niuserre at Abusir, together with the eastern store-room first found in the pyramid of Isesi. These features alone make it impossible to date the pyramid other than to Menkauhor, successor of Niuserre and predecessor of Isesi.

However, its chronological position is further assured by reference to the complex of Teti directly to the west, where the upper end of the causeway most unusually joined the mortuary temple at the southern extremity of its façade (Lauer and Leclant 1972: 10–12), clearly to allow the upper end of the causeway to bypass the southern face of L.XXIX.[5] The pyramid of Teti is also orientated eleven degrees away from the cardinal points (in contrast to the properly orientated L.XXIX), clearly because of the need to fit it into the otherwise unsuitable location required to allow the upper causeway to follow the desired line.

To judge from the angle at which it left Teti's mortuary temple, this first section of causeway ran parallel with the side of L.XXIX, and over part of the site of an earlier large stone mastaba,[6] probably late 3rd or 4th Dynasty (Quibell 1907: 1–2, pls. III–IV, VI; cf. Smith and Jeffreys 1978: 11), which lies close to the south-east corner of L.XXIX (see further below). However, any traces of the actual causeway in this area will have been lost as a result of Middle Kingdom, New Kingdom and Late Period construction work (Porter and Moss 1974–81: 558–90; Jeffreys and Smith 1988: 40–1).

While these arrangements could simply have been to allow the causeway of Teti's pyramid to avoid L.XXIX on its way down to the cultivation, the slightly earlier case of Niuserre's appropriation of the lower part of the causeway of Neferirkare at Abusir comes to mind. In this case the usurping king's mortuary temple layout also had to be adapted to allow the upper causeway to be aligned with the lower section of Neferirkare's. Given the relatively steep descent to the cultivation at this point (similar in profile to that for the putative causeway of Userkaf), it is likely that Teti's architect would have been keen to use a pre-existing structure that would presumably have already taken the optimum line off the plateau.

Unfortunately, no certain traces of any Old Kingdom causeway(s) leading on down to the edge of the cultivation have been recorded by any of those who

5   Some confusion continues to arise from Perring's erroneous identification (1842: pl. VII) of the walls of the Bubastieion as a causeway (cf. p. 12, above), implicitly that of Teti (e.g. Awady 2009: 114).

6   Cf. Quibell 1907: 1, who notes that the north-east corner always seems to have been exposed, owing to the differential patination as compared with the rest of the mastaba masonry.

have excavated in the area (for whom, see Jeffreys and Smith 1988: 1–2). The aforementioned buried mastaba has a section of a later linear feature of massive limestone adjacent to its north-west corner (Quibell 1907: ii; Jeffreys and Smith 1988: fig. 59; Hawass 2010: fig. 3), with 'underpinnings [that] deepen further east down the slope, presumably to create a gentler gradient' (David Jeffreys, personal communication, 3 September 2014): at first sight, this might seem to be the foundations of a causeway (as suggested in Jeffreys, Bourriau and Johnson 2000: 9). However, the feature's orientation does not line up with either the entrance to Teti's mortuary temple or any credible course of an upper cause-way from the actual entrance. It is also too far south-west to be associated with a causeway of L.XXIX and, indeed, apparently wrongly orientated to be the foundation of any part of that complex, as was observed by Jean-Philippe Lauer (Jeffreys, personal communication).

One wonders whether the lower end(s) of the L.XXIX/Teti causeway(s) might have coincided with any of the 'ways' dating from the Late to Ptolemaic Period that rose up through the Anubieion in a combination of ramps and stairs (Jeffreys and Smith 1988: fig. 62). The easternmost, Way 3, gave access to the Serapeum Way, which continued across the Saqqara plateau, and the place-ment of the valley building of Teti on such an axis might explain the large gap between his pyramid and those of his family, the two groups of monuments thus flanking the causeway where it crested the top of the escarpment. On the other hand, to reach this axis, the middle part of the causeway would have had to cut across the slope at an extreme angle, in contrast to Way 1, which lies between the axes of the Teti and L.XXIX pyramids and might thus be the most likely relict of the ancient axis (if any relict indeed remained within the layout of the Late to Ptolemaic Period).

Despite this lack of identifiable remains, it seems nevertheless clear that these Old Kingdom causeway(s) – or rebuildings thereof – formed a major means of access to the Saqqara plateau during the late Old, Middle and New Kingdoms, to judge from the concentration of tombs of these periods around Teti's pyramid, whether or not they were associated with that king's cult (Porter and Moss 1974–81: 508–73).

The pyramid complex of Unas

It is instructive that the major groups of New Kingdom tombs known at Saqqara all lie close to the probable course of an Old Kingdom pyramid causeway. The largest of these lie south of the causeway of Unas, a king whose whole complex is an illustration of the problems of building a pyramid of post-3rd Dynasty type at Saqqara-North. First, the causeway (Porter and Moss 1974–81: 417; Labrousse and Moussa 2002; Awady 2009: 110–14) needed to connect a viable building spot to the edge of the cultivation three quarters of a kilometre long, around twice the length of the second longest causeway, that of Pepy II. Second, that viable pyramid building spot was actually the 2nd Dynasty precinct adjacent to the Step Pyramid, requiring the demolition of the superstructures of these ancient monuments to make way for the pyramid and mortuary temple; many lesser tombs were also dismantled or buried under the course of the causeway itself. Third, a need or desire to keep within the predetermined bounds of this precinct meant that the pyramid of Unas was constrained within dimensions some 25 per cent smaller than the preceding and succeeding pyramids.

A cemetery of mastabas was erected south of the causeway of Unas (demolished in whole or part when New Kingdom tombs were built in the area – cf. Martin 1989: 133–4), but it is unclear whether this represented a new foundation following the opening-up of the area by the building of the causeway, or whether they were a continuation the 2nd Dynasty private necropolis mentioned above, presumably accessed like it via the Abusir Wadi.

The access route provided by the Unas causeway is likely to be a reason for the use of the area of the king's mortuary temple for large shaft tombs of the late 26th to early 27th Dynasties (Porter and Moss 1974–81: 648–51). It is likely that similar considerations applied at Giza, where a number of tombs of the period concentrate on the causeway of Khaefre (Porter and Moss 1974–81: 289–91; Sadeek 1984: 103–48; Hawass 2007).

It may thus be seen that a consideration of the modes of approach to the Saqqara necropolis can provide useful insights into the chronological and spatial relationships between monuments at the site and contribute to their individual characterisation. This emphasises the importance of zooming out from a particular monument to look at its relationship with other monuments and the overall landscape within which they were constructed – and also at changes in that landscape over time (cf. Graham 2010).

Acknowledgement

I am most grateful to Dr David Jeffreys for discussing his 1970s discoveries and their implications with me.

References

Awady, T. el (2009), *Abusir XVI: Sahure – The Pyramid Causeway: History and Decoration Program in the Old Kingdom* (Prague: Charles University).

Bárta, M. and Vachala, B. (2001), 'The Tomb of Hetepi at Abusir South', *Egyptian Archaeology* 19, 33–5.

Davies, S. and Smith, H. S. (2005), *The Sacred Animal Necropolis at North Saqqara. The Falcon Complex and Catacombs: The Archaeological Report* (London: Egypt Exploration Society).

Gould, D. (2003), 'A study of the relationship between the different dynastic factions of the Early Dynastic Period and of the evidence for internal political disruptions', in S. Bickel and A. Loprieno (eds.), *Basel Egyptology Prize 1: Junior Research in Egyptian History, Archaeology, and Philology* (Basel: Schwabe), 29–53.

Graham, A. (2010), 'Islands in the Nile', in M. Bietak, E. Czerny and I. Forstner-Müller (eds.), *Cities and Urbanism in Ancient Egypt: Papers from a Workshop in November 2006 at the Austrian Academy of Sciences* (Vienna: Verlag der Österreichischen Akademie der Wissenschaften), 125–43.

Hawass, Z. (2007), 'The discovery of the Osiris shaft at Giza', in Z. A. Hawass and J. E. Richards (eds.), *The Archaeology and Art of Ancient Egypt: Essays in Honor of David B. O'Connor*, I (Cairo: Conseil Suprême des Antiquités de l'Égypte), 379–97.

—— (2010) 'The excavation of the headless pyramid, Lepsius XXIX', in Z. A., Hawass, P. Der Manuelian and R. B. Hussein (eds.), *Perspectives on Ancient Egypt: Studies in Honor of Edward Brovarski* (Cairo: Conseil Suprême des Antiquités de l'Égypte), 153–70.

Jeffreys, D. (2001), 'High and dry? Survey of the Memphite escarpment', *Egyptian Archaeology* 19, 15–16.

Jeffreys, D., Bourriau, J. and Johnson, W. R. (2000), 'Fieldwork, 1999–2000: Memphis, 1999', *Journal of Egyptian Archaeology* 86, 5–12.

Jeffreys, D. G. and Smith, H. S. (1988), *The Anubieion at Saqqâra*, I (London: Egypt Exploration Society).

Labrousse, A. and Lauer, J.-Ph. (2000), *Les complexes funéraires d'Ouserkaf et de Néferhétepès* (Cairo: Institut Français d'Archéologie Orientale).

Labrousse, A. and Moussa, A. (2002), *La chaussée du complexe funéraire du roi Ounas* (Cairo: Institut Français d'Archéologie Orientale).

Lacher, C. (2008), 'Das Grab des Hetepsechemui/Raneb in Saqqara: Ideen zur baugeschichtlichen Entwicklung', in E.-M. Engel, V. Müller and U. Hartung (eds.), *Zeichen aus dem Sand: Streiflichter aus Ägyptens Geschichte zu Ehren von Günter Dreyer* (Wiesbaden: Harrassowitz), 425–51.

Lacher-Raschdorff, C. M. (2014), *Das Grab des Königs Ninetjer in Saqqara: Architektonische Entwicklung frühzeitlicher Grabanlagen in Ägypten* (Wiesbaden: Harrassowitz).

Lauer, J.-Ph. and Leclant, J. (1972), *Le temple haut du complexe funéraire du roi Téti* (Cairo: Institut Français d'Archéologie Orientale).

Martin, G. T. (1989), *The Memphite Tomb of Horemheb, Commander-in-Chief of Tutankhamūn*, I (London: Egypt Exploration Society).

Maragioglio, V. and Rinaldi, C. A. (1970), *L'architettura delle Piramidi Menfite*, VII (Rapallo: Officine Grafische Canessa).

Mathieson, I. (2000), 'The National Museums of Scotland Saqqara Survey Project', in M. Barta and J. Krejčí (eds.), *Abusir and Saqqara in the Year 2000* (Prague: Czech Institute of Archaeology), 33–42.

Mathieson, I., Bettles, E., Clarke, J., Duhig, C, Ikram, S., Maguire, L., Quie, S. and Tavares, A. (1997), 'The National Museums of Scotland Saqqara Survey Project 1993–95', *Journal of Egyptian Archaeology* 83, 17–53.

Mathieson, I., Bettles, E, Dittmer, J. and Reader, C. (1999), 'The National Museums of Scotland Saqqara Survey Project: earth sciences 1990–1998', *Journal of Egyptian Archaeology* 85, 21–43.

Mathieson, I. and Tavares, A. (1993), 'Preliminary report of the National Museums of Scotland Saqqara Survey Project', *Journal of Egyptian Archaeology* 97, 17–31.

Munro, P. (1993), 'Report on the work of the Joint Archaeological Mission Free University of Berlin/University of Hannover during their 12th campaign (15th March until 14th May, 1992) at Saqqâra', *Discussions in Egyptology* 26, 47–58.

Perring, J. S. (1842), *The Pyramids of Gizeh, from Actual Survey and Admeasurement*, III: *The Pyramids to the Southward of Gizeh and at Abu Roash* (London: J. Fraser).

Porter, B. and Moss, R. L. B. (1934), *Topographical Bibliography of Ancient Egyptian Hieroglyphic Texts, Reliefs and Paintings*, IV: *Lower and Middle Egypt* (Oxford: Clarendon Press).

—— (1974–81), *Topographical Bibliography of Ancient Egyptian Hieroglyphic Texts, Reliefs and Paintings*, III: *Memphis*, 2nd edn by J. Málek (Oxford: Griffith Institute).

Quibell, J. E. (1907), *Excavations at Saqqara (1905–1906)* (Cairo: Institut Français d'Archéologie Orientale).

Reader, C. (2004), 'On Pyramid Causeways', *Journal of Egyptian Archaeology* 90, 63–71.

Regulski, I. (2009), 'Investigating a new Dynasty 2 necropolis at South Saqqara', *British Museum Studies in Ancient Egypt and Sudan* 13, 221–37.

—— (2011), 'Investigating a new necropolis of Dynasty 2 at Saqqara', in R. F. Friedman and P. N. Fiske (eds.), *Egypt at its Origins 3: Proceedings of the Third International Conference 'Origin of the State: Predynastic and Early Dynastic Egypt', London, 27th July – 1st August 2008* (Leuven: Peeters), 293–311.

Sadeek, W. el- (1984), *Twenty-Sixth Dynasty Necropolis at Gizeh* (Vienna: AFRO-PUB).

Smith. H. S. and Jeffreys, D. G. (1978), 'The North Saqqâra temple-town survey: preliminary report for 1976/77', *Journal of Egyptian Archaeology* 64, 10–21.

Spencer, A. J. (1974). 'Researches on the topography of North Saqqâra', *Orientalia* 43, 1–11.

Swelim, N. (1983), *Some Problems on the History of the Third Dynasty* (Alexandria: The Archaeological Society of Alexandria).

—— (1988), 'The dry moat of the Netjerykhet complex', in J. Baines, T. G. H. James, A. Leahy and A. F. Shore (eds.), *Pyramid Studies and Other Essays Presented to I. E. S. Edwards* (London: Egypt Exploration Society), 12–22.

—— (1991), 'Some remarks on the great rectangular monuments of Middle Saqqara', *Mitteilungen des Deutschen Archäologischen Instituts, Kairo* 47, 389–402.

Wetering, J. van (2004), 'The royal cemetery of the Early Dynastic Period at Saqqara and the Second Dynasty royal tombs', in S. Hendrickx, R. F. Friedman, K. M. Ciałowicz and M. Chłodnicki (eds.), *Egypt at its Origins: Studies in Memory of Barbara Adams. Proceedings of the International Conference 'Origin of the State: Predynastic and Early Dynastic Egypt', Kraków, 28th August – 1st September 2002* (Leuven: Peeters), 1055–80.

2

The Sacred Animal Necropolis at North Saqqara: narrative of a ritual landscape

Paul T. Nicholson

Professor Rosalie David has done more than perhaps any other Egyptologist of recent times to make her subject accessible to the public and in particular her interest in mummies – animal as well as human – and the religious rites associated with them. This chapter will attempt to incorporate some of those interests and to provide a short summary view of the Sacred Animal Necropolis at North Saqqara for those unfamiliar with it.

In 1974 Professor Harry S. Smith published his *A Visit to Ancient Egypt*, which he described, with typical modesty, as 'popular rather than scholarly' (Smith 1974: unpaginated). Though it was aimed at general readers it was based on much research, and its final chapter, arguably the most 'popular', offered what might be described as one of the first examples of modern 'archaeological narrative' (see Pluciennik 1999; Joyce 2002) in Egyptology.

Although the term 'narrative archaeology' is used in a variety of ways, all share the desire to put together facts about a place or period into a series of meaningful statements which in some measure help to explain it. Traditional scholars of archaeology have generally seen this as a way of popularising their views on a site or period, an opportunity to write more freely than the measured confines of academia sometimes allow. However, in setting down their work in this way they often provide the most succinct and accessible views of their subject, and even if those views subsequently change they provide a valuable 'snapshot' of their thinking on that subject at a given moment in time.

The landscape of North Saqqara as seen today is a sandy plateau, dominated by the Step Pyramid and pock-marked by the depressions of numerous tomb shafts from many different periods. Among and around these shafts are the remains of other structures – tomb superstructures, temples, processional ways and the like. It is clear to the archaeologist, but not to the casual visitor, that North Saqqara was once a very different place from the quiet and desolate plateau it now is.

This chapter attempts to give an overview of how North Saqqara might have looked and functioned at the time the Sacred Animal Cults were at their height from the Late Period (664–332 BC) into Ptolemaic times (332–30 BC) (see Figure 2.1). In so doing it will not be confined to reporting on one particular animal temple or catacomb but will try to look at all of them within their landscape and consider where the animals, found buried in such great numbers, came from, and how they were processed and by whom. In summary, the chapter will try to give a picture of what an observer might have seen at North Saqqara during the Late to Ptolemaic Period. Such a picture will already be familiar to scholars working at Saqqara, but the aim of this Chapter is to provide an overview. It is hoped that future work, currently being undertaken by Scott Williams, a doctoral student of Cardiff University, will elucidate some of the reasons behind the locations of particular monuments.

North Saqqara today

The area under consideration is that north of the Step Pyramid itself; indeed only the southern wall of the Bubastieion extends significantly south of the line of the north wall of the Step Pyramid enclosure. The area extends as far north as the end of the Saqqara plateau, though in considering it in its ancient context one should include the now dried-up lake of Abusir, probably to be identified with the ancient 'Lake of Pharaoh' (see Figure 2.1).

The modern visitor reaches the plateau via an asphalt road which runs along the eastern edge of the plateau before turning towards the west and passing the Bubastieion (see also Dodson in Chapter 1 above). Most visitors will then head south-west to visit the Step Pyramid complex and perhaps the area around the Unas pyramid. The more dedicated visitor may go a little north to the tomb of Mereruka and the pyramid of Teti. The Serapeum, once on the itinerary of most visitors, has only just been reopened after extensive renovation, and it remains to be seen whether it regains its former place in tourist itineraries. One thing that is clear from a study of early travellers' accounts and later tourist guides to Saqqara is that various monuments rise and fall in popularity, some to the extent that they are entirely lost to view – as was the case with the Ibis Catacombs, known at the time of the Napoleonic expedition but lost by the late nineteenth century.

Most modern visitors are not permitted to go further north than the tomb of Ti and will reach it from the west side of the plateau. As a result the rest of the plateau appears to them only as a confusing 'moonscape' of mounds and

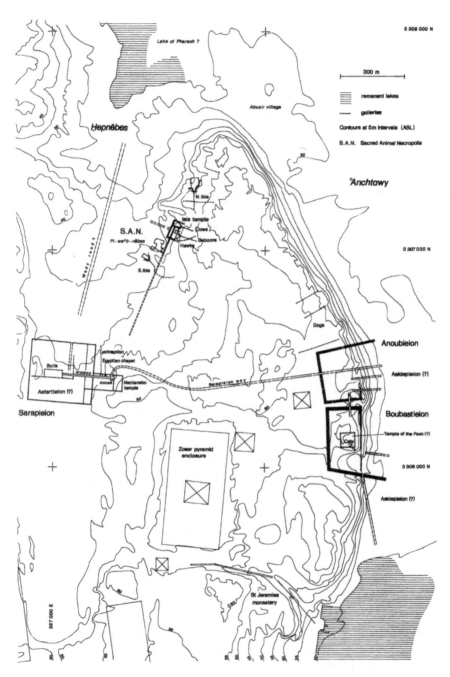

The necropolis of North Saqqara.

2.1 The necropolis of North Saqqara. (Courtesy of Dorothy Thompson.)

hollows which only the best informed realise are largely the result of excavation
and of tomb robbery over centuries.

The overall impression of Saqqara is one of quiet desolation, a place where
kings and a few selected officials were buried on the high desert. For most there
is no suggestion that this is a place where people could actually have lived. Yet
were visitors allowed to wander north of the Teti pyramid and towards the 1st
Dynasty tombs on the east of the plateau they would pass a village, settled by the
descendents of Qifti workmen, along with (until recently) the excavation house
of Firth and Gunn which served as the *Taftish*, the local office of the Supreme
Council of Antiquities (SCA). Settlement on the plateau may not be obvious,
but it is present and was still more prominent in antiquity.

A brief landscape narrative for North Saqqara

Here it is possible to do little more than to introduce the landscape of North
Saqqara in the Late to Ptolemaic Period to the general reader. There is not
space to try to reproduce, as Smith did so eloquently, the landscape surrounding a particular event but rather to draw attention to features of the landscape
which can then be used in such a narrative reconstruction, a process which can
itself raise new questions and generate new interpretations. In attempting this
I have made particular use of the work of Smith (1974, 1975), Ray (1972, 1978,
2002) and Thompson (2012), and the reader is directed to those accounts for a
more polished approach. It must be remembered too that ancient visitors would
have had their own pre-conceptions relating to the site and would not necessarily see as significant those things which we consider noteworthy today. Many
would have personal histories bound up in the landscape and would visit shrines
of those deities who they believed had benefited them in the past or places with
which they had ancestral links (e.g. Smith 1974: 74). As Tilley (1994: 16–17) has
put it, landscapes provide 'a sacred, symbolic and mythic space replete with
social meanings wrapped around buildings, objects and features of the local
topography, providing reference points and planes of emotional orientation for
human attachment and involvement'.

The visitor approaching Saqqara during the Late to Ptolemaic Period may
have had a choice of routes; as Thompson (2012: 18) states there were probably a number of paths leading up the escarpment, though there were perhaps
two main routes. The first is that used for dragging the large sarcophagi of the
Apis bull and his mother and was probably around the northern end of the
plateau and along its west side, with the Catacombs of the Mothers of Apis
being an eastward turn from this course, while the Serapeum would have been
straight ahead and could have been entered from its north gate. This is the
route suggested by Dodson (Chapter 1 above) as well as indicated as the 'wady

road' by Davies (2006: fig.1; Thompson 2012: fig. 4; see Figure 2.1) and has the advantage, particularly for those charged with moving sarcophagi, of being a relatively gentle gradient for most of its course. This route would pass through the area of the site known as *Hp-nb=s* (Hepnebes) (Davies 2006: 3), covering the area roughly between the Lake of Pharaoh in the north and the north side of the Serapeum in the south (Thompson 2012: 26–7). The actual funeral procession of the Apis would have passed through the Anubieion and headed west along the Serapeum way, the sarcophagus having already been installed in the catacomb having reached it by the wadi route.

Alternative routes would have been via the east side of the plateau, and pilgrims[1] may have entered onto it via the great southern gate of the Bubastieion (Smith 1975: 420; also Thompson 2012: 19) or perhaps the Anubieion's east gate. In the case of the latter this route would lead one up the escarpment from the valley floor and along the Serapeum Way. This ran across the plateau and descended on the west to the Serapeum Temple and Catacomb, the area of *Pr-Wsir-Hp* the 'House of Osiris-Apis' (see Ray 1972). However, there would have been much to see before embarking on the *dromos* itself.

The Anubieion was the site of at least three temples (Smith 1975: 420; Jeffreys and Smith 1988), one of them being for Anubis himself. It is likely that some of the dogs sacred to Anubis and serving as his representatives lived at the temple itself and would have been mummified here. It is also suggested that the temple enclosure served as a centre for mummification generally, though given the scale of the animal cults alone at Saqqara, let alone the need for human mummification, this was certainly not the only site for embalming, and one must assume that there were numerous other workshops for the mummification of animals, and humans, at Memphis (Thompson 2012: 27) and around it. It is likely that a visitor to Saqqara during the Late Period to Ptolemaic era would have passed by some of these when approaching the Anubieion site. It is also likely that here on the flood plain, as well as in and around Memphis, were institutions which specialised in the breeding of dogs and cats for the cults of Anubis and Bastet respectively. The great number of animals present in these catacombs would preclude all of them having been reared in the respective temples (Nicholson *et al.* 2013: 87; Nicholson, Ikram and Mills 2015).

Within the walls of the Anubieion was a settlement, to the west of the main sanctuaries (Jeffreys and Smith 1988: 25; Martin 2009: 47–8) and perhaps beginning in the third century BC (Jeffreys and Smith 1988: 21). It is uncertain,

---

1   There is no ancient Egyptian term for 'pilgrim' and the word carries Western connotations. It is used here simply to mean a pious visitor and is used interchangeably with 'visitor'. Kessler (1989) places less emphasis on the cults as popular, seeing them as part of a royal cult, but this view is not shared by the writer.

however, whether earlier intra-mural settlement at the site also existed. Some of these buildings may have housed low-ranking temple officials as well as those involved in mummification and in the general maintenance of the building. Interpreters of dreams and scribes who could write questions for consideration by the deity may also have been present.

However, while it is clear that settlement existed within the Anubieion wall it is less clear what may have existed outside it. Caches of bronze objects are well known from the Sacred Animal Necropolis (see Insley Green 1987; Nicholson and Smith 1996; Nicholson 2005), and such pieces, which include numerous bronze *situlae* as well as figures of deities dedicated by pilgrims, must have been locally manufactured. While major temples frequently had workshops, the nature of many of the dedicated bronzes suggests a series of minor workshops which must have been located in Memphis and, perhaps more likely, on the fringes of Saqqara itself. A likely location for these may have been close to the Anubieion, Bubastieion and Serapeum but this must remain speculative.

In the view of the writer it is likely that pilgrims to Saqqara bought votive bronzes and dedicated them at the shrines (although Kessler 1989 sees such bronzes as part of the royal cult). A flavour of the likely pressure to purchase and dedicate objects is given by Smith (1974), and the animal cults probably played a role in the 'economic policy' (Smith 1975: 416) of the time. In order to purchase such objects there must have been vendors of bronzes around the temples and perhaps at intervals along the sacred ways, and one might imagine a scene not unlike that around many ancient sites today where stalls selling reproductions of deities and other trinkets are located. It is apparent that Saqqara would not have been the largely silent and deserted place which we see today. The presence of a detachment of police at the Anubieion (Thompson 2012: 23) as well as the representative of the local governor (*strategos*: Thompson 2012: 23) suggests that the area may have been a good deal less than silent.

The burial catacombs for the animals sacred to Anubis lay immediately north of the Anubieion Temple complex and would no doubt have been connected to it by a *dromos*. There are two 'dog catacombs' immediately next to one another but their chronology is so far uncertain.

Immediately next to the Anubieion, on its south, was the Bubastieion. Thompson (2012: 19) describes this as having two or three stone temples within it as well as the 'Temple of the Peak' (*Thn(yt)*), which was located within or nearby. This location is also noted by Price (in press), who suggests that the temple served several animal cults within the one temple and is known from priestly records (see also Thompson 2012: 19). Perhaps more controversial is the location of the Asklepion (*Pr-'Iy-m-ḥtp*), which evidently 'bordered the temple of the Peak to the North' (Thompson 2012: 19) and was a temple of Imhotep, himself identified by the Greeks as their god Asklepios. Wherever this was located it would have been a focus for those seeking cures for all manner of afflictions.

Within the Anubieion there was also a sanctuary of Bes, the so-called 'Bes chambers', where pilgrims might spend a night in the hope of receiving prophetic dreams whose purpose might be to promote fertility and virility. Bes was a long-established protector of women in childbirth and 'brought luck and prosperity to married couples' (Hart 1986: 60) and as such commonly featured within the temple enclosures of many deities. The inclusion of Bes within the landscape of the Late to Ptolemaic Period at Saqqara, a place associated with popular cults and pilgrimage, is predictable.

In passing one might note that as well as the comings and goings of priests and pilgrims within the *temenoi* of the Anubieion and Bubastieion one must assume that numbers of cats and dogs were allowed to wander within the compounds, or at least within areas of them. These would not have been quiet places, and if mummification was conducted within the Anubieion on any but the smallest scale one might also be justified in assuming that it was not particularly fragrant. Within the precinct walls of these gods the scene was very different from the solemn and incense-scented one so often portrayed by Hollywood.

Leaving this busy scene the pilgrim might pass through the west gate of the Anubieion along the sacred way (*dromos*) leading towards the Serapeum. Strabo in his *Geography* notes that this was lined with sphinxes. These were probably the work of Nectanebo I, who seems to have remodelled the Serapeum Way (Smith 1975: 418). The route would also have been lined with small shrines, and it is not unlikely that some of these would have been the recipients of votive bronzes purchased by pilgrims. There may indeed have been sellers of such items along the route itself.

The visitor walking along the sacred way might have been conscious of some of the Old Kingdom mastaba tombs, although some of these would have been partly or wholly obscured by drifted sand. De Morgan's *Carte de la nécropole de la memphite* (1897) indicates several tombs and shrines of his 'Grecque' era close to or connected with the *dromos*. The desire to be buried close to the Osiris-Apis may account for some of these (Smith 1975: 420), though one should also take into account the likelihood that in tracing the course of the *dromos* most excavation work probably took place close to it and that there may be other late burials further to the north and south. Indeed Late Period burials are known from the area around the Unas causeway as well as on either side of the Serapeum Way (Smith 1975: 416), some re-using earlier tombs. It is well known that burials of particular periods are often clustered together, but given the popularity of the animal cults and the presence of temples for them to the north of the sacred way it would be surprising if more burials were not made around them, though possibly without any tomb superstructure.

As the visitor came to the end of the *dromos* and neared the Serapeum itself he or she would first see the Temple of Nectanebo and immediately to its west, from the time of Ptolemy I, a hemicycle of statues of Greek philosophers (Smith 1975: 421; Ashton 2003: 15–24, 89–95). These statues would not have seemed so incongruous to the Ptolemaic visitor as they do to many modern tourists, not least since they would already have encountered much similar statuary, some of it connected to Dionysiac rites along the Serapeum Way itself (Thompson 2012: 25). In modern times this area of Saqqara has become a sand-trap, and the hemicycle frequently needs to be cleared of drifts. It is likely that a similar problem may have been encountered in ancient times.

From here what might be called the *dromos* proper led straight to the entrance of the Serapeum vaults. This is the area depicted in the famous drawing by Barbot (reproduced as Ray 1976: pl. I; see Figure 2.2). To its north was the 'Egyptian Chapel', a small building which housed a statue of the Apis bull (for plan of this area see Kessler 1989: Abb. 5) probably to be dated to the reign of Nectanebo I and next to it a Corinthian-style building which inscriptions tell us was the *lychnaption*, the 'headquarters of those responsible for the lamps of the god and was also known as the 'Greek Serapis Temple' (Thompson 2012: 25). Here too to the south of the *dromos* is the likely area of the Astartieion. Astarte had been adopted from the Canaanites during the 18th Dynasty and came to be identified as a daughter of Ptah (Hart 1986: 35), hence her placing near the Apis bull, the *ba* of Ptah. It was within her shrine that, in the second century

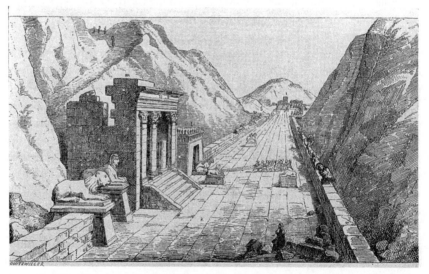

2.2 Looking East from the Serapeum. (After Barbot, reproduced courtesy of the Egypt Exploration Society.)

BC, Ptolemaios the *encatachos* lived and served as an interpreter of dreams (Thompson 2012: 26; Wilcken 1927).

Had our visitor been permitted to go further along the *dromos*, heading due west, he or she would have passed through a gateway surmounted by two lions and erected by Nectanebo I and thence downwards into the burial vaults. In practice this would not have been possible for the average pilgrim. Instead, after paying homage to the Apis at the appropriate shrine(s) he or she may have headed north from the Serapeum, where there was a settlement which may have included 'guest houses' (*Katamulata*) (Smith 1975: 421) where pilgrims might be housed and refreshment provided. Doubtless such buildings did not stand in isolation but would have been surrounded by food stalls, vendors of bronzes and other votives and perhaps even workshops. The location of such guest houses here may be significant since they could serve those who crossed the plateau from the east along the Serapeum Way and those who had come from the north along the wadi road. On the west side of this roadway there were probably tombs of officials who wished to be buried near to the deceased Apis, as Smith (1975: 420) has suggested. Any surface trace of these has now been lost through sanding of the wadi but their presence is to be expected.

After rest or refreshment the visitor might progress roughly north-north-east along the route leading to the temple terrace of the Sacred Animal Necropolis. To the west of this route is the Southern Ibis Catacomb. Today its main courtyard and entrance (Martin 1981) have disappeared beneath the sand but may have been visible to our pilgrim (depending on the date of the visit). It was from here that the archive of the temple official Hor of Sebennytos was recovered (Ray 1976; Ray 2002: 148–52). From this area and extending towards the temple terrace come a number of phallic votives (see Martin 1981) which Smith (1975: 423) associates with the procession of the *Pamyles*, an event associated with Osiris and a 'popular cult' which would have drawn pilgrims to the area.

Proceeding along the north-north-easterly route or turning off the wadi road and approaching via the brick-built Pylon of Nectanebo II, the visitor would reach the temple terrace. Here on the edge of the escarpment were shrines to the Falcon, Baboon and Mothers of Apis along with the entrances to their various catacombs. To judge by the cache of bronzes unearthed in 1995 (Nicholson and Smith 1996) and similar finds made by Professor Emery in the 1960s (see Insley Green 1987) these shrines were a focus for the deposition of votive bronzes, perhaps further reinforcing the view that vendors of such items would have been positioned near the Serapeum and along the routeways to and from it. The baboon chapel may have included the shrine of the 'Hearing Ear' (Smith 1975: 422; Smith and Davies 2014). Immediately above it, during Ptolemaic times, pilgrims were leaving votive *donaria* in front of the entrance corridor of the 3rd Dynasty mastaba 3518 (Emery 1971: 3–4) in the hope of receiving cures for various afflictions. Our visitor may well have seen other pilgrims coming to this spot or indeed gone there herself or himself as part of a progress around the necropolis.

The pilgrim might then leave via the pylon gateway to join the wadi road and head north. In the distance flocks of black and white sacred ibis (*Theskiornis aethiopicus*) may have been visible wading on, and flying around, the Lake of Pharaoh. Given that ibises are also noisy and, when *en masse*, not particularly fragrant the colony could also have been noted for its noise and stench. Mathieson and Dittmer (2007: 83) have suggested that the lake may have been little more than a seasonal pool at this time, but coring work by Earl (2011) suggests that it was a 'semi-permanent lake' (2011: 86) suitable for the breeding of ibis. There may also have been booths for embalmers of the ibis in this area. Since the plateau itself has no water it is possible that the lake, along with the Nile and the canal on the east of the plateau, was a source of water for the settlements, in which case water carriers may well have passed along the wadi road too. However, Mathieson and Dittmer (2007) have shown that a concentration of tombs and other buildings stretch across the wadi south of the lake, and they may have obscured the view of it. They suggest (2007: 83) that some of these may be workshops and storage areas, as might be expected given the scale of the cults. A little to the north of the temple terrace (that for the Falcons and Baboons) the pilgrim might have a choice; to head north to the lake shore or turn east around a promontory. If he or she chose the latter then it might easily be possible to make a short southern detour and visit the garden and shrine in front of the entrance to the North Ibis Catacomb. Smith (1975: 419, 422) suggests that this was begun in the 30th Dynasty and was replaced by the Southern Ibis Catacomb not later than the second century BC.

The visitor might then have walked up onto the plateau above the vaulted entranceway to the North Ibis Catacomb and by walking south would have come again to the Serapeum Way. Alternatively, he or she could have walked around the northernmost point of the plateau before turning south and thus have made a complete circuit encompassing all of the animal galleries. Given what is known of festival processions elsewhere in Egypt (cf. Bell 1997) such a circuit may not be improbable.

It should be noted too that our visitor may have seen the entrances to, and shrines associated with, the burial places of the calves of the Apis bull, of the Mendesian Rams and even of lions associated with Sekhmet/Bastet. While evidence of all of these exists in the form of literature and even faunal remains their precise locations remain unknown.

Conclusion

There are at least two kinds of 'narrative archaeology'. One of these looks at the manner in which archaeologists have developed a structured narrative of events, such as the process described by Leriou (2002), while the other looks at the manner in which individuals respond to and interact with elements of landscape and interpret it in particular ways. These interpretations will be shaped by the relationships that those individuals have with the landscape and any 'historical' knowledge they may have of it. In the words of Knowlton, Spellman and Hight (n.d.), 'Imagine walking through the city and triggering moments in time. Imagine wandering through a space inhabited with the sonic ghosts of another era. Like ether, the air around you pulses with spirits, voices, and sounds. Streets, buildings, and hidden fragments tell a story.' This is well exemplified by Jeremy Hight:

> The writer/artist can now read cities, towns, and open spaces. The place has layers to be read, studied, historical events and details, ethnography, geography, geology, etc (the list is quite long and exhilarating). Narrative written utilising gps [global positioning system] and wireless to trigger on a laptop, pda [personal digital assistant] or cell phone moves into a 'narrative Archeology' a reading of physical place as one moves through the world with story elements and sections triggered at specific locations and detail. (Hight n.d.)

This chapter has attempted to examine this second type of narrative by providing the kind of back-drop which visitors to Saqqara need in order to appreciate more fully the landscape they are seeing. Although the main focus of the cults is from the Late Period, aspects of their story extend back to the construction of the Step Pyramid by Imhotep and his subsequent deification, and to the Apis cult (see Ray 1978). At least some of the ancient visitors to Saqqara would have been aware of parts of this connected narrative, and the same is true for some visitors today. The difference is that for the visitor of the Late to Ptolemaic Period many monuments were standing and familiar whereas to the casual modern visitor they are just another set of ruins. The modern visitor may also unsuspectingly carry the mental baggage of a tour itinerary with all that that implies about a partial history of the site.

It is hoped that sufficient has been said to draw the attention of modern visitors to a very different social and landscape context at Saqqara and to point out to the specialist that there is utility in painting a narrative picture of a landscape since this might then be used to generate new archaeological questions and interpretations. This is a way of telling with which Professor David has long familiarity and in which she has made a major contribution to the discipline.

Acknowledgements

I am grateful to Professor Rosalie David for her help and support over many years and hope that this contribution is of interest to her. This chapter has benefited greatly from comments made by Professor H. S. Smith, Sue Davies, Robert G. Morkot and Campbell Price, and I am grateful to all of them for their observations and advice.

References

Ashton, S.-A. (2003), *Petrie's Ptolemaic and Roman Memphis* (London: Institute of Archaeology).

Bell, L. (1997), 'The New Kingdom "divine temple": the example of Luxor', in B. Shafer (ed.), *Temples of Ancient Egypt* (Ithaca: Cornell University Press), 127–84.

Davies, S. (2006), *The Sacred Animal Necropolis at North Saqqara: The Mother of Apis and Baboon Catacombs: The Archaeological Report* (London: Egypt Exploration Society).

De Morgan, J. (1897), *Carte de la nécropole de la memphite: Dahchour, Sakkarah, Abou-Sir* (Cairo: Institut Français de l'Archéologie Orientale).

Earl, E. (2011), *The Ancient Lakes of Abusir* (Cambridge: Unpublished Independent Research Project, Department of Earth Sciences, University of Cambridge).

Emery, W. B. (1971), 'Preliminary report on the excavations at North Saqqara, 1969–70', *Journal of Egyptian Archaeology* 57, 3–13.

Hart, G. (1986), *A Dictionary of Egyptian Gods and Goddesses* (London: Routledge and Kegan Paul).

Hight, J. (n.d.), 'Narrative archaeology: reading the landscape', http://web.mit.edu/comm-forum/mit4/papers/hight.pdf (last accessed 12 August 2014).

Insley Green, C. (1987), *The Temple Furniture from the Sacred Animal Necropolis at North Saqqara 1964–1976* (London: Egypt Exploration Society).

Jeffreys, D. G. and Smith, H. S. (1988), *The Anubieion at Saqqara I: The Settlement and the Temple Precinct* (London: Egypt Exploration Society).

Joyce, R. A. (2002), *The Languages of Archaeology* (Oxford: Blackwell).

Kessler, D. (1989), *Die heiligen Tiere und der König* (Wiesbaden: Harrassowitz).

Knowlton, J., Spellman, N. and Hight, J. (n.d.) '34 North 118 West: mining the urban landscape', http://34n118w.net/34N/ (last accessed 12 August 2014).

Leriou, N. (2002), 'Constructing an archaeological narrative: the Hellenization of Cyprus', *Stanford Journal of Archaeology* 1, 1–32.

Martin, C. (2009), *Demotic Papyri from the Memphite Necropolis.* (Turnhout: Brepols).

Martin, G. T. (1981), *The Sacred Animal Necropolis at North Saqqara* (London: Egypt Exploration Society).

Mathieson, I. and Dittmer, J. (2007), 'The geophysical survey of North Saqqara, 2001–7', *Journal of Egyptian Archaeology* 93, 79–93.

Nicholson, P. T. (2005), 'A hoard of votive bronzes from the Sacred Animal Necropolis at North Saqqara', *British Academy Review* 8, 41–4.

Nicholson, P. T. and Smith, H. S. (1996), 'An unexpected cache of bronzes', *Egyptian Archaeology* 9, 18.

Nicholson, P. T., Harrison, J., Ikram, S., Earl, E. and Qin, Y. (2013), 'Geoarchaeological and environmental work at the Sacred Animal Necropolis, North Saqqara, Egypt', in L. Marks (ed.), *The Memphite Necropolis (Egypt) in the Light of Geoarchaeological and Palaeoenvironmental Studies*, Studia Quaternaria 30 (2), 83–9.

Nicholson, P. T., Ikram, S. and Mills, S. (2015), 'The catacombs of Anubis at North Saqqara', *Antiquity* 89, 645–61.

Pluciennik, M. (1999). 'Archaeological narratives and other ways of telling', *Current Anthropology* 40 (5), 653–78.

Price, C. (in press). 'East of Djoser: preliminary report of the Saqqara Geophysical Survey Project, 2007 season', in P. Kousoulis and N. Lazaridis (eds.), *Proceedings of the Tenth International Congress of Egyptologists, Rhodes* (Leuven: Peeters).

Ray, J. D. (1972), 'The House of Osorapis', in P. J. Ucko, R. Tringham and G. W. Dimbleby (eds), *Man, Settlement and Urbanism* (London: Duckworth), 699–704.

Ray, J. D. (1976), *The Archive of Hor* (London: Egypt Exploration Society).

Ray, J. D. (1978), 'The world of North Saqqara', *World Archaeology* 10 (2), 149–57.

Ray, J. D. (2002), *Reflections of Osiris* (London: Profile Books).

Smith, H. S. (1974), *A Visit to Ancient Egypt* (Warminster: Aris and Phillips).

Smith, H. S. (1975), 'Saqqara: Late Period', in W. Helck and E. Otto (eds.), *Lexikon der Ägyptologie*, V (Wiesbaden: Harrassowitz), 412–28.

Smith, H. S. and Davies, S. (2014), 'Demotic papyri from the Sacred Animal Necropolis at North Saqqara, pleas, oracle questions and documents referring to mummies', in M. Depauw and Y. Brouw (eds.), *Acts of the Tenth International Congress of Demotic Studies* (Leuven: Peeters), 263–317.

Thompson, D. (2012), *Memphis under the Ptolemies*, 2nd edn (Princeton: Princeton University Press).

Tilley, C. Y. (1994), *A Phenomenology of Landscape: Places, Paths, and Monuments* (Oxford: Berg).

Wilcken, U. (ed.) (1927), *Urkunden der Ptolomäerzeit* (Berlin and Leipzig: Walter de Gruyter).

3

The Manchester 'funeral' ostracon: a sketch of a funerary ritual

Peter Robinson

I am delighted to offer this contribution for Rosalie David. Rosalie was instrumental in transforming my boyhood interest in 'mummies, tombs and pyramids' into disciplined study, through attendance at some of her many inspiring public lectures, and on the Certificate in Egyptology course at the University of Manchester Extra-Mural Department. It was after one of these lectures that I 'discovered' the ostracon that is the subject of this chapter, in one of the side cabinets at Manchester Museum.

In 1913, Sir Alan Gardiner published a brief paper about an object that he had bought from an antiquities dealer in Gurna, Luxor (Gardiner 1913: 229). This object, an ostracon of white limestone, bore a sketch of what Gardiner described as a 'burial of the humbler kind'. Gardiner subsequently donated the ostracon to add to the collection of the then recently expanded Manchester Museum, where it was entered under the catalogue number 5886. For much of the time since then, the ostracon has been on display to the public in the museum's Egyptology galleries. Although there have been a number of subsequent images and line drawings reproducing the sketch (e.g. Schäfer 1986: 126; Duquesne 2001: 15), Gardiner's is the only publication to date to have described the sketch and ostracon as a whole.

The ostracon

Made of white limestone, the ostracon consists of a single flake measuring 10.2 cm wide by 11.7 cm long (Plate 1). It is lenticular in cross-section with a thickness of approximately 2 cm at its greatest extent, and with a number of flakes chipped off the sides and edges. A sketched image of a tomb shaft and a number of figures drawn in black ink cover much of the surface of the recto (Figure 3.1a). The verso of the flake is uninscribed other than the modern accession number '[5886]', which is written in large red characters. Although this author has carried out no chemical analysis on the verso of the flake, there is a slight greasy deposit on the corners and edges of the flake that may perhaps have resulted from its earlier handling, either in ancient times or subsequent to its modern discovery. The top half of the verso is covered with a slightly yellowish patina. It is unclear whether this patina is of the original geological matrix from which the flake had been extracted, or whether it has resulted from exposure to the air, subsequent to the flake's extraction, use or discovery.

The sketch on the recto seems to be the only ancient drawing upon the flake's surface and it may be concluded that the drawing was made upon a fresh flake rather than re-using a cleaned palimpsest flake. No inscription survives in the composition and so it is now virtually impossible to identify the original owner or producer of the sketch, nor can anything be used to date the piece with any certainty, given its unprovenanced acquisition by Gardiner (1913: 229; McDowell 1999: 27). It may be due to the lack of writing that Gardiner described the piece only briefly and that it is relatively unknown within academic literature.

In order to investigate the nature of the sketch, we must understand the nature of ostraca and their role in the material culture left to us by the ancient Egyptians. Ostraca can be defined as 'sherds of pottery or flakes of limestone bearing texts or drawings, commonly consisting of personal jottings, letters, sketches or scribal exercises' (Shaw and Nicholson 1995: 216).

As well as the many texts and images found on ostraca recording the daily activities of the ancient Egyptians, we have many sketches of scenes from after-life texts, some of which may be initial drafts of scenes for tombs or temples (Robins 1997: 191). Perhaps, then, the Manchester ostracon could be the initial sketch of a funeral for some purpose other than simply *reportage* of an event.

Breaking down the image

The majority of surviving ostraca from Thebes, and especially the New Kingdom workmen's village of Deir el-Medina, carry jottings, texts and images, many of which are apparently non-religious in content (De Garis Davis 1917: 235–6; McDowell 1999: 4). The image on the Manchester ostracon, however, depicts the rare theme of a funeral. There are no parallel examples of such a theme on ostraca known to the writer, and as a result, any interpretation may at first sight be difficult and complex. One way to attempt to understand this image is by breaking it down into its component parts. The following analysis takes this approach, selecting the key elements in turn.

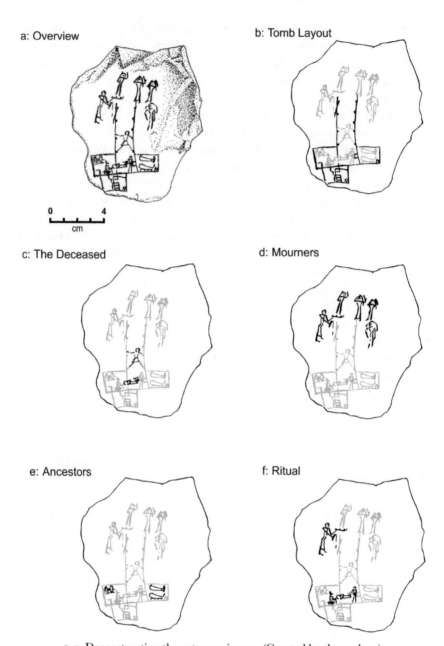

3.1 Deconstructing the ostracon image. (Created by the author.)

The tomb layout (Figure 3.1b)

Layouts of built structures in ancient Egyptian art and their interpretations can be somewhat problematic (Schäfer 1986: 129–31). Depictions of buildings in reliefs are usually shown as a combination of elevation and plan, where rooms may be shown stacked, one upon another, in a somewhat contradictory arrangement that appears obscure to modern interpretation. The Manchester ostracon shows the structure of the tomb shaft and chambers in a moderately ambiguous architectural arrangement, though it is possible to get a reasonable idea of the tomb's layout because of its simple structure.

The tomb, as depicted, appears to consist of a simple vertical shaft, with a number of chambers at its lower end. These are entered by doorways. One of the chambers appears to be at a lower level and contains what may be a single vessel. This lower chamber is approached by a short stairway from the burial chamber above. The shaft entrance lacks any indication of a chapel on the surface, or any other distinguishing marker such as a stela. The means of descending the burial shaft is indicated by small projections (or perhaps cut notches) spaced at intervals down the shaft walls.

Tomb layouts have survived on the 'Turin Royal Tomb Plan' papyrus and also the Cairo ostracon CG 25184. Both of these, however, represent the more formal layouts of royal tombs of the later Ramesside rulers in the Valley of the Kings, arranged as architectural plans, rather than the less formal smaller tombs of the non-royal elite (Carter and Gardiner 1917). Both the Papyrus Turin and the Cairo ostracon include detailed hieratic descriptions of the tombs, their measurements and their parts. Furthermore, it has been suggested that the Papyrus Turin, showing the tomb of Ramesses IV, KV 2, was an archive copy depicting the burial of the dead pharaoh within his sarcophagus, while the Cairo ostracon is assumed to be a working drawing used during construction since it was drawn on more durable limestone (Kemp and Rose 1991: 123).

There are also representations of tombs in a number of spells from the Book of the Dead. Chapter 151 (rubricated as a 'Spell for the Head of Mystery') includes a vignette depicting the plan of the burial chamber itself, within which lies the coffin, accompanied by Isis and Nephthys, the necropolis god Anubis and the deceased's *ba* bird (Naville 1903: 107).

Another image of the tomb appears in the vignette to Chapter 1 of the Book of the Dead. Here, the spell is often accompanied by a scene showing the events at the tomb entrance, including the bringing of offerings to the tomb, scenes of mourning and the ritual of the 'Opening of the Mouth' (see further below).

The deceased (Figure 3.1c)

On the Manchester ostracon, a representation of the deceased appears in the burial chamber. In this part of the image, however, the wall of the burial

chamber and perhaps a doorway are drawn in rough lines of varying thickness, overlapping part of the deceased's recumbent form, and it is difficult to
distinguish between a coffin or simply a masked mummy. However, if the lines
represent part of the burial chamber and a doorway, then the deceased is probably depicted enclosed in a coffin. It is also difficult to determine the gender of
the deceased, but there may be a slight indication of a beard to indicate that the
deceased was male.

The deceased's apparent coffin appears to be anthropoid in design, with its
'head' to the left of the chamber. The coffin lies flat and is neither supported on
an embalming bed nor on any form of bier. The later section of Chapter 1 of the
Book of the Dead is concerned with 'permitting the deceased to descend to the
Netherworld on the day of interment' (Faulkner 1985: 35). Near the bottom of
the burial shaft, the ostracon depicts a male figure, legs and arms outstretched,
straddling the width of the shaft. Gardiner (1913: 229) identifies this figure as '[s]
ome male relative'.

The mourners (Figure 3.1d)

Around the entrance to the tomb, an officiant and a number of other figures
stand, four of whom appear to be women, with their arms raised in an act
of mourning. Similar scenes occur in other representations of the funeral in
tomb reliefs and funerary papyri (Naville 1896: pls. II–IV). The priest stands
at the shaft entrance holding an incense burner in his left hand and pouring
water from a jar in his right. Many New Kingdom Books of the Dead illustrate
similar scenes, such as that of the papyrus of Hunefer in the British Museum
(EA 9901/5), where a *sem*-priest, clad in a panther skin, burns incense from an
arm-shaped burner and pours water over a pile of offerings (Faulkner 1985: 54).
In the Manchester ostracon, however, there is no indication of what the priest
is pouring water over.

The 'ancestors' (Figure 3.1e)

In the tomb chamber to the right of the burial shaft lie two anthropoid coffins,
laid flat and aligned in the same direction as the main coffin in the burial chamber. Because of the roughness of the sketch, it is not possible to discern much
detail from the image, although the lower of the two coffins may sport a divine
beard. It is possible, therefore, that these may be the parents of the deceased,
who is being buried in a family tomb. Although there is no indication of scale,
the two coffins, along with a vessel, a domed object and another indeterminate
object, seem to fill the adjoining side chamber. Maybe these three objects were
funerary offerings previously left for the two occupants of the coffins.

In the burial chamber itself, in the left-most corner, squat two figures. As
the three coffins and two figures all face to the right (and therefore probably the

living world of the east), we might consider that the figures are in the west of the tomb, and conceivably therefore may represent some metaphysical aspect of the occupants of the coffins in the side chamber, such as their *akh*-personas, now residing in the western world of the dead. Alternatively, the figures could represent images of the tomb owner and spouse painted upon the walls of the chamber, but given the lack of other indications of such funerary depictions, this is uncertain.

The ritual (Figure 3.1f)

As well as the purification ceremony and mourning around the tomb shaft entrance, there is a ritual of some kind taking place in the burial chamber. Gardiner suggested that the figures around the coffin were those of an embalmer wearing a jackal-headed Anubis mask, and a son of the deceased or his deputy. In Chapter 151 of the Book of the Dead, Anubis is, however, accompanied by 'the Two Sisters', Isis and Nephthys, who stand or sit at either end of the coffin. In the vignette to this chapter, Anubis is the deity 'who is in the place of embalming' and is usually shown with the deceased's corpse under the embalming tent or *per wabet* (Wilkinson 2003: 188). In addition, other than being in the presence of Isis and Nephthys, in the Chapter 151 vignette, Anubis is shown working alone in performing an 'Opening of the Mouth' ritual. The Anubis character in the Manchester ostracon, however, is accompanied by another male officiating over the deceased's coffin in an otherwise empty burial chamber.

Assmann's explanation of the roles of various priests in the funerary ritual can perhaps explain the personnel depicted on the ostracon (Assmann 2005: 302–3). A New Kingdom funeral was a complex undertaking requiring a number of participants. It is perfectly conceivable, of course, that such a funeral would have been an expensive affair, requiring some form of 'payment in kind' to all the participants. For those families who could not afford a costly funeral, one would expect that 'cost savings' could be made by employing fewer participants, maybe from the deceased's own family or relatives, who would undertake a number of roles in the ritual. Assmann suggests that those taking the roles of *sem*-priest and lector priest could participate in other activities within the funeral. In the discussions above, we have already seen the *sem*-priest at the entrance to the burial shaft as he purifies the area around the tomb entrance by burning incense and pouring water. The *sem*-priest and the chief lector priest participate in the 'Opening of the Mouth' ritual, usually at the entrance of the tomb, where they may be joined by 'the embalmer', wearing an 'Anubis mask'. Is it possible that these three are indicated on the ostracon, with the chief lector priest, reading from sacred texts, and 'the embalmer', both of whom are in the burial chamber with the deceased's mummy?

The jackal-headed participant at the head of the deceased's coffin appears to hold a horizontal staff in one hand and a vertical staff in the other. Both staffs seem to be forked or cleft sticks, rather than in the 'classic' adze design which appears in scenes of the 'Opening of the Mouth' ritual. The staff held horizontally appears to have a bulbous top with 'ears', but the thickness of the ink line and the small scale of the image make it difficult to interpret its actual form. It could be a jackal-headed staff. Alternatively, it could be a serpent-headed *wr-ḥk3w*, which was another implement used the 'Opening of the Mouth' ritual (Strudwick 2009: 221–5), as shown in the papyrus of Hunefer. The participant at the coffin's foot may be holding a long staff or rod that extends over the foot of the coffin.

A Book of the Dead parallel: the papyrus of Nebqed

Most vignettes associated with Chapter 1 of the Book of Dead show many of the key elements of the funeral, including the bringing of the coffin to the tomb upon a sledge drawn by men and oxen, individuals bringing goods and chattels to be placed in the tomb, mourners and rituals at the entrance of the tomb (Taylor 2010: 88). In most examples, the events of the vignette take place above ground, with the key ceremonies taking place at the tomb entrance. The papyrus of Nebqed, dating to around the mid-18th Dynasty, however, unusually includes a representation of events below ground, in the stairway to the burial chamber, as well as the burial chamber itself (Figure 3.2a; Naville 1896: pl. IV). As well as the detail of the funerary procession and an illustration of the 'Opening of the Mouth' by a *sem*-priest upon Nebqed's coffin, accompanied by a female mourner at the entrance to his tomb, the papyrus depicts stylised features of the tomb itself, including a descending stairway and a number of rooms beyond the lower end of the stairway. Descending the stairway, between the tomb entrance and the burial chamber, there is the clear depiction of a human-headed *ba* bird, wings spread as if in the act of flying down the stairway. Immediately at the bottom of the stairway, in the antechamber to the burial chamber, the papyrus's artist has drawn a chair and offering table. In the burial chamber itself, Nebqed lies within his anthropoid coffin, upon a bier, his name written above, and surrounded by braziers and jars containing offerings. In a side chamber, we see the grave goods in a box, the deceased's sandals and another offering table, ready to receive offerings. Finally, above the image of the burial chamber, the deceased appears to be standing in the sunlight, as part of his abilities, rubricated in Chapter 1, of 'going out [of the tomb] into the day' (Faulkner 1985: 34).

The image of the tomb depicted in Nebqed's papyrus shares a number of similarities with the Manchester ostracon (Figures 3.2b and 3.2c). We see ritual

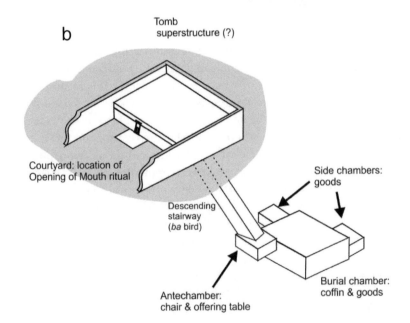

3.2 Tombs in the Papyrus of Nebqed and Manchester 'funeral' ostracon compared:
(a) Vignette from Chapter 1 of the *Book of the Dead of Nebqed*. (Created by the author
after Naville 1896: pl. IV.) (b) Interpretation of the architecture of the tomb of
Nebqed. (Created by the author.) (c) Interpretation of the architecture of the tomb of
Manchester 'funeral' ostracon. (Created by the author.)

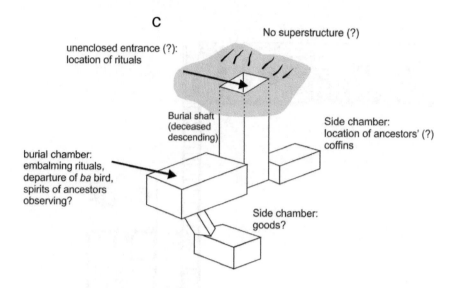

around the entrance to the tomb, where an officiant is accompanied by one or more mourners. The burial chamber of the tomb is approached by a descending corridor or shaft. The subterranean part of the tomb consists of a number of chambers, one or more of which contain objects. There are, however, differences between the two images. Nebqed's funeral and indeed his tomb in general seem to be more generously equipped, with a stairway, superstructure and more grave goods, whereas the Manchester ostracon shows a poorly equipped funeral, with a single jar of offerings and the deceased interred in an already occupied tomb. One could even argue that while Nebqed's coffin is shown on a bier, that in the ostracon does not appear to be supported on a bed, bier or other form of staging, and that after the funeral was complete, one might expect the coffin to have been placed in the side chamber to accompany the other two coffins, if space permitted. While Nebqed's *ba* is descending into his tomb in bird form, it is possible that the figure descending (or climbing up) the burial shaft of the ostracon may represent some aspect of the deceased's post-mortem persona, related, perhaps, to the theme of Chapter 1 of the Book of the Dead.

Tombs at Deir el-Medina

Although Gardiner could not ascribe a precise provenance to the ostracon, nonetheless it is typical of the inscribed material that has been found in and around Deir el-Medina. The earliest tombs of the village, cut into the hill to the east, date to the reigns of the Tuthmoside kings. Although these tombs often contained personal possessions of the tomb owner, providing us with information about the status of the village inhabitants, we have virtually no written material from this period of the village's occupation that can tell us more about the workmen's community (McDowell 1999: 18–19). On the opposite side of the village, in the Western Cemetery, the tombs are mostly of a later Ramesside date and arranged in a series of terraces up the side of the valley. Those tombs dating from the reign of Ramesses II are especially grand and richly decorated.

The tomb of Sennedjem (Theban tomb no. 1) is typical of Ramesside tombs in the Western Cemetery (Bruyère 1959: 5). It consists of a number of subterranean chambers beneath an open-air courtyard on the surface. A tomb chapel lay at the far end of the courtyard, above which was a small, brick-built pyramid topped by a stone pyramidion. The entrance to the subterranean chambers was at the bottom of a vertical shaft that opened from the courtyard rather than from within the tomb chapel. Footholds were cut into the mudbrick-rendered walls of the shaft, to allow the tomb's builders to pass down into the tomb chambers (Figure 3.3a; Bruyère 1959: 6–7). It is apparent that Sennedjem's tomb was similar to the tomb depicted upon the ostracon. Of course the ostracon shows no superstructure or chapel, unlike Sennedjem's, but from the viewpoint of the courtyard in front of Sennedjem's chapel, the two tombs exhibit similar shafts and subterranean chambers (Figure 3.3b).

Sennedjem's tomb appears similar in design to that of the Manchester ostracon and was found to contain twenty bodies, many of which seemed to be members of three generations of Sennedjem's own family. As some of these bodies were deposited in the tomb without coffins, but wrapped in simple bandages and shrouds, the excavators believed that later burials were meagre and the family did not have sufficient funds for anything but simple burials (Bruyère 1959: 2–3). Cooney (2011: 5–8) has suggested that by the 20th Dynasty, most people in Thebes could not afford to commission their own tombs and therefore cut corners or re-used pre-existing tombs in the necropolis. Furthermore, as the security of the necropolis sites broke down during the 21st Dynasty, coffins began to be systematically taken from earlier tombs and re-used, sometimes even two or three times (Cooney 2011: 31). Thus, earlier tombs became stripped of their coffins, perhaps explaining this lack of a full set of funerary equipment for all of Sennedjem's family. Whether this relates directly to the lack of objects and the re-use of the tomb on the ostracon, of course, is difficult to determine for certain.

Sennedjem's tomb is just one of many in the Theban necropolis. The tomb itself was one of the most intact in the area on its discovery, and one whose

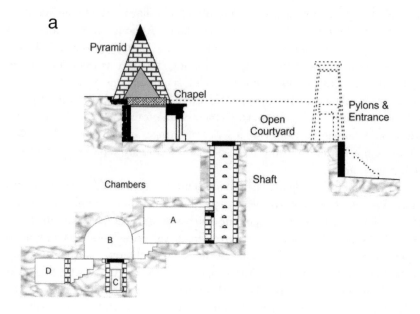

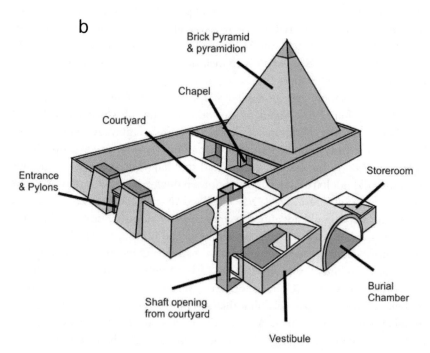

3.3 The tomb of Sennedjem: (a) Cross-section of the tomb of Sennedjem. (Created by the author after Bruyère 1959: pl. VII.) (b) Interpretation of the architecture of the tomb of Sennedjem. (Created by the author after Siliotti 1996: 133.)

excavation has been well documented. However, although it is unlikely that this tomb is the one depicted on the ostracon, it may be representative of the type of tomb shown, as well as one that gives us a good parallel with the funerary rituals and processes taking place for the families of artisans and craftsmen occupying the middle strata of New Kingdom Theban society.

Conclusion

The impression given by the image on the Manchester ostracon is one of a poorly furnished tomb and meagre funeral. The tomb appears cramped and already in use, perhaps by members of the deceased's family. There are few grave goods stored in the tomb chambers. The burial shaft is descended not by stairs but by notches cut into the sides, which gives an impression of a less ornate and more 'economical' tomb, though the example of Sennedjem's tomb with its brick-cut footholds within the burial shaft, used by a number of generations, was richly decorated and contained a wealth of funerary objects (Siliotti 1996: 134). We could also suggest that the various participants depicted on the ostracon had multiple roles in the rituals taking place within and around the tomb. Despite an uncertain date and provenance for the ostracon, and the lack of any ancient textual information about it, the fact that it was purchased in Luxor and affinities between the sketch and New Kingdom tombs lead us to suggest that the scene represents a funeral taking place in the Theban necropolis.

The ostracon's scene raises many more questions than can easily be answered from a simple initial analysis. Close examination of this object, as we have seen, can lead us down a number of avenues of enquiry. For a start, what was the purpose of the ostracon? If, as Gardiner seems to suggest, the scene was *reportage* of a funeral, why do we have a 'humbler' example of a funeral illustrated, when in other examples of Egyptian funerary art, the depiction of the deceased and aspects of their funeral always seem to be of perfection and order, with a well-furnished ritual and an abundance of offerings, celebrants and family? In addition, if this were a report of a funeral, who would the expected audience be? Should we see this ostracon in much the same way, therefore, as we would nowadays view a set of photographs or a video taken at the wedding or some other 'life event' of a family member or friend? Or was the intended audience not within the deceased's immediate or extended family?

It is unlikely that the ostracon represents an accurate plan for a tomb architect. There are no measurements or indications of scale for measuring out the tomb, or any description of the tomb other than the drawing itself. Indeed, the drawing with its depiction of a funerary ritual taking place would imply a tomb already excavated and previously occupied, as indicated by the other coffins shown in the side chamber.

The papyrus of Nebqed is the only known example of the detail of a tomb substructure known in a vignette of the funeral and its ritual from the Book of the Dead, Chapter 1. It would appear, therefore, that the recording of a tomb's burial chamber made while events were taking place at the moment of burial is somewhat rare, and not part of the normal illustrative programme of Chapter 1. To return to Sennedjem's tomb, however, there is an interesting illustration within the burial chamber that may perhaps shed some light on this ostracon (Figure 3.4). This image depicts the lone god Anubis, or a jackal-masked priest, bending over the deceased Sennedjem, who lies in his coffin on an embalmer's lion-headed bed within the *per wabet*. Although this may be a reference to the Chapter 151 discussed above, there are texts to the side of and below the vignette which form part of the textual element to Chapter 1 of the Book of the Dead. Contextually, therefore, this suggests a connection between the ostracon's image and Chapter 1 of the Book of the Dead. It could be argued thus that this ostracon was a rough trial piece to conceptualise the design for a vignette for part of this chapter, which eventually was not incorporated in a finished Book of the Dead manuscript, or for an as yet undiscovered or now lost manuscript. We should note, however, that

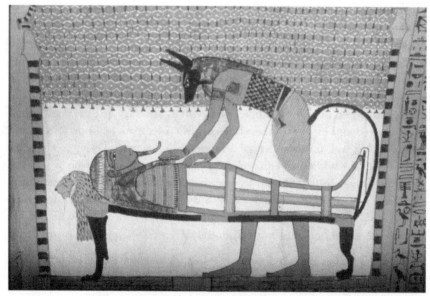

3.4 Anubis tends to Sennedjem. (Photograph © R.B Partridge, Peartree Design.)

the figures depicted on the ostracon do not conform to a standard canon of proportions, nor appear neatly drawn, as would be expected for a final draft of a vignette.

Baines has noted that much of the ritual of Egyptian religion was not depicted, yet must have been discussed among its participants (Baines 1989: 476). This may be another credible explanation for the purpose of this ostracon. Instead of this image providing a physical record or memento of a completed funeral, retained within the deceased's family, or a trial piece for building the tomb or illustrating a funerary text, we may see it in a more mundane sense as illustrating roles for an intended funeral, used as a 'discussion document'. One can imagine the key participants allocating who was to do what and where during a funeral for a recently departed family member, with a sketched jotting drawn rapidly upon a limestone fragment, picked casually up off the ground or from a pile of nearby debris. Once the roles had been decided upon or explained, and the funeral verbally rehearsed by its participants, this ephemeral ostracon could have been quickly discarded among the detritus and rubble, where it was eventually to be found in the modern era. Sadly, we do not have the details of an exact find-spot, as Gardiner purchased the ostracon from a dealer. Without this firm provenance, therefore, we may never know the circumstances of the object's location, which would have given clues as to its purpose and use.

The ostracon can pose other questions, focusing on the production of the image, such as the order of drawing the various figures and features, or an analysis of the inks and brushes used to create the image. Even the pressure applied to the brushes used when it was drawn, and any emphasis given to particular features or parts of the image, can all give an indication of the artist's state of mind, or graphical abilities and experience, when he was producing the sketch. These questions, however, are beyond the scope of this present chapter, and so have not been addressed.

Even the most mundane or ephemeral of objects within museum collections can often provide the scholar with a rich mother-lode of source material for analysis, even though such objects may previously have gone unnoticed or unexamined, eclipsed by the richer or more familiar material on display. It is therefore hoped that this chapter has shed some light upon an otherwise little-known object that may offer an insight into the rituals and architecture from the Theban necropolis and the funerary aspirations of an otherwise unnamed and unknown resident of Thebes, some three millennia ago.

Acknowledgements

I gratefully acknowledge the assistance of Dr Campbell Price and the staff of Manchester Museum, Department of Egypt and the Sudan, for permission to

investigate and photograph this ostracon at close hand. I wish to thank the
editors and anonymous reviewers for their suggestions on earlier drafts of this
chapter. In addition, I wish to thank Peartree Design for the permission to use
the photograph in Figure 3.4, originally taken by Robert B. (Bob) Partridge
(1951–2011), who I am sure would also have wished to offer a chapter for this
volume.

References

Assmann, J. (2005), *Death and Salvation in Ancient Egypt*, trans. David Lorton (Ithaca and
     London: Cornell University Press).
Baines, J. (1989), 'Communication and display: the integration of early Egyptian art
     and writing', *Antiquity* 63, 471–82.
Bruyère, B. (1959), *La tombe N°1 de Sen-nedjem à Deir el Medineh* (Cairo: Institut Français
     d'Archéologie Orientale).
Carter, H. and Gardiner, A. H. (1917), 'The tomb plan of Ramesses IV and the Turin
     plan of a royal tomb', *Journal of Egyptian Archaeology* 4, 130–58.
Cooney, K. M. (2011), 'Changing burial practices at the end of the New
     Kingdom: defensive adaptions in tomb commissions, coffin commissions, coffin
     decoration, and mummification', *Journal of the American Research Center in Egypt* 47,
     3–44.
De Garis Davis, N. (1917), 'Egyptian drawings on limestone flakes', *Journal of Egyptian
     Archaeology* 4, 234–40.
Duquesne, T. (2001), 'Concealing and revealing: the problem of ritual masking in
     ancient Egypt', *Discussions in Egyptology* 51, 5–30.
Faulkner, R. O. (1985) *The Ancient Egyptian Book of the Dead*, ed. Carol Andrews (London:
     British Museum Press).
Gardiner, A. H. (1913), 'An unusual sketch of a Theban funeral', *Proceedings of the Society
     of Biblical Archaeology* 35, 229.
Kemp, B. and Rose, P. (1991), 'Proportionality in mind and space in ancient Egypt',
     Cambridge Archaeological Journal 1 (1), 103–29.
McDowell, A. G. (1999), *Village Life in Ancient Egypt* (Oxford: Oxford University
     Press).
Naville, E. (1896), *Das aegyptische Todtenbuch der xviii. bis xx. Dynastie* (Berlin: Ascher).
Naville, E. (1903), 'The Book of the Dead', *Proceedings of the Society of Biblical Archaeology*
     25, 105–10.
Robins, G. (1997), *The Art of Ancient Egypt* (London: British Museum Press).
Schäfer, H. (1986), *Principles of Egyptian Art*, trans John Baines (Oxford: Griffith
     Institute).
Shaw, I. and Nicholson, P. (1995), *The British Museum Dictionary of Ancient Egypt* (London:
     British Museum Press).
Siliotti, A. (1996), *Guide to the Valley of the Kings* (Vercelli: White Star).
Strudwick, N. (2009), 'True "ritual objects" in Egyptian private tombs?', in B. Backes,
     M. Müller-Roth and S. Stöhr (eds.), *Ausgestattet mit den Schriften des Thot* (Wiesbaden:
     Harrasowitz), 213–38.

Taylor, J. H. (2010), 'The day of burial', in J. H. Taylor (ed.), *Ancient Egyptian Book of the Dead* (London: British Museum Press), 82–103.

Wilkinson, R. H. (2003), *The Complete Gods and Goddesses of Ancient Egypt* (London: Thames and Hudson).

4

The tomb of the 'Two Brothers' revisited

Steven Snape

In 2007 I was involved, in a small way, with the publication of Rosalie's book on the 'Two Brothers' (David 2007), the important Middle Kingdom tomb group from Rifeh. In this chapter I hope to shed some light on the original home of this famous pair of long-term residents of the Manchester Museum while doing honour to another, Rosalie herself.

Rifeh is one of the most archaeologically under-explored of the regional cemeteries of large rock-cut elite tombs of the Middle Kingdom in Upper Egypt. Lacking the high-quality decorated walls of roughly contemporary cemeteries, for instance Beni Hasan, Meir or Qubbet el-Hawa, it did not attract the concentrated attention of early archaeologists. As F. Ll. Griffith put it in 1889, 'Champollion and Lepsius passed by and left them to the tender mercies of later Egyptologists hurrying up the river to Thebes' (Griffith 1889a: 121). Perhaps also, when compared with other sites of a similar nature, it represented too daunting a task; the necropolis at Rifeh is vast and relatively complicated in its physical layout. When compared with, for instance, Beni Hasan, the rock-cut tombs at Rifeh are not arrayed in one neat terrace of a relatively limited number of major tombs, but both are much greater in number and have much greater variability in size, and are spread over the eastern face of the Gebel Durunka mountain in a more irregular fashion (Figure 4.1). In this respect, Rifeh is, unsurprisingly, most similar to the necropolis at Asyut, which has both a similarly complex layout and underdeveloped archaeological history, and which has only recently been the subject of a focused archaeological project after more than a century of neglect and inaccessibility (see e.g. Kahl 2007).

Part of the problem for early explorers of the site was the nature of Deir Rifeh itself. The term 'Deir' refers here to a cluster of Coptic dwellings and religious structures which grew up around the large tombs at the northern end

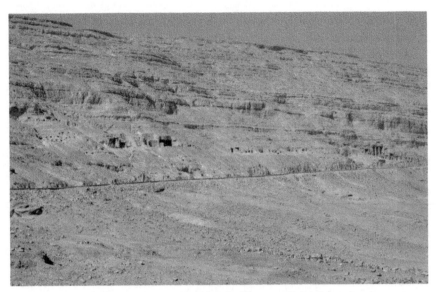

4.1 The necropolis at Deir Rifeh. (Photograph by the author.)

of what might be thought of as the greater Rifeh cemetery. Many of the largest and most immediately interesting of the Rifeh tombs (i.e. those numbered III–VII by Griffith) were within the 'Deir', and the written accounts of Griffith, W. M. F. Petrie, P. Montet and M. Pillet (see below) make it clear that they were still being occupied by Coptic villagers during their work at the site.

Griffith at Deir Rifeh

The first significant fieldwork to be carried out at Rifeh was Griffith's epigraphic work, which had come about through chance (for his account see Griffith 1889a). In 1886–87 he and Petrie undertook a trip to 'many an-out-of-the-way and unexplored corner of Upper Egypt' including the 'almost unknown tombs cut in the Western Cliff at the Coptic village of Dêr Rifeh' which had been recommended to them by Archibald Sayce. Petrie and Griffith spent 31 December 1886 'completely exploring the hill above the town' of Asyut. The following day they walked from the cliff above Asyut to Deir Rifeh and, on arriving at the latter, quickly copied some of the accessible texts in what were to be assigned the designations Tombs I and II. Griffith returned to Deir Rifeh in May 1887, when he spent a week revising and adding to his copies of the texts in the tombs. In the winter of 1887–88 Griffith returned again to Asyut and Deir Rifeh, intending to work at the latter in January–February 1888, but in the event he was too busy at Asyut to be able to do so. Griffith did not provide a location map of the Deir

Rifeh tombs he examined, although he did give sketch-plans of Tombs I and II
(Griffith 1889b: pl. 16).

Griffith numbered the Rifeh tombs from south to north, Tomb I belonging
to the Middle Kingdom *ḥry-tp* '3 Khnum-Nefer. This tomb Griffith describes
as a very large single chamber of which a substantial portion had been quarried
away, and which 'forms the centre of a large group of about 150 tombs' (Griffith
1889a: 181) which were uninscribed and in several rows on the face of the cliff.
Further north Griffith specifically refers to Tomb II, with its scant ink inscriptions from the New Kingdom, and about 100 yards north of Tomb II a further
set of tombs which were difficult to assess because they were located within the
'Deir'. Those which Griffith was able to access were mainly assigned by him to
the New Kingdom (Tomb III, which he assigned to Rameri and dated to the
late 19th Dynasty, the 'very large' Tomb IV belonging to the *ḥry-pḏt* Tutu son
of Rahotep, Tomb V belonging to the *ḥm-nṯr tp* Nana and the 'great' Tomb
VI), although he recognised that Tomb VII, with its portico with massive
polygonal columns and containing a Coptic church in its main hall, inscribed
for the *ḥ3ty-ʿ* Nakht-Ankh, was clearly Middle Kingdom in date.

Petrie at Deir Rifeh

When Petrie also returned to Rifeh, in 1906, his main concern was the excavation of the cemetery which lay below the rock-cut tombs, and not these tombs
themselves (which he notes were still 'fully occupied': Petrie 1907: 2). However,
he, or rather his assistant Mackay, did work in Tomb II, which was close to,
but not part of the 'Deir', the work resulting of course in the discovery of the
'Two Brothers' group. This work also produced other Middle Kingdom burials:
a group of four box coffins in a chamber similar to that of the 'Two Brothers'
which was 'a little south of this along the edge of the rock terrace', then 'nearby
on the south, was a small tomb, with a box coffin' and finally 'one other tomb'
containing a further box coffin' (Petrie 1907: 12–13). Apart from Tomb II, none of
these tombs is located on Petrie's 1:20,000 site map (Petrie 1907: pl. VIII), which
also gives the approximate locations of Deir Rifeh and Tomb VII, his 'unfinished
tomb' (Figure 4.2) and Tomb I (Khnum-Nefer). Petrie also provided (1907: pl.
XIIIE) 1:200 sketch-plans of another three tombs: Griffith's Tombs I and II
(which he attributes on this plan to Khnumu-Aa) and, in addition, a large tomb
located between these two tombs, which he referred to as an 'unfinished tomb'.

Montet and Pillet at Deir Rifeh

In the period from 1910 to 1914 the site was revisited by Montet and Pillet, the
former to check and add to the epigraphic copies made at Asyut and Deir Rifeh

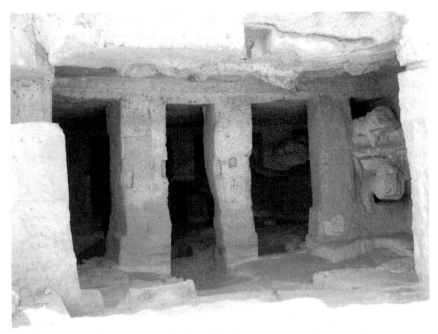

4.2 Petrie's 'unfinished tomb'. (Photograph by the author.)

by Griffith and the latter to carry out a detailed architectural survey of the tombs. Montet's account of his work at Asyut and Deir Rifeh was published in three articles between 1928 and 1936 in the journal *Kêmi* (Montet 1928, 1930s, 1936), in which he followed the numbering of tombs given by Griffith but, curiously, made no reference to the discovery of the 'Two Brothers' burial in 'Tombeau II'.

Pillet's plans of the Rifeh tombs were published at the same time as Montet's 1936 article (the one which is concerned principally with Rifeh rather than Asyut) on his epigraphic work, but in *Mélanges Maspero* (Pillet 1935–38). Pillet described the tombs as extending 'sur un longeur de près de deux kilomètres' with a Coptic church ('couvent') as part of the northern group (Pillet 1935–38: 61). Pillet's general plan of the extended site (1935–38: fig.1) includes not only the northern group of the Deir Rifeh tombs but also the northern part of the eastern face of the Gebel Durunka as far as the necropolis of Asyut and including the unfinished tombs about three kilometres to the north-north-west of Deir Rifeh which had been noted by Petrie. Pillet's work was largely focused on a detailed architectural study of the large Rifeh tombs, and he produced a set of high-quality plans of several of the tombs known and worked on by Griffith and by Petrie. These plans make a real contribution to the recording of the larger and more important tombs at Deir Rifeh, especially in the context of a detailed record of the state of these tombs in 1912. There are, however, a number of peculiarities in Pillet's publication. The most important of these peculiarities is that he makes no reference to earlier work at the site. If he had been unaware of Griffith's 1886–87 work and Petrie's discovery of the 'Two Brothers' in 1906 this in itself would be a little odd, but to show no sign of having subsequently become aware of this work before revising it for publication in 1935–38 seems even odder. This seeming unawareness of the Griffith work at Rifeh is reflected in Pillet's numbering of the tombs in the Deir Rifeh cluster using his own north–south system, even though Montet used the Griffith numbering system in his publication. As far as Petrie's work is concerned, Pillet planned Tomb II in great detail (Pillet 1935–38: fig.9) but did not include the sloping shaft and chamber of the 'Two Brothers' tomb itself. Of the other tombs which he planned in some considerable detail, Pillet was able to identify the owner of the tomb of Tutu (Pillet 1935–38: fig.8), but not that of Nakht-Ankh (which he referred to as 'Tombeau d'Inconnu': Pillet 1935–38: fig.4).

The plans that Pillet published were (i) a main plan of the terrace with the entrances to Tombs I–VI in his numbering system, equating to the tombs between and including those of Tutu (Griffith IV) and Nakht-Ankh (Griffith VII); (ii) a detailed plan of his Tombs VI (Tutu) and VII, which allows his Tomb VII to be connected to the main plan by overlap with Tomb VI; (iii) a detailed plan of his Tomb I (i.e. Nakht-Ankh, Griffith Tomb VII); and (iv) a detailed plan of Tomb II (unnumbered on his system), which cannot be directly connected to Pillet's main plan (although the main plan is annotated to state that this tomb is approximately 160 m south of the tomb of Tutu).

The Liverpool–Asyut Deir Rifeh Project

In the past century little scholarly attention has been given to the site of Deir Rifeh. Part of the reason for this has been the significant military presence in the area of the Gebel Durunka, which has made archaeological activity impossible. In recent years this restriction has eased. However, much work has been carried out since 1912 by the Antiquities Service at Deir Rifeh itself, most notably the removal of the remains of the abandoned Coptic occupation, revealing even further, relatively small, rock-cut tombs, and sets of rock-cut stairs leading to the larger tombs (Figure 4.3). However, the site is still important to the local Coptic population, especially one of the tombs (Pillet Tomb IV, not numbered by Griffith), which is still active as the 'host' of a Coptic chapel dedicated to the Virgin Mary and Saint Teodros, and Tomb VII, which still contains an operating church within its hall.

In October–November 2010, as part of the preliminary stages of the development of a fieldwork project between the universities of Liverpool and Asyut

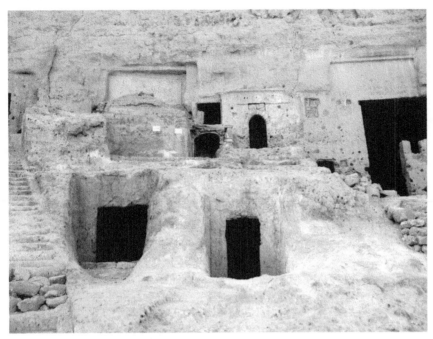

4.3 View of the central part of the Deir Rifeh group in 2012.
(Photograph by the author.)

focused on the Deir Rifeh necropolis, a reconnaissance survey was made in the necropolis. The purpose of this reconnaissance survey was to (i) locate the tombs which were known from the publications of work carried out over 100 years before, (ii) reconcile the various accounts of the specific locations of those tombs and (iii) assess the potential of the necropolis of rock-cut tombs, which is very extensive and packed with rock-cut tombs. This work was carried out by members of the joint Liverpool–Asyut project, specifically Dr Steven Snape and Dr Ashley Cooke (Liverpool) and Dr Osama Sallama (Asyut). In July 2012 a further visit was made to the Deir Rifeh tombs to carry out checks on data collected in 2010, and to add to the photographic record of the Rifeh necropolis. The Liverpool–Asyut team is grateful for assistance provided by the Ministry of Antiquities, local representatives of the Egyptian Armed Forces and the Thames Valley Ancient Egypt Society.

The plan of the site presented as Figure 4.4 represents an initial attempt to produce a location map of those tombs which were the subject of the work by Griffith, Petrie, Montet and Pillet, based on a number of sources. These sources include (i) Survey of Egypt maps, including the recent 1:50,000 series, (ii) Pillet's plan of the Deir Rifeh tombs, (iii) GPS readings taken by the Liverpool–Asyut

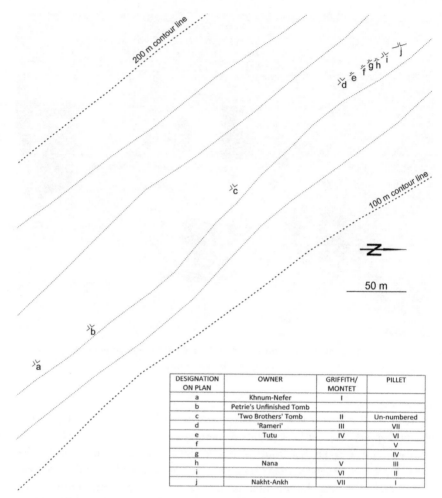

DESIGNATION ON PLAN	OWNER	GRIFFITH/ MONTET	PILLET
a	Khnum-Nefer	I	
b	Petrie's Unfinished Tomb		
c	'Two Brothers' Tomb	II	Un-numbered
d	'Rameri'	III	VII
e	Tutu	IV	VI
f			V
g			IV
h	Nana	V	III
i		VI	II
j	Nakht-Ankh	VII	I

4·4 Preliminary Plan of the Necropolis at Rifeh. (Created by the author.)

team and (iv) line-and-compass measurements taken by the Liverpool–Asyut team to connect the northern cluster with the 'Two Brothers' tomb, Petrie's 'unfinished tomb' and the tomb of Khnum-Nefer.

It must be stressed that this is a preliminary plan of the site pending future detailed work. It does not attempt to record even in general terms the very great number of visible rock-cut tombs which have not been the subject of earlier work. It also does not fully reconcile the relative positions of the tombs on this plan (which can be regarded with some confidence having been checked on the ground by the Liverpool–Asyut team) with other published topographic data for the region. It does, however, represent a step forward in understanding the nature and extent of this important necropolis and the position within it of the tomb of the 'Two Brothers'.

References

David, A. R. (2007), *The Two Brothers: Death and the Afterlife in Middle Kingdom Egypt* (Bolton: Rutherford Press).

Griffith, F. Ll. (1889a), 'The inscriptions of Siût and Dêr Rîfeh', *The Babylonian and Oriental Record* 3, 121–9, 164–8, 174–84, 244–52.

Griffith, F. Ll. (1889b), *The Inscriptions of Siût and Dêr Rîfeh* (London: Trübner and Co.).

Kahl, J. (2007), *Ancient Asyut: The First Synthesis after 300 Years of Research* (Wiesbaden: Harrassowitz).

Montet, P. (1928), 'Les tombeaux de Siout et de Deir Rifeh', *Kêmi* 1, 53–68.

Montet, P. (1935), 'Les tombeaux de Siout et de Deir Rifeh (suite)', *Kêmi* 6, 45–111.

Montet, P. (1936), 'Les tombeaux de Siout et de Deir Rifeh (troisième article)', *Kêmi* 6, 131–63.

Petrie, W. M. F. (1907), *Gizeh and Rifeh* (London: British School of Archaeology in Egypt and Quaritch).

Pillet, M. (1935–38), 'Structure et décoration architechtonique de la nécropole antique de Deïr-Rifeh (province d'Assiout)', in *Mélanges Maspero* (Cairo: Institut Français d'Archéologie Orientale), 61–75.

5

A review of the monuments of Unnefer, High Priest of Osiris at Abydos in the reign of Ramesses II

Angela P. Thomas

Unnefer was the High Priest or First Prophet of Osiris at Abydos for a substantial part of the long reign of Ramesses II, and was the fourth member of a family who held this office. An ancestor, To, served in the reign of Horemheb and possibly that of Ramesses I; he was followed by Hat, his brother-in-law, in the reign of Sety I, and then Hat's son Mery continued in the post into the reign of Ramesses II and was succeeded by his own son, Unnefer (Kitchen 1985: 170–1). Unnefer was followed by his son Hori, then by another son, Yuyu, before the end of Ramesses II's reign, and then by Siese, son of Yuyu, after the reign of Merenptah (Gaballa 1979: 46). Another son of Yuyu, Unnefer II, was High Priest of Isis (Frood 2007: 105). Monuments of the latter are also known from Abydos, and as he bore the same name as his grandfather, this gave rise to confusion about the family genealogy in some earlier publications (cf. Petrie 1902: 46–7). The first Unnefer had important connections, naming Prehotep and Minmose on inscriptions as 'brothers' (*snw*), although this denotes either a political or family relationship, a kinship through marriage or through a marriage in a previous generation. These relationships have been discussed and the details debated, but the fact that Unnefer at times states them appears to indicate their significance to him as part of his identity and wider, official position (Raedler 2004: 354–75; Moreno García 2013: 1038). Prehotep I was Northern Vizier during part of Unnefer's pontificate, and a second Prehotep was Northern Vizier later, then High Priest of Memphis and Heliopolis and Governor of Upper Egypt, unless as some have suggested this was the same man, and Minmose was High Priest of Onuris in Thinis during the whole of Unnefer's career (Kitchen 1985: 240–3).

Monuments and objects relating to Unnefer were discovered at Abydos in early work by collectors or their agents or in excavations by Émile Amélineau in 1895–98, by Auguste Mariette in 1858–76 and by Petrie and others between 1899 and 1926 (Richards 2005: 126–8). Unnefer's monuments are well known,

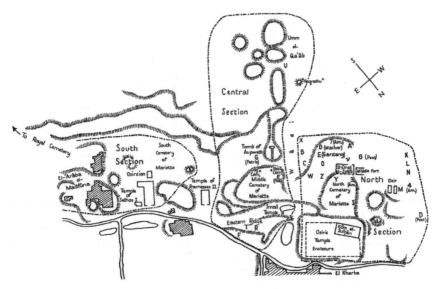

5.1 Plan of Abydos. (Porter and Moss 1937. Courtesy of the Griffith Institute, Oxford.)

as are their inscriptions. His items are all certainly from Abydos, whether these are provenanced or now unprovenanced; the unprovenanced material will be discussed, but where a precise site provenance at Abydos is recorded, this reveals that Unnefer is associated with the North and Central Sections. This includes in the North Section the Osiris Temple Enclosure and its surroundings, and in the Central Section the Small Temple investigated by Mariette, Cemetery G of Petrie and the tomb of Djer at Umm el-Qaab, which was identified as the tomb of Osiris (Figure 5.1). These areas are connected with Unnefer's responsibilities and activities in life as High Priest in the service of his god and king and his place in death and in the afterlife. More recent and continuing excavations at Abydos have contributed valuable information about some of these areas, and further work and publication will add to our knowledge of the cult of Osiris at Abydos in general and during this period in particular.

North Section: Osiris Temple Enclosure

Amélineau carried out some brief excavations and Mariette also undertook work at Kom es-Sûltân in the north-eastern part of the enclosure, but Mariette in addition investigated to some extent the temple enclosure (Amélineau 1899a: 7–8; Mariette 1880a: 26–35). Mariette clearly could not determine the site of the Osiris Temple, nor could he discover whether the tomb of Osiris might lie here, but he did note the Portal Temple of Ramesses II. Petrie was engaged in more extensive excavations, but his general plan and that of Garstang reveal the extent of the site and its difficult nature and indicate that its history was likely to be a complex one (Petrie 1903: pl. XLIX; Garstang 1901: pl. XXXVII). Petrie's summary of his results notes the early worship of Wepwawet and Khentiamentiu, the latter being absorbed by Osiris (although Wepwawet retained a role in the mysteries and festivals of Osiris), and states that Osiris, although known in the Late Old Kingdom through the Pyramid Texts, appears to come to prominence at Abydos by the Middle Kingdom. Petrie also refers to 'the ten successive temples', which he had cleared (1903: 47–9). Petrie's results and his interpretation have been the subject of debate over a long period. Excavations by the University of Pennsylvania Museum and Yale University began in 1967, establishing that the Portal Temple of Ramesses II was not only a gateway but a temple, and it was intended to investigate the Osiris Temple Enclosure (O'Connor 1967: 10–21). Since 1995 excavations have been continued by the Institute of Fine Arts, New York University, in various areas and are still in progress (O'Connor 2013–14: 2). The detailed history of the modern excavations is not relevant here but recent work suggests that Petrie's excavations in the Osiris Temple Enclosure included earlier Ka chapels and some cultic buildings but perhaps not the main temple (Klotz 2010: 134–5). Two phases of a major temple are being excavated, possibly the cult temple of Osiris, the later phase being of the 30th Dynasty and the earlier of the New Kingdom.

The recent work and its implications are important with regard to the monuments of Unnefer discovered in the Osiris Temple Enclosure; whether these were in their original position or moved and whether they had once been in the cult temple or in one or more other buildings are difficult to assess. Monuments of Unnefer discovered in the enclosure comprise fragments of an inscription of a hymn or prayer to Osiris naming Ramesses II together with a group of sculptures found near the causeway (Petrie 1903: 36, 45–6, pl. XXXVIII; Legrain 1909: 212, doc. 11): a granite squatting statue of Unnefer in poor condition, of which only the head was recovered, from near the temple of Nectanebo (Petrie 1902: 31, 44, pl. LXV, 5–7; Legrain 1909: 213, doc. 12; Figure 5.2); a granite double statue of Unnefer and his wife Tiy from near the enclosure wall, but probably from the temple of Nectanebo (Petrie 1902: 31, 44, pl. LXV, 9–10; Legrain 1909: 212, doc. 10); and two fragments of basalt statuettes (Petrie 1902: 31, 46, pl. LXVII; Legrain 1909: 212, doc. 8).

North Section: Shûnet ez-Zebîb

In 1921–22 Petrie carried out excavations in the area of the funerary enclosures, often referred to as funerary palaces, of the kings of the 1st and 2nd Dynasties

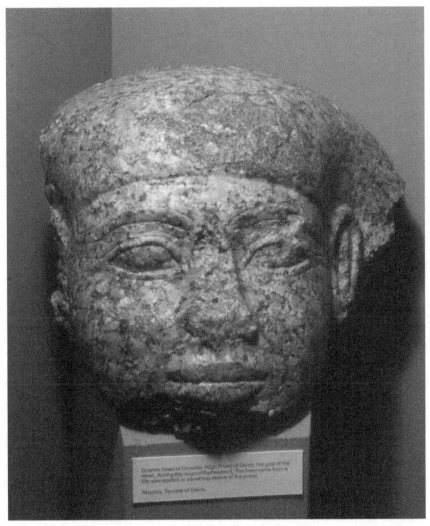

5.2 Granite head of Unnefer from the Osiris Temple Enclosure, 1903.46.9. (Courtesy of Bolton Museum, © Bolton Council, from the collections of Bolton Museum.)

whose tombs lay away to the south at Umm el-Qaab. He excavated graves surrounding certain enclosures, those of Djer, Djet and Merneith, and commented that they might surround a ceremonial area. He did not find any walls of these enclosures, although he was aware of the enclosure or fort of Peribsen, and that of Khasekhemui (the Shûnet ez-Zebîb, the best preserved of the enclosures), but without knowing their real purpose (Ayrton, Currelly and Weigall 1904: 1–5, pls. V–VIII; Petrie 1925: 1–3). Among the various later finds were fragments of a shrine which had been ornamented with ebony inlays, these comprising inscribed strips, girdles of Isis and flat thin figures of Unnefer with incised decoration (Petrie 1922: 35, 37; Petrie 1925: 11–12, pls. XXX, nos. 11, 12; XXXI, no. 5). These were found between the south enclosure walls of the Shûnet ez-Zebîb and not far from the enclosure of Djer. Recent excavations have revealed more about the structures and identified further enclosures (Bestock 2009: 51–61). However, given the use of parts of this area from the Middle Kingdom and later, it is not clear what the state of overall preservation and status of the early funerary enclosure zone was in the time of Unnefer, and therefore the fragments of his found here seem to be in the nature of a stray find which had originally been elsewhere.

Central Section: the Small Temple

This temple to the south of the Osiris Temple Enclosure was called 'le petit temple de l'ouest' by Mariette. He described the temple as ruined and reduced to ground level. Mariette employed many people and engaged in work on various sites at which he and his deputy Jean Gabet were not always present, but it appeared that the construction was of a thick core of mud brick faced with thin panels of limestone (Mariette 1869: 4). No dimensions or layout are given, and thus the position of any finds is unknown. Some items were left in situ as their condition was poor and material was damaged. Mariette was uncertain as to the dedication of the temple, but this would appear to have been to the Osirian family – Osiris, Isis and Horus. Items, those left on site and those removed to Cairo, included relief offering scenes of Tuthmosis IV and Ramesses III, a lintel of Ramesses II, part of a lintel of Psamtek I and Nitocris, the base of a naophorous statue of Ramesses III, a triad of Osiris, Isis and Horus, remains of granite naoi of Nectanebo I and Nectanebo II, part of a stela with a hymn to Osiris and buried in sand a limestone stela of Unnefer (Mariette 1869: 4–5; Mariette 1880a: 36–7; Mariette 1880b: cat. nos. 76, 354, 1053, 1126, 1129, 1289, 1424; Porter and Moss 1937: 70–1). The stela is an important monument of Unnefer, dated to year 42 of the reign of Ramesses II with the king offering to Osiris, Isis and Horus on the upper register, and below Unnefer and his wife Tiy adoring and the inscription referring to him as 'the servant of the god in his going out, in his day as Horus' and with Prehotep and Minmose mentioned as 'brothers' (*snw*) (Mariette 1880a: pl. 41; Legrain 1909: 209–10, doc. 4).

Nothing of a date earlier than the 18th Dynasty was found at the temple site. The temple may have been founded before then, or perhaps was established in the 18th Dynasty and continued until the 30th Dynasty. Nectanebo I and II undertook quite extensive restoration and building work after the Persian

Period, and at Abydos this included the Small Temple as well as the Osiris Temple. Material from Abydos was removed before the nineteenth century for re-use, and elements were utilised in the White Monastery Church of Saint Shenoute at Sohag and are also found in the monastery remains. A fragment of a naos of Nectanebo I has been recorded in the Yale White Monastery Project as lying in the church narthex after a previous repaving of the nave (Klotz 2011: 38). This is suggested as being from the Osiris Temple, and is compared to the naoi from the Small Temple, although the latter are implied wrongly to be from the Osiris Temple (Klotz 2011: 42).

Unprovenanced material

Legrain records five monuments of Unnefer in Athens, Paris and Cairo, which are unprovenanced, but which are certainly from somewhere at Abydos, and which were in their respective museum collections by the time of his publication (1909: 202–12, docs. 1, 2, 5, 6, 7). The most magnificent of these is the pillar or column statue of Unnefer in granodiorite in the Musée du Louvre, Paris, whose form suggests that it was an architectural element from a building, as indeed does the upper part of the pillar statue in the National Archaeological Museum, Athens, also granodiorite. To these has been linked a part of such a statue in the Egyptian Museum, Cairo (JE 35258), with relief figures in siliceous limestone (Frood 2004: 133–5). Mariette had been informed by local sources that about forty years previously, namely in about the early 1820s, material had been taken by collectors and the agents of consuls from the Small Temple area, and he surmised that this included the pillar statue of Unnefer and a naophorous statue of his son Yuyu, which he knew were in the Louvre (Mariette 1880a: 36). Giovanni Anastasi, Giovanni d'Athanasi on behalf of Henry Salt, Giuseppe Passalacqua, and Père Ladislaus on behalf of Bernardino Drovetti were all active at that period, and all acquired items from Abydos (Bierbrier 2012: 19–20, 28, 484–5, 418, 306, 161–2).

The pillar statue of Unnefer was in the Louvre in 1827 as it was on display in the Salle Civile, one of the four rooms for Egyptian antiquities whose exhibitions opened on 15 December 1827 with a catalogue prepared by Champollion (1827: 66–7, no. 50). At this stage there were some items in the museum which had been acquired at a rather earlier date, but the first major collection, that of Durand, who obtained material in Europe, had been purchased in 1825 (Detrez 2014: 47–8). The second collection of Salt had been bought in 1826 and Drovetti's second collection in 1827. However, comparison between Champollion's catalogue and inventory transcriptions of exhibits slightly later, when some material was in store, reveal that Durand's and Salt's collections were on display in 1827 and the Salt collection had included twenty-eight statues, and therefore this pillar statue (Buhe 2014; Bénédite 1923: 165–6). Drovetti's collection clearly arrived slightly later, and among it was the naophorous statue of Yuyu. The fragment of the pillar statue in the Athens National Archaeological Museum was originally recorded as having been found in Greece (Porter and Moss 1975: 403). It was not noted as a Greek find by Pendlebury (1930: 77–8). Legrain's statement that it had been found recently in Greece was misleading, for what he meant was that it had entered the collections of the Athens museum not long before he wrote his article, and probably as part of the collection donated by Alexandros Rostovitz in 1904 (Legrain 1909: 202–3, doc. 1; Bierbrier 2012: 475). The Athens pillar statue fragment includes a Hathor head; Hathor is a deity on the niche stela described below, associated with Isis, and can be associated with the djed-pillar (van Dijk 1986: 9).

The site provenance of these three pieces remains uncertain, but the Small Temple has been viewed as a likely provenance, as it was on the processional route from the Osiris Temple to Heqreshu Hill and thence to Umm el-Qaab (Frood 2004: 134–5). The other two unprovenanced pieces are the sandstone stela in Cairo (JE 32025) and the niche stela in the Louvre (C97) (Gaballa 1979: 45–7; Boreux 1921–22: 49–50, fig. 6). The Cairo stela is of a similar width to the one from the Small Temple, but only the upper register survives with a fragment of text below. The scene shows Unnefer adoring the seated Osiris with Isis, Nephthys and Anubis standing behind his throne and is inscribed for the benefit of the Ka of Unnefer. The niche stela depicts on the upper part figures of Osiris, Re, Isis and Hathor and on the lower part Unnefer, his wife and his parents. Both these pieces are of a funerary nature and perhaps came from his tomb or funerary chapel.

Central Section: Cemetery G of Petrie

Arriving at Abydos on 29 November 1895, Amélineau spent a few days in the North Section before going over to the Central Section to the south of the wadi and to the area south of the Small Temple and south of the Middle Cemetery of Mariette leading towards Umm el-Qaab. This was on the advice of a former *reis* of Mariette. The Middle Cemetery covered an extensive area with elite and non-elite tombs of earlier and later dates, and, aside from the activities of collectors, various excavations took place here after Mariette's and Amélineau's work (Snape 1986: 8–18). Amélineau discovered bricks of the ruined tomb chapel and enclosure of Minmose, High Priest of Onuris, with a later tomb above or partly over it. The shaft at the north of the tomb chapel was fifteen metres deep, was lined with bricks and led to what Amélineau described as five underground chambers. These were rock-cut and undecorated and had not been completely cleared, with fragments of statuettes and large vases being found. In the great chamber was the lid of a granite sarcophagus. Among the debris of the tomb was found the upper part of a stela of Minmose, with fifty-three fragments of limestone relief decoration recovered from the brick chapel above ground. No human or coffin remains were found underground, and there was evidence of material having been burnt (Amélineau 1899a: 9–12). Investigations nearby revealed nothing promising but about twelve metres away the tomb of Iuput A, the second son of Shoshenq I, was found, though this had apparently not been completed or used (Amélineau 1899a: 14–23). However, there had clearly been elite tombs in this area.

Amélineau listed later in his publication the fifty-three mixed fragments of relief from the ruined chapel of Minmose (1899a: 37). Though this was a relatively detailed recording, the fragments were not in order and thus not in a reliable context. Some of the fragments obviously related to Minmose as might be expected, but a number also related to Unnefer, including seven fragments of cornice with his name and titles, listed as one item (Amélineau 1899a: 37–45, nos. 1, 6, 7, 8, 15, 25, 36, 51; Porter and Moss 1937: 74). Of the statuettes listed, three were ushabtis of Minmose and one of Unnefer, although Amélineau records that three further ushabtis and a squatting statue, which Porter and Moss note as apparently from the tomb of Minmose, were from his work at Kom es-Sûltân (Amélineau 1899a: 49–51). The tomb of Minmose was, however, reinvestigated in 1900 by John Garstang and numbered G. 100. Working for Petrie's Egyptian Research Account in the North Section in Cemetery E, Garstang went over to the Central Section as there were reports that a previous excavator had left a granite statue in the tomb. In fact this was the granite lid of the sarcophagus of Khnumais, which Amélineau had intended to remove in a following season, but this he had not done. Garstang drew a plan and section of the tomb, which showed part of the enclosure wall, the shaft leading to two chambers, a passage, the burial chamber and a smaller chamber off it, which contained a limestone sarcophagus, and he cleared a sloping passage from the surface to the burial chamber, which Amélineau had also found. Garstang removed the lid, which went to the Egyptian Museum, Cairo, and also mentions some ushabtis of Minmose, fittings and small fragments of jewellery, although only a drawing of the inscription of a lower part of an ushabti and a fitting are illustrated (Garstang 1901: 11, 21, pls. XV, XVI, XXXIII).

This cemetery area was part of Petrie's concession, but as Petrie admitted it was not worked in a continuous way nor was it particularly worth excavating, though workmen could be placed here when not required elsewhere (Petrie 1902: 1). The tombs which he records are mainly 'late' in date (Petrie 1902: 34–40). However, a number of limestone reliefs were described as found by him or under his direction, three with year dates from the 'tomb of Unnefer' and a granite double statue of Unnefer and his father Mery, possibly from the

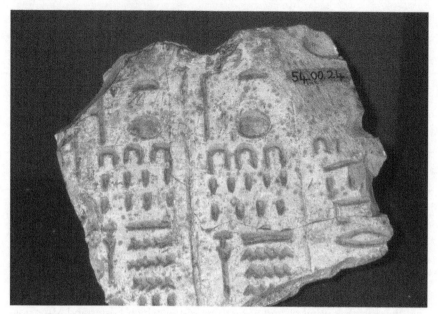

5.3 Fragment of limestone relief with years 38 and 39 of the reign of Ramesses II from the tomb chapel of Unnefer, 1900.54.24. (Courtesy of Bolton Museum, © Bolton Council, from the collections of Bolton Museum.)

same source. Details are regrettably lacking and the pieces were published by Randall-MacIver and Mace (1902: 85, 95, pls. XXXIV, XXXVII). The three fragments with no name surviving refer to the dedication of statues or offerings made in years 21 and 33, and a date probably after 33; and in 38, 39, a lost date, possibly 40, 47 and possibly 48 in the reign of Ramesses II (Randall-MacIver and Mace 1902: pl. XXXIV; see Kitchen 1985: 170; Figure 5.3). It seems perhaps likely that the tomb of Unnefer was next to or close to that of Minmose, or that they had a double chapel; both were ruined and some of the reliefs and the ushabtis were scattered and thus found by Amélineau. The underground chambers would indicate a tomb, but a funerary chapel has also been suggested (Effland and Effland 2004: 7–15).

Central Section: Umm el-Qaab

The tomb of Djer at Umm el-Qaab would seem to have been identified and venerated as the tomb of Osiris from perhaps the late Middle Kingdom or early in the Second Intermediate Period with processions being made to it, ceremonies conducted for the resurrection of the god and offerings consecrated and left there. Aside from investigating the original tomb, Amélineau discovered the granite sarcophagus or bed of Osiris, which dated to the 13th Dynasty and

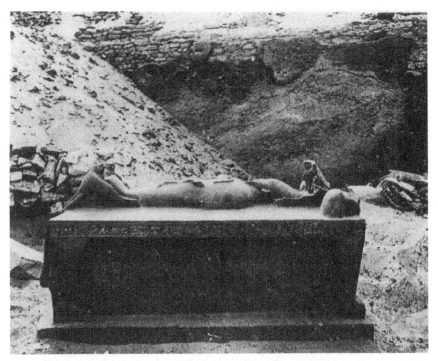

5.4 Granite sarcophagus of Osiris discovered at the tomb of Djer. (Reproduced from Amélineau 1899b: pl. III.)

was the major element of the shrine (Amélineau 1899b: 109–15, pls. III–IV; Ryholt 1997: 217; Figure 5.4). He also discovered many of the offerings, which were mostly pottery, including those naming Minmose and Prehotep and also Unnefer, who was named on a statuette (Amélineau 1899b: 44–6; Amélineau 1904: 49, 279, 289–90, pl. XXXV, 3, 7, 8; Porter and Moss 1937: 79–80). However, Amélineau also cleared away votive deposits, and the investigation of the dumps and debris in the area relating to the cult of Osiris is a research project of the Deutsches Archäologisches Institut. In recent work, items of Minmose have been found at Umm el-Qaab and Heqreshu Hill (Effland and Effland 2004: 9–10). Excavation, documentation and publication are still in progress (Effland, Budka and Effland 2013: 1–9).

The number of surviving monuments of Unnefer at Abydos is perhaps not surprising given that he held the post of High Priest or First Prophet of Osiris for a period of nearly thirty years or more. Ramesses II visited Abydos in the first year of his reign, and it might be assumed that he was not very pleased to find that buildings of previous kings were neglected and works had not been completed. More particularly work on the temple of his father Sety I remained unfinished, and clearly he intended that this should be accomplished as a mark of his piety towards his father and so that Osiris would favour him with a long life (David 1973: 10). Consequently, he gave orders for the completion of the temple, for the celebration of its services and offerings and for the provision of its lands and endowment, and he also ordered that restorations should be carried out where required in the cemetery, namely the royal cemetery (Kitchen 1985: 45–6). These works were probably undertaken when Unnefer's father, Mery, was the High Priest, although they may have extended into the period when Unnefer became High Priest. No monument of Unnefer has come from the South Section of the site or from the royal cemetery. A naos of his son Yuyu and his son Unnefer II was found near the pylon in the enclosure of the Osireion, but perhaps this was not its original location (Caulfeild 1902: pls. XXI, XXII; Legrain 1909: 217, doc. 23; Porter and Moss 1937: 90). It would appear that Unnefer had no role in terms of the royal cemetery where the structures were concerned with the cults of rulers. Unnefer's monuments are all apparently connected with the North and Central Sections at Abydos. This would imply that his administrative and religious responsibilities were devoted to the cult temple of Osiris, to the North votive zone, concerning which a project was initiated in 1996 and is ongoing, to the festivals of Osiris and to the procession to the so-called tomb of Osiris and the ritual activity there.

The inscriptions of Unnefer record his titles and details of his family including his father Mery, High Priest of Osiris, and his mother Maiany, songstress of Osiris. His wife Tiy was the daughter of Qeni, Chief of the Granaries of the North and South, and his wife Uay, along with Tiy, was a 'great one of the harem' of Osiris and songstress of Osiris. The year dates of Ramesses II's reign recorded on the limestone relief fragments from Unnefer's tomb chapel relate to religious dedications but perhaps also to significant events in the reign such as the treaty with the Hittites and the celebrations of jubilees (Kitchen 1985: 171). The stela of year 42 from the Small Temple refers to his family and his connection with Prehotep and Minmose and emphasises his skill in his role (Frood 2007: 100–1). The inscriptions on the pillar statue in the Louvre again record his family, parents and wife, and Prehotep and Minmose, but those on the back pillar refer to his role in the mysteries of Osiris, the festival and the procession to the tomb of Osiris and in carrying out everything with success (Frood 2007: 97–9). Thus he perhaps felt assured of his position not only in life but also in the afterlife.

References

Amélineau, É. (1899a), *Les nouvelles fouilles d'Abydos 1895–1896* (Paris: Ernest Leroux).
Amélineau, É. (1899b), *Le tombeau d'Osiris: monographie de la découverte faite en 1897–1898* (Paris: Ernest Leroux).

Amélineau, É. (1904), *Les nouvelles fouilles d'Abydos 1897–1898*, Part I (Paris: Ernest Leroux).

Ayrton, E. R., Curelly, C. T. and Weigall, A. (1904), *Abydos*, Part III: 1904 (London: Egypt Exploration Fund).

Bénédite, G. (1923), 'La formation du Musée égyptien au Louvre', *La revue de l'art ancien et moderne* 43, 161–72.

Bestock, L. (2009), *The Development of Royal Funerary Cult at Abydos: Two New Funerary Enclosures from the Reign of Aha* (Wiesbaden: Harrassowitz).

Bierbrier, M. L. (ed.) (2012), *Who was Who in Egyptology*, 4th rev. edn (London: Egypt Exploration Society).

Boreux, C. (1921–22), 'La stèle-table d'offrandes de Senpou et les fausses portes et stèles votives à representations en relief', *Fondation Eugène Piot: monuments et mémoires publiés par l'Académie des inscriptions et belles-lettres* 25, 29–51.

Buhe, E. (2014), 'Musée Charles X: inventory transcriptions of the Durand, Salt, and Drovetti collections of Egyptian antiquities', in E. Buhe, D. Eisenberg, N. Fischer and D. Suo, 'Sculpted Glyphs: Egypt and the Musée Charles X', *Nineteenth-Century Art Worldwide* 13 (1), www.19thc-artworldwide.org (last accessed 6 October 2014).

Caulfeild, A. St G. (1902), *The Temple of the Kings at Abydos* (London: Bernard Quaritch).

Champollion, J.-F. (1827), *Notice déscriptive des monuments égyptiens du Musée Charles X* (Paris: L'Imprimerie de Crapelet).

David, A. R. (1973), *Religious Ritual at Abydos (c. 1300 BC)* (Warminster: Aris and Phillips).

Detrez, L. (2014), 'Edme Antoine Durand (1768–1835): un bâtisseur de collections', *Cahiers de l'École du Louvre: recherches en histoire de l'art, histoire des civilisations, archéologie, anthropologie et muséologie* 4 (April), 45–55, www.ecoledulouvre/cahiers-de-l'ecole-du-louvre/numero4avril2014/Detrez.pdf (last accessed 2 October 2014).

Effland, U., Budka J. and Effland, A. (2013), 'Abydos, Umm el-Qaab: Osiriskult in Abydos', *Deutsches Archäologisches Institut, Jahresbericht 2012* (Berlin: Deutsches Archäologisches Institut), 1–9.

Effland, U. and Effland, A. (2004), 'Minmose in Abydos', *Göttinger Miszellen* 198, 5–17.

Frood, E. (2004), 'Self-Presentation in Ramessid Egypt' (DPhil thesis, University of Oxford).

Frood, E. (2007), *Biographical Texts from Ramessid Egypt* (Atlanta: Society of Biblical Literature).

Gaballa, G. A. (1979), 'Monuments of prominent men of Memphis, Abydos and Thebes', in G. A Gaballa, K. A. Kitchen and J. Ruffle (eds.), *Glimpses of Ancient Egypt: Studies in Honour of H. W. Fairman* (Warminster: Aris and Phillips), 42–9.

Garstang, J. (1901), *El Arábah: A Cemetery of the Middle Kingdom. Survey of the Old Kingdom Temenos; Graffiti from the Temple of Sety* (London: Bernard Quaritch).

Kitchen, K. A. (1985), *Pharaoh Triumphant: The Life and Times of Ramesses II*, 3rd corrected impression (Warminster: Aris and Phillips).

Klotz, D. (2010), 'Two studies on the Late Period Temple at Abydos', *Bulletin de l'Institut français d'archéologie orientale* 110, 127–63.

Klotz, D. (2011), 'A Naos of Nectanebo I from the White Monastery Church (Sohag)', *Göttinger Miszellen* 229, 37–52.

Legrain, G. (1909), 'Recherches généalogiques II: les premiers prophètes d'Osiris d'Abydos sous la XIXᶜ Dynastie', *Recueil de travaux* 31, 201–18.

Mariette, A. (1869), *Abydos*, I (Paris: Librairie A. Franck).

Mariette, A. (1880a), *Abydos*, II (Paris: L'Imprimerie Nationale).

Mariette, A. (1880b), *Catalogue général des monuments d'Abydos découverts pendant les fouilles de cette ville* (Paris: L'Imprimerie Nationale).

Moreno García, J. C. (2013), 'The 'other' administration: patronage, factions and informal networks of power in ancient Egypt', in J. C. Moreno García (ed.), *Ancient Egyptian Administration* (Leiden: Brill), 1029–65.

O'Connor, D. (1967), 'Abydos: a preliminary report of the Pennsylvania-Yale Expedition, 1967', *Expedition* 10, 10–21.

O'Connor, D. (2013–14), 'The Abydos project of the Institute of Fine Arts', *IFA Archaeology Journal* 2, 2.

Pendlebury, J. D. S. (1930), *Aegyptiaca: A Catalogue of Egyptian Objects in the Aegean Area* (Cambridge: Cambridge University Press).

Petrie, W. M. F. (1902), *Abydos*, Part I: *1902* (London: Egypt Exploration Fund).

Petrie, W. M. F. (1903), *Abydos*, Part II: *1903* (London: Egypt Exploration Fund).

Petrie, W. M. F. (1922), 'The British School in Egypt', *Ancient Egypt* 2, 33–9.

Petrie, F. (1925), *Tombs of the Courtiers and Oxyrhynkhos* (London: British School of Archaeology in Egypt).

Porter, B. and Moss, R. L. B. (1937), *Topographical Bibliography of Ancient Egyptian Hieroglyphic Texts, Reliefs, and Paintings*, V: *Upper Egypt: Sites* (Oxford: Oxford University Press).

Porter B., and Moss, R. L. B. (1975), *Topographical Bibliography of Ancient Egyptian Hieroglyphic Texts, Reliefs, and Paintings*, VII: *Nubia, the Deserts and Outside Egypt* (Oxford: Griffith Institute).

Raedler, C. (2004), 'Die Wesire Ramses' II: Netzwerke der Macht', in R. Gundlach and A. Klug (eds.), *Das ägyptische Königtum im Spannungsfeld zwischen Innen-und Außenpolitik im 2. Jahrtausend v. Chr.* (Wiesbaden: Harrassowitz), 354–75.

Randall-MacIver, D. and Mace, A. C. (1902), *El Amrah and Abydos 1899–1901* (London: Egypt Exploration Fund).

Richards, J. (2005), *Society and Death in Ancient Egypt: Mortuary Landscapes of the Middle Kingdom* (Cambridge: Cambridge University Press).

Ryholt, K. S. B. (1997), *The Political Situation in Egypt during the Second Intermediate Period 1800–1550 BC* (Copenhagen: Museum Tusculanum Press).

Snape, S. R. (1986), 'Mortuary Assemblages from Abydos' (PhD thesis, University of Liverpool).

van Dijk, J. (1986), 'The symbolism of the Memphite Djed-pillar', *Oudheidkundige Mededelingen uit het Rijksmuseum van Oudheden te Leiden* 66, 7–20.

6

Thoughts on Seth the con-man

Philip J. Turner

The great Sethian scholar Herman te Velde, after examining Seth's attributes, alluded to him as a trickster and concluded that Seth had five elements in common with tricksters of other cultures, namely that he was disorderly and uncivilised, and he was a murderer, a homosexual and a slayer-of-the-monster (te Velde 1968). This chapter offers thoughts on another aspect of his role as a trickster, what may be termed in modern parlance a 'con-man'. Other early tricksters include Loki in Norse mythology (Ricketts 1993) and Satan in Christian mythology (De La Torre and Hernandez 2011). A comparable role for Seth as a trickster may be seen in his part in the death of Osiris, a narrative pieced together from various accounts, and his use of 'trickery' during his subsequent 'contendings with Horus', as described in the New Kingdom Papyrus Chester Beatty I and by Plutarch. Other examples of his confidence tricks include those described in the Ptolemaic Papyrus Jumilhac. These apparently negative aspects of Seth's character, fitting the nuances of the modern term 'con-man', appear not to have been an obstacle to his worship for much of Pharaonic history.

The *Collins English Dictionary* (2000: 339) defines a con-man as follows: '1; a person who swindles another by means of a confidence trick or 2; a plausible character.' A con-man requires a number of attributes; first among these is the power of persuasion. The con-man must persuade his intended target to trust him. The con-man also needs to be likeable and persuasive, as the former con-man Simon Lovell puts it: 'many men have kissed the Blarney Stone, a con-man has swallowed it' (Schrager 2014).

So how can we compare Seth with other con-men? The latter certainly possess the power of persuasion, and Seth also possessed this quality, as can be seen by his ability to persuade Osiris initially to attend the magnificent party that he held in his honour (Babbit 2003: 35, 13). The fact that Osiris attended this festivity even though, as Plutarch tells us, he knew that Seth was not to be trusted is testament to Seth's powers of persuasion. Following on from this, Seth then persuades Osiris to lie in the coffin that he has had made and springs his trap, slamming the lid and fastening it shut before setting it adrift in the river Nile (Babbit 2003: 37, 13). Seth's power of persuasion is also shown in the Papyrus Chester Beatty I account of 'The Contendings of Horus and Seth' in the passage that describes how Seth asks Horus to 'Let us pass a happy day together in my house' (Simpson 1973: 119–20; Lichtheim 1976: 219). Horus agrees to this even though earlier in the account Seth had attacked Horus and blinded him.

A con-man also needs to be likeable. In the Dream Book of Qenherkhepshef the dreams of at least two categories of individuals are described, the final section being headed: 'Beginning of the dreams of the followers of Seth' (Szpakowska 2003: 73). Included in this section is a description of this type of man. Szpakowska describes the Sethian man thus:

> A man with curly hair, possibly naturally red in colour who is potentially vio-
> lent, decadent and debauched and a womaniser. He often drinks to excess and
> when he does, his Sethian character takes control. Whilst he may be a member
> of the royal classes, his tastes and manners are unrefined, unrestrained and
> earthy, like those of a commoner. (Szpakowska 2003: 73)

While in many ways this is not a flattering description, these roguish traits in a person have attracted followers in many times and places. Con-men are invariably likeable, in some sense, for otherwise men and women would not fall for their schemes, and Seth shows this particular characteristic never more than when he manages to elicit the support of Re during his contending with Horus over the throne of Egypt. Re says to Horus: 'You are feeble in thy limb, and this kingly office is too great for you, child, the taste of whose mouth is bad' (Lichtheim 1976: 216). Even at the conclusion of the Chester Beatty tale, when Horus has been awarded the throne, Re requests that Seth should be given to him so that he can live with him as his son, and he will be the thunder in the sky and that men will fear him (Simpson 1973: 123–5; Lichtheim 1976: 222), implying some appreciation of Seth's strength.

A con-man must also possess skills as a conversationalist. Seth shows this time and time again in the account of 'The Contendings of Horus and Seth', appearing to bounce back from each set-back and attempting to persuade the Company of Heaven that he is the one to rule Egypt. Argument vacillates between the two contending parties: it is not simply that Horus is the righteous heir; Seth persuades some of the gods of his claim too. Thus, Banebdjedet, replying to Thoth's declaration 'Shall the office be given to a brother on the side of the mother, while a son of the body is yet alive?', then states, 'Shall the office be given to this child, while Seth, his elder brother is yet alive?' (Simpson 1973: 113; Lichtheim 1976: 216; Morgan 2005: 306). Banebdjedet appears to support Seth's arguments as to why he should be the legitimate heir to the throne.

The ability to adopt many guises is another attribute that the ideal con-man requires, and Seth certainly demonstrates this. In Papyrus Jumilhac, Seth changes his appearance to that of a crocodile (Vandier 1961: 74) and that of Anubis (Vandier 1961: 104) in order to attempt to achieve his aim of destroying or despoiling the body of Osiris (Pinch 2002: 80). Then when he fails in this endeavour he flees from the real Anubis and Thoth to the region of the gebel, where he transforms himself into a panther (Vandier 1961: 104). In another story recounted in the papyrus, Seth turns himself into a bull in an attempt to copulate with Isis (Vandier 1961: 110).

Despite Seth's widely known negative character traits, his worship continued until the Roman Period, and he maintained an important position in both personal religious piety and state ideology. It is likely that the Egyptians wanted to see in their king a combination of the attributes of both Horus and Seth. Thus Hatshepsut recorded upon her obelisk at Karnak Temple: 'as I wear the White Crown, as I appear in the Red Crown, as Horus and Seth have united for me their two halves, as I rule this land like the son of Isis [i.e. Horus], as I have become strong like the son of Nut [i.e. Seth]' (Sethe and Helck 1906: 366; Breasted 1906: 133). Strength and cunning go together.

Assmann (2006: 44) makes the point that the contrast between Seth and Horus symbolises a change from old disorder to new stability, one of reconciliation. In the mythic version of this change as described in 'The Contendings of Horus and Seth', order triumphs over chaos, rule over anarchy and law over force. But the alternatives to order are not ignored or demonised; rather they are seen as a necessary part of the whole. Life must have both positive and negative aspects. The king must demonstrate the faithfulness and respect for his parents shown by Horus on the one hand, and also the brute strength, bloody-mindedness and cunning of Seth on the other (Turner 2013: 69).

It seems probable that during the Early Dynastic Period Seth was regarded as a benevolent god by a large part of the population, especially those around the site of Nubet, in the Delta, and perhaps also at the oases of the Libyan Desert, where he was later known as the 'Lord of the Oases' (te Velde 1967: 115). Possibly because of this latter role, he also became known as the god of the eastern deserts and came to be associated with all the frightening elements that the Egyptians believed emanated from the desert: wind, rain, storm and thunder. By extension, Seth also added 'Lord of Foreign Lands' to his titles (Turner 2013: 69).

In his role of 'Lord of Foreign Lands', Seth was still very much viewed as an Egyptian god, one might say as a Foreign Minister rather than a Foreign

Ambassador to put things into modern diplomatic vernacular. This is important as it means that his first accountability was towards Egypt rather than
towards foreigners. It was in this role that Seth was identified during the Hyksos
Period, and this may explain why on their expulsion he was not vilified. To the
Egyptians, he had carried out his role as Foreign Minister and, while being associated with the foreigners, he had protected Egypt's privileged position within
the universe. One can imagine that the Egyptians would have realised that in
order to do this his guile would have been very useful; the ability to ingratiate
himself and the art of persuasion represent the diplomatic skills necessary for the
holder of the post of Foreign Minister.

All this supports the idea that the Egyptians could see Seth in two lights.
Te Velde (1967: 27–63) sees Seth as an evil figure, citing not only his murder
of Osiris but also the circumstances of his birth (where he burst through his
mother's side) and his attempted rape of Horus (see my comments on this latter
matter in Turner 2013: 22) as evidence of this. However, Kemboly (2010: 244)
believes that the Egyptians saw Seth as someone who challenged authority, the
establishment, the status quo, social convention and so on – one could say a
typical description of a con-man – or even a loveable rogue. Kemboly's view
suggests that Seth represented a principle through which society kept itself open
to critique in order to improve and to be able to tolerate a certain amount of
disorder.

Much of the demonisation of Seth came in the first millennium BC, when
the name of the god was attacked or written without the chaotic Seth animal
determinative (e.g. Soukiassian 1981: 59–68). At this time, as David Klotz has
recently remarked (Klotz 2013: 176), the traditional Seth animal was considered
suitable only for Seth as a villain, but was no longer deemed appropriate for an
object of worship. Thus, according to Klotz, Seth was not demonised so much
as he was emasculated or disarmed. A catalyst may have been the invasion of
the country by the Assyrians, which saw Thebes itself sacked for the first time
(Kitchen 1973: 394), when the Egyptians may have observed that Seth had failed
in his role of Foreign Minister. As te Velde puts it:

> In late times, the Egyptians were faced with the enigma that the chosen
> country could yet be occupied and plundered by foreigners. Their dread and
> discontent were uploaded not upon the whole pantheon, but upon the tradi-
> tional god of foreigners, who had always had a special and precarious place in
> the pantheon. (Te Velde 1967: 143)

Seth as 'Lord of Foreign Lands' now has negative connotations: a foreign
ruler who has been defeated but is planning a new invasion which includes
wreaking havoc amongst the temples of Egypt. This is illustrated particularly
in the Early Ptolemaic Papyrus Louvre 3129 (Schott 1930: 18–24; Turner 2013:

52–3), which describes how Seth has turned once more to Egypt and has come to plunder the land, destroy holy sites, tear down chapels and make uproar in the temples. He catches sacred fish, pursues animals and fowl, performs bad deeds in the embalming house, sets fire to sacred trees and generally desecrates all the temples, as the papyrus concludes: 'suffering reigns in the place where he abides' (Assmann 2006: 390–2).

This represents the point at which Seth perhaps reaps his just rewards for his character but one cannot help thinking that this character was what perhaps endeared him to the Egyptians, who could probably see aspects of themselves within him. His quarrelsome nature, his strength and might and, indeed, his liking for drink and sex were all things that they could readily identify within themselves and are likely to have contributed to his popularity.

References

Assmann, J. (2006), *The Mind of Egypt* (London: Harvard University Press).

Babbit, F. C. (ed. and trans.) (2003), *Plutarch's Moralia* (Cambridge, MA: Harvard University Press).

Breasted, J. H. (1906), *Ancient Records of Egypt*, II, reprinted 2006 (Chicago: University of Illinois Press).

Collins English Dictionary (2000) (Glasgow: Harper Collins).

De La Torre, M. and Hernandez, A. (2011), *The Quest of the Historical Satan* (Minneapolis: Fortress Press).

Kemboly, M. (2010), *The Question of Evil in Ancient Egypt* (London: Golden House Publications).

Kitchen, K. A. (1973), *The Third Intermediate Period in Egypt (1100–650 BC)* (Warminster: Aris and Phillips).

Klotz, D. (2013), 'A Theban devotee of Seth from the Late Period – now missing: ex-Hannover, Museum August Kestner Inv. S. 0366', *Studien zur altägyptischen Kultur* 42, 155–80.

Lichtheim, M. (1976), *Ancient Egyptian Literature: The New Kingdom* (Berkeley: University of California Press).

Morgan, M. (2005), *The Bull of Ombos: Seth and Egyptian Magick* (Oxford: Mandrake and Mogg Morgan).

Pinch, G. (2002), *Egyptian Mythology* (Oxford: Oxford University Press).

Ricketts, M. L. (1993), 'The shaman and the trickster', in W. J. Hynes and W. G. Doty (eds.), *Mythical Trickster Figures: Contours, Contexts, and Criticisms* (Tuscaloosa: University of Alabama Press), 87–105.

Schott, S. (1930), *Urkunden mythologischen Inhalts* 6 (Leipzig: G. Steindorff).

Schrager, A. (2014), *How to Cheat at Everything*, www.moreintelligentlife.co.uk/story/how-to-cheat-at-everything (last accessed 15 January 2015).

Sethe, K. and Helck W. (1906), *Urkunden des ägyptischen Altertums* 4 (Leipzig: Hinrichs).

Simpson, W. K. (ed.) (1973), *The Literature of Ancient Egypt* (New Haven: Yale University Press).

Soukiassian, G. (1981), 'Une étape de la proscription de Seth', *Göttinger Miszellen* 44, 59–68.

Szpakowska, K. (2003), *Behind Closed Eyes: Dreams and Nightmares in Ancient Egypt* (Swansea: The Classical Press of Wales).

Te Velde, H. (1967), *Seth, God of Confusion: A Study of his Role in Egyptian Mythology and Religion* (Leiden: Brill).

Te Velde, H. (1968), 'The Egyptian god Seth as a trickster', *Journal of the American Research Center in Egypt* 7, 37–40.

Turner, P. J. (2013), *Seth: A Misrepresented God in the Ancient Egyptian Pantheon?* (Oxford: Archaeopress).

Vandier, J. (1961), *Le Papyrus Jumilhac* (Paris: Musée du Louvre).

7

A Psamtek ushabti and a granite block from Sais (Sa el-Hagar)

Penelope Wilson

Herodotus's account of the temples at Sais represents a point of departure for most discussions of the topography of the 26th Dynasty city, the temples and the royal tombs within the enclosure (Leclère 2008: 159–96). Herodotus provided a detailed description of the Royal Tombs in the precinct of the temple of Athene-Neith, near the sanctuary on the left of the entrance. The tomb of Amasis was a little further from the sanctuary and the tombs of the Saite ancestors, but was still within the temple court (Herodotus, *Histories*, II, 169; Godley 1966: 483). Furthermore, the tomb of Amasis seems to have lain through a portal which was approached by a palm-capital colonnade. The structure may have been a ground-level tomb chapel or funerary temple. Unfortunately, nothing is left of the temple and its ancillary buildings (Wilson 2006: 99–115), and the ruina-tion of Sais seems to have begun with the Persian invasion, for the statue of Udjahorresnet alludes to renovations that were necessary in the temple of Neith in the 27th Dynasty (Lloyd 1982). Further large-scale destructions, evident at the site from the Ptolemaic and Roman Periods in the form of pottery dumps and a bath-house (Wilson 2006: 130–42), meant that when Western travellers arrived there in the nineteenth century, the ruins represented a small part of what had once existed. For example, in 1828, Champollion recorded a 'great enclosure', in the middle of which were a 'memnonium' or necropolis approxi-mately 300 m long to the west and another enclosure with two hills, which could have been the tombs of Amasis and Apries, as well as a mound just north of the village of Sa el-Hagar, itself upon a mound (Champollion 1833: 49–53). His published plan, however, does not contain so much detail. Later, from visits in 1821 and 1833, John Gardner Wilkinson made a topographical map showing the central east–west structure and also a western north–south enclosure within the Northern Enclosure, published to accompany a commentary on Herodotus (Rawlinson 1862: 218). By the end of the nineteenth century, not only had the enclosure wall and '*qasr*' to the north been removed, but the mound to the south of the site adjacent to the village had also gone (Foucart 1898: 168–9, fig. 19), creating the 'Great Pit' and liberating statuary, bronzes and other treasures for museum and private collections. However, few objects that could be associated with the Royal Tombs have been recognised, suggesting that they have been destroyed and lost.

Barbotin (2000) published part of what could be a royal sarcophagus in the Musée du Louvre, Paris (E32580), and in many ways the Louvre granite fragment represents the sad history of the Sais tombs. The block came from a private collection, and it is not clear how long ago it came out of Egypt. The fragment is slightly curved on the back, which is otherwise uncarved, but has a sunk relief image of a ram-headed form of Re in the sun barque on the front. The scene is from the *Amduat*, and the date of the fragment is provided by a cartouche of Psamtek II Neferibre. If the sarcophagus did not come from this king's tomb, it must have belonged to someone else of royal status. The likely large scale, the material – red granite – and the subject matter indicate, however, that the granite fragment was from something that belonged to the king or a very close relative. The two known queens' sarcophagi of the 26th Dynasty are both also made of granite, but were found at Athribis (Adam 1958) and Memphis (now in the Hermitage; Buhl 1959: 197).

Barbotin further noted all of the known material that could otherwise have come from the Saite Royal Tombs, including ushabti figures (2000: 37). A heart scarab of Necho II, which was known from the Comte de Caylus collection in 1767, gave rise to the idea that the tomb of Necho II had been discovered in the eighteenth century, but it is not now possible to know the truth of this claim (Barbotin 2000: 38, n. 26).

The mission of the Egypt Exploration Society, Durham University and the Supreme Council for Antiquities at Sais has since 1997 been probing the different areas of the site to understand the archaeological material that is still extant and is able to add a small number of pieces to those already known.

A granite fragment with the Four Sons of Horus

In April 2003, a large fragment of red granite some 1.30 m long and 77 cm wide was found in a cow-shed in the village of Ganag, removed to nearby Sa el-Hagar and subsequently taken for storage to the magazine at Tell Farain (Buto) (Figure 7.1). The back of the granite fragment is slightly convex and the front, flat side is lightly incised with a scene showing a *wadj*-papyrus stem flanked by the Four Sons of Horus, with the jackal- and human-headed sons on the right of the stem and the falcon- and baboon-headed sons on the left. They flank the papyrus column as if in a square or circle around it. The carving is carefully

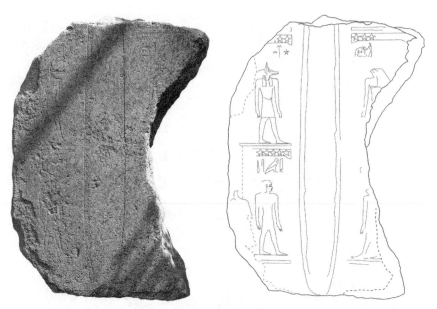

7.1 Granite block from Ganag and drawing of upper face. (Created by the author.)

executed in low, sunk relief, with the interior rounded and pecked, similar to the Louvre fragment. The hieroglyphs are carefully but not deeply incised and the names of the Four Sons are each surmounted by a sunk relief *pt*-sign decorated with raised relief stars. The surface was well smoothed and polished. The subject matter suggests that the fragment is from a funerary context; the scale of the fragment suggests a large wall or object, and the convex back may suggest some kind of box or container, such as a sarcophagus or its lid. There is nothing by which to date the fragment, except perhaps the face of the human-headed Imsety. He is depicted with full cheeks, lidded eyes, rounded nose with fold indicated, pursed lips with drilled corners and a slightly golf-ball-like chin (Figure 7.2). All of these indications would suggest a Late Period to Ptolemaic date (Josephson 1997: 5), with a hint of the so-called 'Saite smile' (Josephson and El-Damaty 1999: 86).

The granite fragment was re-shaped with a hemispherical cut on its left-hand side, perhaps to accommodate a grind-stone, after it was taken from its original location. That the stone fragment originated at Sais is likely, as many other blocks have been traced to surrounding villages and nearby towns over the years (Habachi 1943; Wilson 2006: 203–30) and Ganag is less than 5 km north of Sa el-Hagar. The other alternative as a source of the fragment would be Buto, although it may be just too far away to have supplied villages to the south.

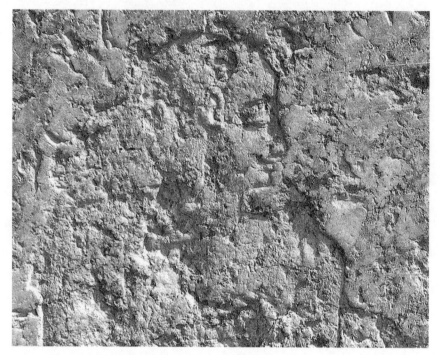

7.2 Detail of the head of Imsety, showing the face. (Photograph by the author.)

Many of the anthropoid sarcophagi lids dating to the Late and Ptolemaic Periods have depictions of the Four Sons of Horus on them, flanking the sides and in the same configuration (for example, Buhl 1959: 59, fig. 25; 125, fig. 75; 137, fig. 79). The *wadj*-papyrus stem, however, seems to be a rare element and may allude to a more Delta-orientated origin or idea. Even on the foot of a sarcophagus of Wahibre, from Kawady, the front cover shows the Four Sons of Horus on either side of bands of text containing their names and in the same grouping as on the granite fragment (Wilson 2006: 211–15). Although none of the known Saite sarcophagi seem to provide a direct comparison with the new fragment, it may still be possible that the fragment came from a royal tomb at Sais and perhaps from the sarcophagus lid of one of the kings.

An ushabti of the King of Upper and Lower Egypt, Psamtek

An object more certainly connected with the Saite Royal Tombs was found in 2007, during excavation of the area for the foundations of the magazine of Durham University and the Egypt Exploration Society at Sa el-Hagar. The mission found a fragment of an ushabti figure with the cartouche of the 'King of Upper and Lower Egypt, Psamtek' (Figure 7.3). The context for the find was the

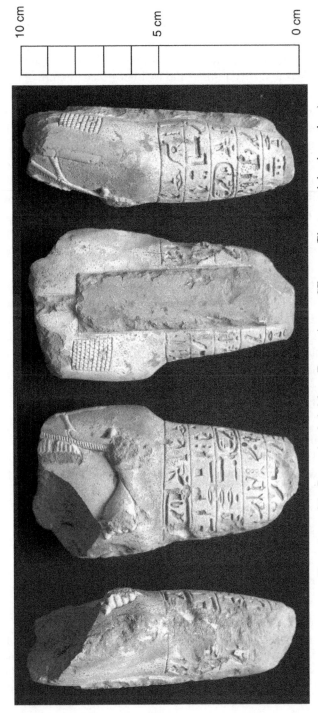

7.3 Four views of the Psamtek ushabti from Excavation 10, SF10.175. (Photograph by the author.)

10 cm

5 cm

0 cm

rubble fill of the foundations of a Late Antique church building on the eastern side of the Great Pit to the south of the main enclosure. A number of other smaller ushabtis and amulets, as well as Saite Period pottery, also came from the fill, but they were mixed together with Ptolemaic and Roman material, showing that the rubble contained a re-used and well-integrated mixture of remains.[1]

The ushabti fragment has a maximum height of 9.8 cm, maximum width of 5.3 cm and maximum thickness of 3.2 cm. It is made of high-quality faience, very fine and dense in composition. Most of the original glaze has been lost, leaving the ushabti mostly white in appearance, with some faint traces of turquoise colour. The back pillar has a brown tinge, suggesting that it could have been a different colour from the rest of the figure or reacted to the deposition conditions differently. The head and feet of the ushabti have been broken away and there is damage to the right-hand side, hands and back of the figure along the bottom edge. The ushabti is shown as mummiform, holding a hoe and a basket in the right hand, and in the left hand there was an unidentified object, lost at the top of the hand and where it rested upon the right shoulder. The rope of the basket is detailed on the front of the figure, and the basket itself is on the back of the ushabti. The ushabti has a blank back-pillar. There are the remains of five horizontal lines of the ushabti spell (Chapter 6 of the Book of the Dead) on the lower part of the figure, underneath the crossed hands, beginning beside the back-pillar on the back and running from right to left across the body and over onto the back, to end at the back-pillar. There are traces of a *nemes*-headcloth on the left-hand side of the figure, and the gathered 'tail' of the covering extends to the top of the back-pillar at the back. The quality of the workmanship is good, with much detail apparent on the tools and headdress. The figure was found in good condition, but, in places, the surface was a little powdery. It was brushed gently with a fine brush to remove dirt after it had dried out slowly. The object was registered by the Supreme Council of Antiquities and Ministry of State for Antiquities.

The preserved text is as follows:

1. *sḫḏ wsir nsw-bity Psmtk...* 'I
2. *wšbty ipn ir ipn ....*
3. *nsw-bity Psmtk mȝ'-ḫrw r irt kȝt ... m*
4. *m ḫrt-nṯr is tw ḥw sḏb...*
5. *r ḫrt[2] m'[k] w*

---

1   I am grateful to Mohamed Rashad, Ahmed Bilal, Said el-Assal, Ibrahim el-Dessouki and Emad el-Shennawi for their cooperation in Excavation 10. A preliminary report on the excavation can be found at www.dur.ac.uk/penelope.wilson/sais.html.

2   *ḫrt* is written with a butcher block sign (Gardiner sign list, T 28), not *ḫ* the placenta (?) (Gardiner sign *Aa* 1).

Translation
1. Illuminating the Osiris King of Upper and Lower Egypt Psamtek …
   forever. O
2. this ushabti, if this one …
3. King of Upper and Lower Egypt, Psamtek, true of voice, to perform (any)
   work
4. in the necropolis land, then you will remove any hindrance …
5. to the desert edges in …

Around twenty-five ushabti fragments are known for the 26th Dynasty kings, and there may be museums and collections all over the world that have yet unidentified or unpublished pieces in their stores. Aubert and Aubert (1974) and Schneider (1993) reviewed the evidence and noted only a few ushabtis with provenance, including one from Memphis. There were, at that time, ten Psamtek ushabtis, mostly from collections in Europe, but with one in the Egyptian Museum, Cairo, from Memphis (JE 86759, Aubert and Aubert 1974: 212). In addition, three further ushabtis have since been published elsewhere so that the Sais fragment makes a total of fourteen examples. The other 26th Dynasty kings have even fewer ushabtis attributed to them, with Necho I or II having two ushabtis, both in museum collections; three ushabtis of Apries are known – including one also found at Sais by Daressy on the western side of the Great Pit and one found as an *ex-voto* at Saqqara (Cairo CG 48516) – and for Amasis there are five. So far, only one possible canopic fragment of Apries from Saqqara has been reported (Emery 1971) and there are no known vessels or jewellery that may have a connection with the Saite royal burials.

Although the ushabti figures with the name Psamtek clearly belonged to a king, it is not immediately clear to which of the three kings called Psamtek they can be attributed. The name 'Psamtek', which is usually the nomen of the Saite kings concerned, is preceded by 'King of Upper and Lower Egypt' and has thus become the prenomen of the kings to whom the ushabtis belonged (Aubert and Aubert 1974: 211; Reeves 1996: 95). The transposition of prenomen and nomen may be due to the fact that Psamtek I was the founder of the new dynasty and that there was no reason to differentiate him from any other Psamtek. It is, therefore, very likely that the ushabtis bearing the name 'Psamtek' can be attributed to Psamtek I 'WahibRe' (664–610 BC). In addition, the practice of the use of only the nomen on ushabtis was followed in the 25th Dynasty, thus this tradition continued unbroken. It can also be noted that the nomen of Apries (589–570 BC), WahibRe, was used on his ushabtis. As this was the prenomen of Psamtek I, it seems that Apries was both following the tradition of using the nomen only as well as highlighting his link with the dynastic founder Psamtek I. Furthermore, it has been suggested that the relatively short reign of Psamtek II may be a factor in the lack of funerary equipment attributable to

Table 7.1 Details of the Psamtek ushabtis from published accounts and museums

Museum details	Height (cm)	Width (cm)	Depth (cm)	Head-dress	Colour	Date and provenance	Notes	Published
Berlin, Ägyptisches Museum und Papyrussammlung 4254	17.5, complete				brown	1857, Anastasi collection	formerly in Charlottenburg Museum	Kaiser 1967: 96
Berlin, Ägyptisches Museum und Papyrussammlung 8085	9.5, part					at the museum by 1899	formerly in Charlottenburg Museum	Kaiser 1967: 96
Berlin, Bode Museum							lost?	Schneider 1993: 155
Cairo, Egyptian Museum JE 86759	c.14, part			nemes	beige	Memphis excavation	limestone?	Badawi 1984: 12, pl. 3
Cairo, Egyptian Museum?	9.8, part	5.3	3.2	nemes	light green	2007, Sa el-Hagar excavation		Wilson forthcoming
Copenhagen, Nationalmuseet AEIN 1460	11.24, no head	5.67	3.5	nemes	blue	1911, Valdemar Schmidt collection		Aubert and Aubert 1974: 212
Myers Museum, Eton College ECM 1709	17.0, complete			nemes	black			Reeves 2008: 95
Paris dealer, Hôtel Drouot						Pozzi Collection 1970		Aubert and Aubert 1974: 212
London, British Museum EA 21922	15.2, part	5.4	–	nemes	pale green	1887, Chester collected		Hall 1931

Location	No.	Height		Headdress	Colour	Provenance / notes	Reference
London, Petrie Museum of Egyptian Archaeology, UCL 40317	13.2, part	5.9	—	nemes	light green	Petrie	Petrie 1935: pl. 43
London, Petrie Museum of Egyptian Archaeology, UCL				bag-wig		Wellcome collection	Schneider 1993: 155
Stockholm, Gardell private collection		18	—		pale green	On loan to the Medelhavs-museet until 2008	Peterson 1977: 13–14
Tübingen, Ägyptisches Sammlung der Universität Tübingen 899	9.5, part			nemes		Sieglin expedition 1898–1914; Lindenmuseum, Stuttgart	Brunner-Traut and Brunner 1981: 280–1
Vienna, Kunst-historisches Museum 8354				nemes	pale green	acquired before 1952	Satzinger 1994: 109

him. If the Louvre sarcophagus fragments did come from his tomb furniture, however, this may not then be the case and an ushabti head from a Paris private collection could have had both prenomen and nomen inscribed upon it, as it is slightly different to the other Psamtek ushabtis (Aubert and Aubert 1974: 211).

A closer analysis of the Psamtek ushabtis (see Table 7.1) shows that, when the provenance of the objects is known, they are attested in museum collections during the nineteenth century, often having been bought through dealers (as probably those of Petrie), and donated by travellers to Egypt including Greville Chester in 1887 (British Museum), Anastasi in 1857 (Ägyptisches Museum und Papyrussammlung, Berlin) and the Sieglin Expeditions in 1898–1902 and 1909–14 (Linden-Museum, Stuttgart). This timing corresponds to periods of intense *sebakhin* digging at Sa el-Hagar in the latter part of the nineteenth century (Foucart 1898). The ushabtis could have been found by *sebakhin* at Sa el-Hagar and entered the general dealer market during the nineteenth century, when many of them were acquired. Some examples took longer to be declared in collections such as that in the Nationalmuseet, Copenhagen (1911).

The example in the British Museum (EA 21922) lacks only its feet and base and gives a good indication of the original appearance of the complete figures. The ushabti has the same form as the Sais fragment, with two hoes held in the hands and the basket held with a hoe in the left hand. The back pillar is also blank. The face of the figure seems to be extremely distinctive and beardless, and Hall compared it to the face of Psamtek I on the famous intercolumnar screen-wall slab, also in the British Museum. He concluded that the two were not alike, especially when it came to Psamtek I's 'thin lips'. Although it did not compare well to a possible colossal head of Psamtek II (EA 1238) either, Hall (1931: 12) was inclined to attribute the ushabti to Psamtek II. Schneider (1993: 154–5) was equally circumspect in attributing the Psamtek ushabtis to any of the known kings of that name. He did note, however, that the ushabti in the Petrie Museum of Egyptian Archaeology at University College London (UCL) (ex-Wellcome collection) wears a bag-wig rather than a *nemes*-headdress. Although such a feature may distinguish the ushabti as belonging to a different king from those of the *nemes*-headdress figures, it is not such a distinctive guide, because ushabti figures can vary in their headgear, especially in royal groups.

When the location[3] of the king's name is compared on the Psamtek ushabtis, there is a noticeable difference between the exact position of the text

3 Positions are described from the viewpoint of the ushabti, and thus 'right-hand side' means the left-hand side from the viewer's perspective.

as far as can be judged from published photographs. Using a central vertical axial line from the place where the hands of the figure cross, on the
British Museum example, the cartouche is situated in a central position on the
figure, while the new Sais example has the 'King of Upper Lower Egypt' title
more centrally placed and the cartouche offset to the right-hand side of the
figure. In fact, the other complete examples in the Kunsthistorisches Museum,
Vienna, and the Myers Museum, Eton College, and the fragments in UCL and
Copenhagen all have a more centrally placed cartouche. On the other hand,
the ushabti fragment in Stuttgart has the cartouche placed between the Sais
example's cartouche and the central position. The difference in location of
the cartouches suggests that different moulds were used in the manufacture of
the ushabtis. The details of the hands, rope holding the basket and the hoe, as
well as the basket on the back, all seem to be broadly similar, but the position
of those attributes relative to each other is different, again as can be judged
from photographs. The Eton example seems to have very high-relief hands
and the ends of the hoe and rope seem to extend into the hieroglyph band
below. In the British Museum, Sa el-Hagar and Vienna examples the ends
of the rope and hoe are clear of the text, and in the UCL 40317 and Stuttgart
examples the ends of the tools are well clear of the text. The lines of text on
the Stuttgart and the Vienna ushabtis are both sloping down to the left hand
side of the ushabti whereas on the others, the text is relatively horizontal. The
four examples with intact faces also show differences, although there is wear-
and-tear and damage to most of them. The Eton and British Museum figures
have prominent and detailed ears and well-rounded cheeks, the Stuttgart face
seems leaner, but also has detailed ears while the Vienna example has long
ears and a narrower face than the British Museum and Eton examples. The
Stuttgart example also has a vertical incised line to the left of the back pillar,
which is not present on the Sa el-Hagar example. If the moulds used were
individually different or made in batches, then the small number of surviving
ushabtis may be too limited to supply examples of every batch of figures. Petrie
had noticed that among the 399 ushabti figures of Hor-wedja from Hawara,
dating to the 30th Dynasty, there were at least seventeen different identifiable
styles of figure, perhaps from one large workshop (Petrie 1935: 13; Janes 2012:
392–434).

The content of the text is exactly the same in all cases, but the colour of
the faience glaze where it survives varies from light green to turquoise-green.
The black Eton ushabti is once again more of an outlier than the others in this
respect. Inevitably, the conditions of preservation of the figures and the way in
which they have been stored may account for some colour change, but if the
ushabtis were made in different batches, then there may have been variations
in the glaze colour.

The size of the complete figures is more or less the same, ranging between 17.0 and 18.0 cm in height. The discrepancy in the exact measurements may be due to individual measuring errors, and until they can all be measured by the same person in the same way, it is difficult to know whether this is significant. The same problem applies to width, with a range from 5.3 to 5.9 cm.

Schneider (1993: 165) suggested that, because of the find-spots of some of the 26th Dynasty royal ushabtis in general, some may have been specifically made in Memphis originally and never reached Sais or were removed from Sais and taken to Memphis in the first Persian or Ptolemaic Period as *ex-voto* offerings. One example, Cairo JE 86759, was found at Kom Fakhry, Mit Rahineh, in the embalming house of the Apis bull along with alabaster measures, an alabaster stand inscribed for Amasis, an alabaster ushabti mould of Late Period type and a duck mould. This interesting group may have been brought to the embalming house specially. The material of the ushabti seems to be limestone; hence its designation as an *ex-voto*, but the type is similar to that with the cartouche in central position on the body. It should be noted that the other faience examples are made from extremely high-quality material so the Memphis example could benefit from a further careful examination. The survival of complete examples may also suggest that some did have a function as dedicatory offerings and perhaps also explain the slight differences between the figures, particularly in the shape and detail of the faces. Until more figures with provenance are known, it is difficult to be certain about the way in which the ushabtis came into circulation, and there is even a possibility that they could all be *ex-voto* offerings.

The Royal Tombs

The discovery of the Sa el-Hagar ushabti figure in contexts with other Saite material re-used as fill for later, Roman buildings suggests that by that time Sais was already in a very ruined state. Furthermore, Roman pottery dumps from the first to second century AD lying over a disassembled limestone monumental structure of the Pharaonic Period and fragments of crushed granite and orthoquartzite, the favourite hardstones in the Saite Period, re-used in the floor of a bath-house at Sais from the first century BC to the third century AD, all suggest that the city including the temples and, therefore, the Royal Tombs was extensively destroyed by the late Ptolemaic to Roman Period (Wilson 2006: 264–9).

Champollion located the Neith sanctuary in the enclosure north of the village of Sa el-Hagar, west of the 'Memnonium' or palace, and claimed that he had identified two hillocks which could be the tombs of Amasis and Apries. Nothing has been found in that area which relates to the Royal Tombs, although

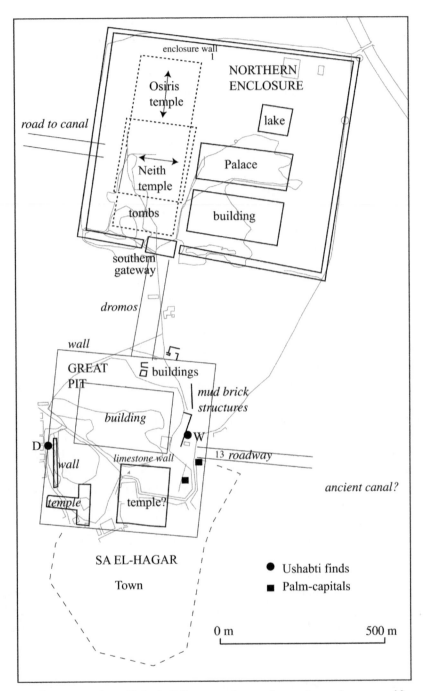

7.4 Reconstruction of Saite buildings superimposed over the modern area of Sa el-Hagar. (Created by the author.)

it was already denuded of stone buildings by the nineteenth century. The ushabti of Apries found by Daressy and that found in Excavation 10 have both
come from the 'Great Pit' area north of the village of Sa el-Hagar. The pit was
covered by a mound or kom in the mid-nineteenth century, when Wilkinson
visited between 1821 and 1833, and first appears in maps or accounts by the
beginning of the twentieth century (Daressy 1901). Between those two periods
the Great Pit was created by *sebakhin* digging, and many objects must have been
found there, judging by the Egyptian antiquities authorities' interest in the site
between 1890 and 1902.[4] In 1891, a hoard of bronzes was found in the 'Great
Pit' area, and Alexandre Barsanti was sent to Sais in 1894 (Daressy 1917) and
Daressy in 1901 to discover their exact provenance and uncover more. Around
the edges of the pit there are substantial amounts of Saite destruction material
remaining. There are indications of monumental buildings inside the pit, and
the limestone 'pylon' base at the south of the pit suggests that the old centre of
the village is upon part of the ancient site. The most recent assessment of the
site by François Leclère proposed that the Great Pit was the suburbs of the city,
with the Northern Enclosure containing the temple of Neith and Royal Tombs
(Leclère 2008: 196, pl. 3.6.c; Figure 7.4).

It is worth considering, however, how the two ushabtis excavated at Sais
came to be found in the Great Pit area and not in the Northern Enclosure. A
large temple building could certainly have been accommodated in the space
occupied by the Great Pit, and, indeed, the only surviving monumental masonry
at Sais stands at the southern edge of the pit. In comparison to the Northern
Enclosure, where settlement is almost continuous down to the Predynastic
Period, concomitant with the presence of an ancient cult centre in the Great
Pit, the Saite to Roman Period is well represented as well as the Predynastic
and Neolithic Periods, with no evidence from the intervening periods yet found.
The situation suggests that at the end of the Saite Period the city shrank back to
the Great Pit area and material was brought there to build new structures, using
stone and rubble from the mounds to the north. The portability of the ushabtis
means that they cannot be relied upon as in situ finds and, during the destruction phase, they could have been mixed with material brought to the edge of the
town situated upon the southern mound.

On the other hand, the presence of at least one, if not more, monumental
perhaps temple structures in the southern area, later the Great Pit, is indicated
by several features. The bath-house at Sais in the south-east corner of the Great
Pit is a typical *tholos*-type, dating from the first century BC to second century

---

4   Decrees were issued in 1893 and 1897 to prevent the extraction of *sebakh* from
    archaeological tells and sites, but enforced by another decree only in 1909, by which
    time it was almost too late for many sites (Anonymous 1909).

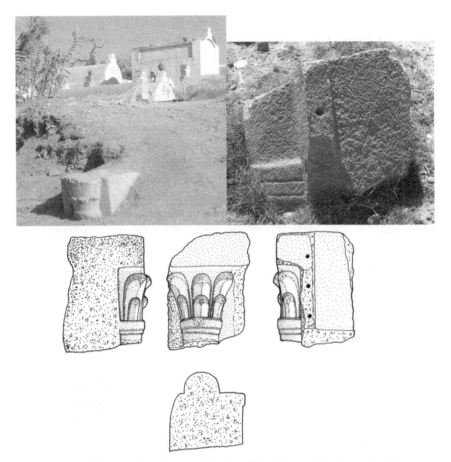

7.5 Three granite palm-capitals from Sais. (Created by the author.)

AD. It incorporated large granite blocks in the structure's foundations, and
smashed fragments of granite, quartzite and basalt were also used as irregular
aggregate for the floor. The location of bath-houses near or next to temples
has been most recently demonstrated at Karnak, with the discovery of a bath-
house of *tholos*-type from the Hellenistic to Roman Period, to the south of the
main pylon of the temple. A remark of Strabo that a tomb of Osiris lay 'above'
the sanctuary of Neith has been interpreted by Woodhouse to suggest that an
Osiris necropolis or temple lay south of the main cult area. Woodhouse (1997:
132–51) suggested that the village of Asdymeh was a possible candidate for the
location of the tomb (cf. Leclère 2008: 183, n. 171), but, in fact, the area where
the limestone wall fragment lies would be a better candidate, perhaps linked to
the Neith sanctuary by a *dromos*.

A further footnote to the evidence of the Royal Tombs is the remark by Herodotus that the funerary temples built above the tombs had palm capitals. In fact, at least three palm-capital blocks have been found at Sa el-Hagar (Wilson 2006: 227, fig. 83; Figure 7.5). They are all made of red granite and are what might be called half-monumental size; that is, they were not as massive as for a large temple, but perhaps in scale with something smaller, but no less important. One complete capital was brought to the Supreme Council for Antiquities office at Sa el-Hagar in 1992. With a height of 87.5 cm, width 73 cm and depth 73 cm, it has three holes drilled down one side for attachment purposes. An almost identical capital fragment was found embedded in the modern cemetery mound at the south-east corner of the Great Pit, close to the monumental wall and to the bath-house. Another fragment of a palm capital lies among a collection of blocks near the bath-house. It is almost certain that the palm-capitals are not in their original position, and they may have been brought to the eastern side of the Great Pit together to be re-used, not far from where the ushabti fragment was found. A small concentration of material, perhaps connected with the Royal Tombs, could suggest that the structures were taken to pieces at the same time and that the debris from them was removed in one batch to the place where they were found in recent times. If the material was removed together then there may have been an attempt later in the Ptolemaic or Roman Period to establish some kind of memorial to the Saite kings and an interest in preserving the small fragments. In subsequent developments, including the closure and dismantling of the temples, these already fragile remains would have been further scattered and lost, leaving the site over the succeeding centuries as useful chunks of hard stone.

While it is certain that the Royal Tombs at Sais have been destroyed and gradually reduced to small pieces, chance finds at Sa el-Hagar and in its environs will continue to add slowly to the fragmentary evidence concerning them. It is to be hoped that it will not be another century before the next fragment is found.

Acknowledgements

I first saw Rosalie David on television in the documentary about mummy 1770 at the Manchester Museum, when I was still at school. I was inspired to follow a career in Egyptology by her care in bringing to life a seemingly unpromising set of remains. I am grateful to Mohamed Rashad, Ahmed Bilal, Said el-Assal, Ibrahim el-Dessouki and Emad el-Shennawi for their cooperation in Excavation 10. A preliminary report on the excavation can be found at www.dur.ac.uk/penelope.wilson/sais.html (last accessed 31 July 2015). I am most grateful to Claus Jurman for information about Cairo JE 86759 and for assistance with bibliographical references, as well as to Carolin Johansson in Stockholm and Tine Bagh in Copenhagen.

References

Anonymous (1909), 'Liste de tells et koms à sebakh', *Journel official du gouvernement égyptien*, 12 February, 1–5.

Adam, S. (1958), 'Recent discoveries in the Eastern Delta, 2: Athribis', *Annales du Service des antiquités de l'Égypte* 55, 303–4.

Aubert, J.-F. and Aubert, L. (1974), *Statuettes égyptiennes: chaouabtis, ouchebtis* (Paris: Librairie d'Amérique et d'Orient).

Badawi, A. M. (1984), *Pages from Excavations at Saqqarah and Mit Rahinah* (Cairo: Dar al-Maaref).

Barbotin, C. (2000), 'Un bas-relief au nom de Psammétique II (595–589 av. J.-C.), une récente acquisition du Louvre', *La revue du Louvre et des musées de France* 5, 33–8.

Brunner-Traut, E. and Brunner, H. (1981), *Die ägyptische Sammlung der Universität Tübingen* (Mainz: Philipp von Zabern).

Buhl, M.-L. (1959), *The Late Anthropoid Stone Sarcophagi* (Copenhagen: Nationalmuseet).

Champollion, J.-Fr. (1833), *Lettres écrites d'Égypte et de Nubie en 1828 et 1829* (Paris: Firmin Didot).

Daressy, G. (1901), 'Rapport sur les fouilles à Sa el Hagar', *Annales du Service des antiquités de l'Égypte* 2, 230–9.

Daressy, G. (1917), 'Alexandre Barsanti', *Annales du Service des antiquités de l'Égypte* 17, 246–60.

Foucart, G. (1898), 'Notes prises dans le Delta', *Recueil de travaux* 20, 162–9.

Godley, A. H. (trans.) (1966), *Herodotus: The Histories* (London: Penguin).

Habachi, L. (1943), 'Saïs and its monuments', *Annales du Service des antiquités de l'Égypte* 42, 369–407.

Hall, H. R. (1931), 'Three royal shabtis in the British Museum', *Journal of Egyptian Archaeology* 17 (1–2), 10–12.

Janes, G. (2012), *The Shabti Collections 5: A Selection from the Manchester Museum* (Cheshire: Olicar House).

Josephson, J. A. (1997), *Egyptian Royal Sculpture of the Late Period, 400–246 B.C.* (Mainz: Philipp von Zabern).

Josephson, J. A. and El-Dalmaty, M. (1999), *Catalogue générale of the Egyptian Antiquities in the Cairo Museum: Nrs 48601–48649 Statues of the XXVth and XXVIth Dynasties* (Cairo: Supreme Council of Antiquities).

Kaiser, W. (1967), *Ägyptisches Museum Berlin* (Berlin: Brüder Hartmann).

Leclère, F. (2008), *Le villes de basse Égypte au Ier millénaire av. J.-C.* (Cairo: Institut Français d'Archéologie Orientale).

Lloyd, A. B. (1982), 'The inscription of Udjahorresnet: a collaborator's testament', *Journal of Egyptian Archaeology* 68, 166–80.

Peterson, B. (1977), 'Gesicht und Kunststil: ein Repertorium der ägyptischen Kunstentwicklung der Spätzeit anhand von Grabfiguren', *Medelhavsmuseet Bulletin* 12, 12–37.

Petrie, W. M. F. (1935), *Shabtis* (London: British School of Egyptian Archaeology).

Reeves, N. (1996), 'An unpublished royal shabti of the 26th Dynasty', *Göttingen Miszellen* 154, 93–7.

Reeves, N. (2008), *Egyptian Art at Eton College and Durham University* (Tokyo: The Tokyo Shimbun).

Rawlinson, G. (1862), *History of Herodotus: A New English Version* (London).

Satzinger, H. (1994), *Das Kunsthistorische Museum in Wien* (Mainz: Phillip von Zabern).

Schneider, H. D. (1993), 'Disparate events of one time: two shabtis of King Necho II, with a repertory of royal funerary statuettes of the Late Period (Dynasties 26, 29 and 30)', in L. Limme and J. Strybol (eds.), *Aegyptus museis rediviva: miscellanea in honorem Hermanni de Meulenaere* (Brussels: Musées Royaux d'Art et d'Histoire), 153–68.

Wilson, P. (2006). *The Survey of Sais* (London: Egypt Exploration Society).

Wilson, P. (forthcoming), *Sais III: The Saite Period at Sa el-Hagar (Sais)*.

Woodhouse, S. (1997), 'The sun god, his Four Bas, and the Four Winds in the sacred district at Saïs: the fragment of an obelisk (BM EA 1512)', in S. Quirke (ed.), *The Temple in Ancient Egypt: New Discoveries and Recent Research* (London: British Museum Press), 132–51.

PART II

Magico-medical practices in ancient Egypt

8

A most uncommon amulet

Carol Andrews

I offer this article to Rosalie on the subject of what I believe to be a unique amulet in the hope that its more curious and contradictory elements will pique her interest sufficiently for her to call into use her extensive knowledge of ancient Egyptian religion and mythology to seek an answer to the questions they pose.

Among the extensive collection of ancient Egyptian amulets in the Department of Egypt and Sudan at the British Museum, EA 26586 is an embellished wedjat eye made of pale green glazed composition (Plate 2). It measures 2.5 cm at its greatest length and 3.1 cm at its greatest height. There is no information on its provenance. The wedjat, especially in this material, is probably the amuletic form to have survived in the greatest numbers to the present day. It was not only worn in life for protection and might be taken to the tomb subsequently for use in the afterlife, but was specifically listed among prescribed amulets to be set on the wrapped mummy. Thus it is found in the pictorial record of amulets to be placed on the body of Osiris himself, depicted on the thickness of a doorway in the western Osiris complex on the roof of the temple of Hathor at Dendera (Andrews 1994: fig. 1). It also occurs in schematic plans of how amulets were to be set on contemporary mummies, found at the end of certain Late Period funerary papyri (Andrews 1994: fig. 2). Examination of Late Period mummies where amulets were still in position has confirmed that the wedjat is almost omnipresent, though rarely in the same place on the body (Petrie 1914: figs. L–LII). However, this particular example of the amulet is embellished with details which render it unique among published examples of wedjats.

The basic amulet resembles a human eye with brow above and markings below, the latter taking the form of a drop shape in front and an up-curling

spiral behind. Since the wedjat is one of the two 'eyes of Horus', the markings
ought to resemble those on the head of the sky-god in falcon form. However,
although the drop shape at the front does indeed imitate the characteristic dark-
coloured feathering at the front of the cheek of the 'Horus falcon' (Houlihan
and Goodman 1986: fig. 61), the up-curling spiral most resembles the lacrimal
line on the faces of big cats, whether lion, leopard or cheetah (Desroches-
Noblecourt 1963: pl. XXVIII). The most likely explanation for this curious
combination has been provided by Westendorf (1963: 138–9).

The piece is pierced horizontally for suspension through the length of the
rectangular box which surmounts the eyebrow. It also has a distinct front and
back. Although by convention the wedjat eye is usually identified as the left
'lunar' eye of the falcon-headed sky-god, damaged or diminished when the
moon waned each month but then healed and made whole ('wedjat') when it
waxed, it is noteworthy that almost as many wedjat eyes as amulets represent
the right 'solar' eye as the left (Andrews 1994: fig. 46). Moreover, the orientation of all the imagery depicted on this piece make it clear that this wedjat was
intended to represent the right 'solar' eye.

Within the thick drop below the eye on both faces, and filling the whole
available space, is depicted a very constricted up-reared cobra wearing a sun
disc with, apparently, the coil of its body behind, arching up to the level of
the head, although this detail is by no means certain. On the back face of the
amulet only, inside the area defined by the up-curling spiral and almost filling
it, is another up-reared cobra, without a sun disc but with a very distinct coil
of the body behind, arching up to the level of its head. Just behind the tip of its
tail three vertical stalk-like stripes, each surmounted by an elongated bud-like
shape, might be intended to represent stylised vegetation of the type where
cobras are sometimes found. All three snakes, whether on the front or back
surface of the amulet, face outwards, that is to the right, thus providing further
confirmation that it is the right eye which is intended. The cobra's connection
with the sun, emphasised by wearing a sun disc, is well established (e.g. Kees
1977: 54); it is particularly obvious when the snake is wrapped around the sun
disc on top of a deity's head. Although there is no reason to assume that the
cobra without a sun disc does not have a solar connection, its presence on this
amulet could just as well be explained as confirmation of one of the functions
of the wedjat itself in a funerary context. The sloughing of a snake's skin and
the emergence of a new reptile from it was considered symbolic of regeneration
and new life. According to the Osiris myth, the offering of his healed eye by
falcon-headed Horus to his dead father Osiris was so powerful a charm that it
restored him to life.

The up-reared cobra or uraeus as goddess was the Eye of the Sun, spitting
fire at enemies when worn on the divine or royal brow and wreaking destruction

at the sun-god's command. But just as important a manifestation of the Eye was any of the various lion goddesses, all of whom had a fierce side to their character: Sekhmet, Menhyt, Mehit, Mut, Tefnut and Wadjyt were among their number. Even the apparently docile cat-headed Bastet, usually depicted with kittens emblematic of her fertility at her feet and sistrum and menyet for music-making and festivity in her hands, had a lion-headed form when she too embodied the sun's vengeful Eye. It is because of this savage aspect of all these goddesses that, even though their usual form might be otherwise, when embodying the Eye they were represented as a woman with maned lion's head: hence their apparently contradictory designation as lion goddesses. That their heads are usually surmounted by a sun disc with uraeus wrapped around it is a further reminder of their connection with the sun-god and his Eye. It is this link which suggests the probable identification of the leonine figure which reclines along the top of this amulet.

The lion, as embellishment, is a rare feature considering the number of wedjats to have survived: only fourteen of this type have been identified (Müller-Winkler 1987: 103). Of these, two are thought to depict a cat rather than a lion in the original publication, and in another of the fourteen the badly damaged figure was originally identified as a bull (Petrie 1914: 33, section 141g). In EA 26586 the lion reclines on top of the rectangular box which surmounts the eye-brow and its body lies to the left, the orientation furnishing further evidence that this is the right 'solar' eye as amulet. However, its head is not forward-facing with the front legs stretched before it, in the posture of all recumbent lion-form amulets, gaming pieces and jewellery elements since the earliest dynasties. This is also the posture from the 4th Dynasty onwards of large scale lion-form sculp-ture in that most characteristic Egyptian hybrid, the human- or animal-headed sphinx. Instead, it is recumbent with its head turned to face the viewer, its front right leg lying nonchalantly over the paw of the left, and, although it is a detail difficult to discern, the underside of the paw of the back left leg appears to be visible behind the right back leg. This is exactly the posture of one of the two red granite Prudhoe lions in the British Museum, the pair being the first ever to exhibit this pose among large-scale lion sculpture, and it occurs extremely rarely subsequently, only in the 30th Dynasty and into the Roman Period, and never on this scale (Kozloff and Bryan 1992: 219, no. 30).

These lions came from the temple of Soleb in Nubia built by Amenhotep III of the 18th Dynasty and would have stood one on either side of the temple's entrance way, hence their mirror-image appearance. The lion on the amulet is identical to the Prudhoe lion which would have stood on the left. It is known that the pair from Soleb represented the eyes of the sun-god, both solar and lunar, and so the lion on the left might be assumed to represent the lunar eye, the entity which the fierce lion-headed goddesses and, in particular, Tefnut embodied. Yet the amulet has been shown to be a right eye. However, texts exist which show that the right and left eyes might be transposed, as for example, Chapter 151 of the Book of the Dead (Allen 1974: 147): 'Thy right eye is the night bark, thy left eye is the day bark.' Perhaps this explains the presence of a lunar manifestation on a right, solar eye.

However, the occurrence of a male lion as the embodiment of a goddess would still need to be explained. In the Heliopolitan cosmogony Tefnut and her partner Shu, as the children of the sun-god, were sometimes represented as a pair of lions; it was in this form that they were worshipped at Leontopolis in the Delta (Kees 1977: 7): here, perhaps, is to be found the explanation. But, with even greater possibility, since Tefnut's savage nature could be illustrated only by a maned lion's head on a woman's body, when she was represented in completely animal form only the lion would suffice. A lioness would not suggest the same destructive potential of an embodiment of the sun's eye. Rather confusingly, although the identification of the recumbent leonine figure on top of this category of wedjat is accepted in the definitive listing of the type as a manifestation of Tefnut, it is always termed there 'Löwin', that is, 'lioness' (Müller-Winkler 1987: 103). Yet in the case of EA 26586 only, there is a possibility that the lion depicted is indeed intended as a manifestation of a male deity.

In spite of their relaxed posture, the Prudhoe lions still manage to embody the creatures' inherent power and strength and were placed before the temple to guard and protect it from enemies, both real and symbolic; the recumbent lion on top of the wedjat surely has the same potential. Perhaps, then, it could represent the sun-god himself since the lion was one of his manifestations: Chapter 62 of the Book of the Dead reveals, 'I am the lion, Re' (Allen 1974: 55). The presence of the lion as guardian and protector is surely necessitated by the first of the two creatures which are uniquely depicted on EA 26586. The recumbent lion on it does not lie directly on top of the eyebrow but on a rectangular box, but whereas in other examples in this category of wedjat surmounted by the leonine figure the box might be decorated with up-reared cobras, in this instance alone the box contains a standing crocodile facing to the right.

The very presence of a crocodile on this amulet, which might be placed on the mummy, is very surprising: Chapters 31 and 32 of the Book of the Dead were specifically directed against malevolent crocodiles in the afterlife (Allen 1974: 41–4). Nor can this be a manifestation of Sobek or any of the other deities who could assume the form of a crocodile: it wears no headdress to define it as divine nor does it stand on a shrine-shaped plinth. When not a divine manifestation, the crocodile was a much-feared denizen of river and marshland and so would be depicted on such a protective amulet as a wedjat only in order to illustrate the very entity which the wearer wished to avoid, its danger negated by apotropaic magic. In mythology, the crocodile was a creature of darkness and so a particular enemy of the sun-god in his passage through the underworld during the hours of night. It is among the animal-form foes that are shown fleeing from the sun's disc in the opening scene to the Litany of the Sun depicted near the entrance to Ramesside royal tombs in the Valley of the Kings at Thebes (Hornung 1982: fig. 77). On the walls of the outer corridor of the temple of Horus at Edfu, in the pictorial account of the myth of the Winged Disc, the crocodile is depicted along with the hippopotamus as defeated enemy of the sun-god. Perhaps then the rectangular box which contains the crocodile on the amulet can be seen as a cage confining it, and the lion reclining on top of it as the sun-god himself acting as guard or even victor over the imprisoned creature. In the same way, the sun-god in the form of his winged disc was shown at Edfu in victory, set over his vanquished crocodile foe. Certainly the imagery recalls that on most Horus cippi on which the figure of the youthful Horus-the-Saviour stands with feet firmly planted on two large crocodiles, and thus negates any danger they might threaten (Saleh and Sourouzian 1987: 261).

Finally, the most inexplicable element of all: within the area delineated by the up-curling spiral, on the front face of the amulet only and facing right, is the most unusual motif. The image is unprecedented on any wedjat, being that of a roaring animal's head with gaping maw, bared canines, bulging eye and flattened ear. At first sight it looks to be the head of a hippopotamus. Such an image of the bellowing male is well established in marsh scenes since the Old Kingdom but its tusks are even more fearsome than those bared here. In any case, it would still be difficult to explain the presence of a roaring male hippopotamus head on a wedjat, especially as the beast was considered the embodiment of Seth, archenemy of the sun-god and Osiris. It was actually the female of the species, whether as Taweret who aided women at childbirth or Ipet bringer of light to the dead, who had a benevolent side to their nature, and they are never depicted with their fearsome jaws agape, only slightly open, sufficiently to show their teeth.

However, closer examination reveals that the neck of the creature bears the stylised markings which by convention denote the hair of a lion's mane. In fact, this lion's head is virtually identical in appearance to a glazed-composition three-dimensional snarling lion's head which was probably once part of a zoomorphic vessel (Bakr, Brandl and Kalloniatis 2014: 237). A catalogue entry for this suggests a likely date in the 26th Dynasty, and may perhaps have some bearing on the date of this amulet, which otherwise is tentatively assigned to the early part of the 22nd to 25th Dynasties in the definitive listing of the category of wedjat to which it belongs (Müller-Winkler 1987: 150). Although the reason for the expression of the vessel's protome is not discussed it must be assumed to be roaring defiance and so furnishing protection. Yet the expression of the lion's head on our amulet bears a very strong resemblance to that of the lion being speared by a Ramesside pharaoh on an ostracon (Peck 1978: fig. 29). Indeed, examination of any New Kingdom lion-hunting scene will elicit at least one beast with the same gaping jaws but the lion in question will invariably be wounded, dying or in the act of being dispatched by the king. So a lion's head with the same expression as the one on this amulet can scarcely be there as a protective element. Indeed, the expression could be seen to denote one of terror rather than one to inspire terror.

It cannot be insignificant that the catalogue entry for the protome suggests it exhibits possible Greek influence, for when Egyptian lions' heads are used in a protective, threatening capacity, as furniture elements, for example, there does not seem to have been a need to have them depicted roaring or snarling. An obvious example is in the lion-headed protomes on the gilded throne from the tomb of Tutankhamun (Desroches-Noblecourt 1963: pl. X). Even lions' heads as waterspouts at the top of temple walls, functioning exactly like gargoyles, do not roar (Wilkinson 2000: 69). So, in the unlikely event that the lion's head on this amulet is to be viewed as protective and, by the magic process whereby the part substitutes for the whole, it represents a complete lion, its presence is redundant: there is already a protective lion reclining along the top of the wedjat. Why this head is depicted, especially in view of its ambiguous nature, is unfathomable.

Without doubt this wedjat is unique and certainly merits further considera-tion if the symbolism of its elements is ever to be more fully understood.

References

Allen, T. G. (1974), *The Book of the Dead or Going Forth by Day* (Chicago: University of Chicago Press).

Andrews, C. (1994), *Amulets of Ancient Egypt* (London: British Museum Press).

Bakr, M., Brandl, H. and Kalloniatis, F. (2014), *Egyptian Antiquities from the Eastern Nile Delta* (Cairo and Berlin: Opaion).

Desroches-Noblecourt, C. (1963), *Tutankhamen: Life and Death of a Pharaoh* (London: George Rainbird).

Hornung, E. (1982), *Tal der Könige* (Zurich and Munich: Artemis).

Houlihan, P. F. and Goodman, S. M. (1986), *The Birds of Ancient Egypt* (Warminster: Aris and Phillips).

Kees, H. (1977), *Der Götterglaube im Alten Ägypten* (Berlin: Akademie-Verlag).

Kozloff, A. P. and Bryan, B. M. (1992), *Egypt's Dazzling Sun: Amenhotep III and his World* (Cleveland: Cleveland Museum of Art).

Müller-Winkler, C. (1987), *Die ägyptischen Objekt-Amulette* (Freiburg: Biblisches Institut der Universität Freiburg).

Peck, W. H. (1978), *Egyptian Drawings* (New York: E. P. Dutton).

Petrie, W. M. F. (1914), *Amulets* (London: Constable).

Saleh, M. and Sourouzian, H. (1987), *The Egyptian Museum Cairo Official Catalogue* (Mainz am Rhein: Philipp von Zabern).

Westendorf, W. (1966), 'Beiträge aus und zu den medizinischen Texten', *Zeitschrift für ägyptische Sprache und Altertumskunde* 92, 128–54.

Wilkinson, R. H. (2000), *The Complete Temples of Ancient Egypt* (London: Thames and Hudson).

9

The sting of the scorpion

Mark Collier

Two notable aspects of Rosalie David's Egyptological work are her sustained engagement with the life sciences over a number of decades and her outreach, particularly in the north-west of England. As an Egyptologist born and based in the north-west, I would like to offer Rosalie the following study which I have tried to write up with such a wider audience in mind, and I will strive to avoid an over-presumption of familiarity with the material I discuss.

I will look here at the occurrence and treatment of scorpion stings among the community of workmen from Deir el-Medina, the workmen who constructed the royal tombs in the Valley of the Kings and the Valley of the Queens during the New Kingdom (*c.*1550–1069 BC).[1] The Deir el-Medina community provides us with the largest body of original textual material which has survived from a single site and period from Pharaonic Egypt and is particularly rich from the second half of the 19th Dynasty through to the end of the 20th Dynasty (the Ramesside Period), a period of about 170 years from very roughly 1240 BC to 1070 BC (dates from Shaw 2000). This material allows us to look in unprecedented detail into the micro-history and life-world context of ancient Egypt.

In terms of occurrence of scorpion stings I will present evidence for the incidence of scorpion stings among the workmen and the period of time they took off work as a consequence. In terms of treatment, although I will utilise the type of 'magical' texts which contain spells against scorpion stings, my main

---

1   Some of the material here was included in a presentation for Egyptology Scotland in August 2002 and the University of Liverpool day school 'Ritual and Magic in Ancient Egypt' in March 2010.

interest will be in the conception of the antagonistic relationship with the venom introduced into the body.

Incidence of scorpion stings and absence from work among the workmen

I will focus on specific examples drawn from records of absence from the work on the royal tombs. I restrict myself to examples where the incidence of scorpion sting is presented in context with an indication of the length of absence of the workman who suffered the sting.

The first example comes from Ostracon BM (British Museum) EA 5634, which carries the comparatively high date of regnal year 40 (which can only be regnal year 40 of Ramesses II during this period). The reign of Ramesses II is currently usually dated to *c.*1279–1213 BC and so his year 40 falls at approximately 1240 BC.

Ostracon BM EA 5634 is a large limestone ostracon, 38.5 cm in height and 33 cm wide, and was acquired by the British Museum in 1823 as part of the Salt collection.[2] The work gang itself (*t3 ist*) was divided throughout its recorded history into two sides, the right (*wnmy*) side and the left (*smḥy*) side (Černý 2001 remains a key resource for the organisation of the gang). This division is reflected in the organisation of the text on the ostracon, which is written on both sides. On the recto is an ordered listing of the names of the workmen of the right side of the gang, written in black ink; on the verso is an ordered listing of the names of the workmen of the left side of the gang, again written in black.[3]

2 The most recent publication is Demarée 2002: 18 (catalogue entry), pls. 25–8 (greyscale photographs and transcription). Demarée reproduces in greyscale the earlier colour transcription from Černý and Gardiner 1957: pls. lxxxiii–lxxxiv (which displays the entries in red ink to better effect and is reproduced at 1:1). Colour images can be accessed from the British Museum Collection Online. No comprehensive English translation has been published in print (but see the British Museum Collection Online entry), although Janssen 1980 provides a comprehensive discussion of the contents of the ostracon. Further data on the ostracon and other source material from Deir el-Medina can be accessed from the online Deir el-Medina Database.

3 At the time of the research reported in Janssen 1980, the organisation of texts of this sort into ordered listing of workmen had not been recognised and so the comments in Janssen 1980: 127–9 and his use of numbering of workmen on p. 130 and throughout his paper would now be updated; hence my extended comments here. Following my work in Collier 2004 I number the workmen by their side (R for right and L for left) along with the position in the ordered listing. So L7 Seba, for example, indicates the workman Seba, who appears as the seventh name in the listing of the left side of the gang.

Following the names of the workmen on each side of the ostracon is the relevant list of dates of his absence, written in black ink. Above these dates are entries in red ink which give a brief label for each absence.

In total there are thirty-nine workmen named (twenty on the right side of the gang and nineteen on the left side).[4] The labels for reasons for absence differ in their level of specificity, and those on the verso are similar to but not exactly the same as those on the recto. However, with a limited amount of consolidation, the following picture of absence can be drawn up.[5] In Table 9.1 the numbers refer to the individual day items listed for relevant workmen: a grand total of 284 absences for thirty-nine workmen, of which but one is due to a workman being stung by a scorpion.

4   The number is usually stated to be forty (e.g. Janssen 1980: 128), but the name 'Nakhy', which appears in Černý and Gardiner's additional line 9a opposite the entry for line 9 for R8 Hehnakhu, is actually a shortened form of the name R5 Amennakht from line 6. So I do not follow Janssen's comments on Nakhy (Janssen 1980: 128, 129 n. 5) nor his numbering of him as his number [38] (Janssen 1980: 130). Such additional entries for certain names, dislocated from the original entry, also occur, with explicit naming, for R3 Siwadjet (main entry line 4, supplementary entries in lines 7a–b) and R4 Horemwia (main entry line 5, supplementary entry labelled 5b). Treating Amennakht and Nakhy as one and the same individual allows for a more direct comparison between the ordered listings of names on Ostracon BM EA 5634 and the slightly later Ostracon DeM [Deir el-Medina] 706, where the name Nakhy appears exactly in the R5 position where the name Amennakht appears on Ostracon BM EA 5634. See Grandet 2000: 2 for the comparison, but note that Grandet does not recognise the equation of Nakht and Amennakht.

5   As Janssen discusses in detail (Janssen 1980: 132–4), the ostracon covers the majority of one calendar year and the start of the next, but lists absences only for days when the workmen were at work (Janssen 1980: 134 suggests that there may have been no more than seventy working days during this period). The ancient Egyptian calendar year was a solar year of 365 days, divided into 360 days plus five extra days at the end of the year. The 360 days were divided into twelve months each of thirty days, themselves organised into three seasons, each comprising four months. The seasons are: *Akhet* (inundation), *Peret* (growing), *Shemu* (harvest). In ancient Egyptian texts dates are usually written by the number of the month within the relevant season and then the specific day. In translation this will be rendered here in the following way: IV *Akhet* 17, which means 'fourth month in the *Akhet* season, day 17'. As Janssen notes, the absence entries on Ostracon BM EA 5634 seem to begin with III *Akhet* and then continue throughout the remainder of the year, with absences from the start of the next calendar year in I *Akhet* occurring at the ends of entries. Incidentally, this accords with the equation proposed here of Nakhy and Amennakht. Two absences in I *Akhet* 14 and 15 are recorded for Nakhy on the additional line 9a. The absences of R5 Amennakht stretch from IV *Akhet* 15 though to III *Shemu* 26 and are recorded over the full length of line 6, even requiring the scribe to utilise the edge of the ostracon. Thus an additional line for Amennakht's I *Akhet* absences is entirely in accord with the practice of the scribe in this early section of the ostracon.

Table 9.1   Absence from work as recorded in Ostracon BM EA 5634

Cause of absence	Right side (20 workmen)	Left side (19 workmen)	Total
Scorpion stung him		1	1
Sick	39	59	98
Suffering with his eyes		4	4
Mother sick	2		2
Absent		5	5
With boss	43	15	58
With scribe	2	7	9
Carrying stone for the scribe	4	3	7
With Aapehty (when he was ill)	13		13
With Horemwia (when he was ill)	9		9
Preparing remedies	14		14
Daughter's menstruation	2	2	4
Wife's menstruation	1	5	6
With his god		1	1
Offering to the god	6	1	7
Burying the god	1	1	2
Pouring water	5	2	7
Passing of family member	4	5	9
Wrapping (body)		2	2
Mourning		1	1
Building work	1	1	2
Brewing	12	5	17
Drinking with Khonsu	1	1	2
His festival		2	2
Unknown	2		2
Total	161	123	284

The two standout categories in terms of numbers of absences are the rather undifferentiated category of being sick (*mr*), including significant sequences of multi-day sickness, and being with the boss (one of the two chief workmen, here referred to as *ḥry* 'boss, superior'). The two sides of the gang show slightly different profiles, but at least part of the difference in total is due to R20 Paherypedjet, who served as the village doctor. He has thirty-nine recorded absences, by some margin the largest number for a single individual, of which fourteen are for preparing remedies (*pẖrt*) and eighteen are for attending workmen (R4 Horemwia and R11 Aapehty) during periods of prolonged illness (entries translated in McDowell 1999: 54 (no. 25) and discussed in Janssen 1980: 137).

Some of the reasons for absence are less well understood, particularly in detail, or require further contextualisation. For example, the entries for absence for brewing show a distinct centring on the *Peret* season, rather than being spread evenly through the year. Similarly, there are specific entries covering menstruation periods of female family members, but at first sight these seem rather selective.[6]

It is the entry for Seba (L7; Seba (iii) in Davies 1999: 10–11 with chart 6) which records him as being absent from work on IV *Akhet* 17 because 'the scorpion stung him' (*psḥ sw t3 wḥ ʿ(t)*). His full list of absences, with labels, is:

Ostracon BM EA 5634, verso 7:

(L7)	Seba:		
IV	*Akhet*	17	the scorpion stung him
I	*Peret*	25	ill
IV	*Peret*	8	his daughter menstruating
I	*Shemu*	25	ill
		26	likewise
		27	ditto
II	*Shemu*	2	ill
		3	ill
		4	ill
		5	ill
		6	ill
		7	ill

Just one recorded scorpion sting in a year of work is hardly a high incidence rate, although by this time in the reign of Ramesses II work on the royal tomb itself (KV 7) would have been at an advanced stage (cf. Janssen 1980: 134 and Černý 2001: 105–6). It is of interest that this is an item isolated out specifically. The importance of this piece of evidence is increased in that it allows us to infer that Seba is recorded as being absent for just one day (IV *Akhet* 17) from this episode. Many of the other reasons for absence involve more than one-day periods of absence and each day is recorded separately, as can be seen from the remainder of Seba's entry provided above.

Of course, the incidence of scorpion stings is contingent on circumstance. So in other bodies of evidence, a higher rate of incidence can be found. A particularly rich body of evidence comes from the absentee records from the reign of the late 19th Dynasty pharaoh Siptah (*c.*1194–1188 BC), during early work on his tomb (KV 47), nearly fifty years later than Ostracon BM EA 5634. The surviving records (Ostracon Cairo CG 25517d & verso, Ostracon Cairo CG

---

6   For this reason Janssen 1980: 141–3 interpreted *ḥsmn* as purification following childbirth. However, Wilfong 1999 has provided a convincing defence of *ḥsmn* as referring to menstruation here, including a reconstruction of the cycles for the relevant women over the period covered by the ostracon, which, interestingly, points to evidence for synchronisation of cycles.

25519 and Ostracon Cairo CG 25521, published in Černý 1935: 15*–17*, 18*–19 and 22*–25 respectively) provide us with a continuous (if occasionally damaged and thus incomplete) record of absences from work for the period from II *Akhet* 12 late in the first regnal year of Siptah to the end of I *Peret*, the first full month of his second regnal year, a period of slightly over three and a half months (for further see e.g. Collier 2004: 34–7 and the Deir el-Medina Database entries for the individual ostraca).

The first incidence in this body of material of a workman being stung by a scorpion is provided by Ostracon Cairo CG 25519, verso 13, in the entry for II *Akhet* 25, where the workman Roma is listed as being absent with the comment *psḥ n wḥʿ(t)* 'sting of a scorpion'. The following day, II *Akhet* 26, Roma is not listed among the workmen absent and so can be inferred to have returned to work. A few days later, Ostracon Cairo 25517, verso 19, records in the entry for II *Akhet* 28 that the workman Hornefer was absent because of being stung by a scorpion. Days 29 and 30 were weekend days (as days 9 and 10 of the ten-day Ancient Egyptian week) and were regular days off for the workmen and so are not recorded on the ostracon. Ostracon Cairo CG 25519 picks up the record with III *Akhet* 1. The entry is damaged with the possible addition of a further name to the eight names of workmen listed as being absent on this day. The name of Hornefer does not appear among these eight, and so the likelihood is that he too recovered quickly from being stung.

Ostracon Cairo CG 25519 is damaged and, in its current state, is incomplete. It records absences during III *Akhet* 1–3 on the recto and IV *Akhet* 6–14 on the verso. The surviving nine days of the verso entries record two incidences of absence from scorpion sting. Ostracon Cairo CG 25519, verso 7, records, in an entry the date of which is not preserved (but may be IV *Akhet* 7), Pamerihu as being absent from a scorpion sting. Ostracon Cairo CG 25519, verso 8, lists the entry for IV *Akhet* 8, and on that date Nebnefer is absent following a scorpion sting. Pamerihu is not listed as being absent and the inference would be that he has returned to work. The following two days, IV *Akhet* 9 and 10, are the decanal weekend days of the ancient Egyptian week and not recorded. The register resumes in Ostracon Cairo CG 25519, verso 8, with IV *Akhet* 11. Nebnefer is not recorded as being absent (nor is he recorded as being absent in the remaining surviving entries), whereas Pamerihu is recorded as being absent 'ill' (*mr*) on IV *Akhet* 11 and continues to be recorded as being absent day by day until the last fully dated entry on IV *Akhet* 14. Fortunately, the absence record is picked up in the more complete Ostracon Cairo CG 25521, which records absences from IV *Akhet* 15 through to the end of I *Peret*. Pamerihu is consistently recorded as being ill through to I *Peret* 22, after which the record is more damaged. Assuming that the entries for early II *Peret* are reasonably complete, he had returned to work by the start of the next month.

Table 9.2   Absence from work as recorded in Ostracon Cairo CG 25521 for the period IV Akhet (A) 23 to I Peret (P) 11

Date	Absent	Scorpion sting	Ill	With chief workman	Making gypsum	Feeding bull
IV A 23	1	1	1	1		
IV A 24			2	1	4	
IV A 27	2	1	2	3		
IV A 28	1		3		4	
I P 4			1	2	2	1
I P 5				1	4	1
I P 6	1		1	1	2	
I P 11			1	1	2	
Total	5	2	11	10	16	2
%	10.9	4.3	23.9	21.7	34.8	4.3

Ostracon Cairo CG 25521, being more complete, allows us to compare the full set of stated reasons for absence during the period IV *Akhet* 23 to I *Peret* 11, a fifteen-day period during which eight days were working days (see Table 9.2). The scorpion-sting entries during this period are both from members of the right side of the gang. Ostracon Cairo CG 25521, verso 2, records that on IV *Akhet* 23 the workman Meryre was absent, having been stung by a scorpion. Meryre is not recorded as being absent on the following day, IV *Akhet* 24, the inference being that he had returned to work.

The entry recorded on Ostracon Cairo CG 25521, verso 3, for IV *Akhet* 27 is more difficult to interpret. On IV *Akhet* 27 Ipuy and Khonsu are recorded as being absent, and then Nebnefer (who is recorded as being ill). Above the name Khonsu an additional interlinear note has been added 'stung by a scorpion' which presumably applies to Khonsu. The entry for the next day is damaged, but the name of Khonsu is not preserved, although the names of both Nebnefer (still ill) and Ipuy (now recorded as being ill) are. Assuming that the scorpion sting incident refers to Khonsu, then this would be another example of a workman returning to work after one day of recorded absence due to a scorpion sting.

The scorpion and its sting

The scorpion remains a hazard to human health in modern Egypt. For a recent study on scorpion venom in Egypt,[7] eight species of scorpions were collected

7   Salama and Sharshar 2013: 77 (see also images on 79–81). Cf. Keenan 1998: 18 who lists *Androctonus australis*, *Androctonus amoreuxi* and *Leiurus quinquestriatus* in his list of dangerously venomous scorpions in Egypt.

from five localities in Egypt (Aswan, Sinai, Baltim, Borg el-Arab and Marsa-Matrouh). The recorded species encountered were *Androctonus bicolor, Androctonus australis, Androctonus amoreuxi, Androctonus crassicauda, Leiurus quinquestriatus, Buthacus arenicola, Orthochirus innesi* and *Scorpio maurus palmatus*. The sting of the scorpion lies in the last articulated segment (the *telson*) of its tail, which ends in a sharp spine (the *aculeus*) with a pore on either side through which the venom is secreted by two glands.[8] The venom is composed of multiple neurotoxin proteins,[9] mucus, salts and various organic compounds.

Keenan distinguishes two categories for the effects of a scorpion sting beyond the immediate, sharp pain at the site of venom injection (Keenan 1998: 25). In the first, symptoms are local and usually transitory and persist for a period from few minutes through to a day or so. The second category includes cases showing the systemic impact of severe envenomation. Keenan tabulates characteristics of severe envenomation by old-world scorpions of Africa and the Middle East and includes (among others): excessive salivation, excessive perspiration, vomiting, diarrhoea, irregular pulse, unstable temperature, respiratory problems, convulsions and blurred vision (see Keenan 1998: 30–1 for the full listing). On occasion the severity of the envenomation can lead to death (particularly with more vulnerable groups such as children), usually through respiratory or cardiovascular complications. The effects are thus systemic, pervading the body and resulting in overt symptoms at numerous locations, including the head (including psychological as well as physical effects) and torso, regardless of the site of the sting.

Body protection texts

As might be expected the ancient Egyptians were quite familiar with the symptoms displayed by victims of scorpion sting. In the textual sources descriptions of symptoms usually occur within the body protection texts, often labelled (sometimes with unfortunate pejorative overtones not appropriate to the original text) as 'magical texts' dealing with scorpion stings. In these texts, and indeed in the absence records from Deir el-Medina, the ancient Egyptian term for the scorpion is *wḥ't*. The action of the sting is referred to with the verb *psḥ*. This word is also used for the bite of a snake, or indeed biting in general including human biting, as for example in eating. The venom itself is usually termed *mtwt*.

---

8   Since I am not an expert in this field, I condense but stick closely to Keenan's text here and in the discussion of symptoms.

9   Salama and Sharshar 2013: 83 refer to there being an estimated 100,000 distinct peptides in scorpion venom, with only a limited number having been described to date.

In these body protection texts, there is often a component projecting the predicament of the victim onto similar problems suffered by the gods (and thus invoking the creative power available to the gods to be deployed for the benefit of the victim), and thus the symptoms are ascribed directly to the suffering god [for a useful collection of scorpion spells in English translation, see Borghouts 1978: 51–85 (nos. 84–123)]. I will focus particularly on Papyrus Chester Beatty VII, which comes from Deir el-Medina:[10]

> From Spell 3 (Papyrus Chester Beatty VII, recto 2.5–2.7):
> (Isis is speaking) 'Ra my lord, Ra my lord, what are you suffering from? Is your face slack (*nn*)? … between your eyebrows (*inḥ*) is sweat (*fdt*).'
> (Ra answers) 'You are Isis, my sister. [Something] has stung me, when I was in the dark(?). [It] is hotter [than] fire, it blazes more than a flame, it is sharper [than a th]orn.'

> From Spell 10 (Papyrus Chester Beatty VII, recto 5.2–5.3):
> (Ra is speaking) 'I have trodden on something which has a hot [sting]. The heart (*ib*) is shocked (*nr*) and my body (*ḥˁ*) is shivering (*ddf*). The most useful part in me (*t3 3ḫt im=i*), it will not listen to me.

Externally, the site of the injection of the venom can itself be engaged with (as part of the overall magical rite):

> From Spell 11 (Papyrus Chester Beatty VII, 6.1–6.2):
> The spell is to be said over the pith of a rush soaked in fermented gruel. To be twisted leftwards, made with seven knots and applied to the mouth of the puncture (*dmw*). This spell is to be said every […].

> From Spell 13 (Papyrus Chester Beatty VII, 6.6):
> To be recited (over) barley-bread crumb, onions and ochre, heated and placed at the site of the sting (*st psḥ*). It can't spread (*ḫnt*).

As the second example shows, part of the intention behind this would seem to be that application of a magically infused poultice might prevent the spread of the venom through the body.

The venom was conceived of as an entity which passes through the body through its own agentive force, settling in and affecting the body's constituent

---

10 Papyrus Chester Beatty VII, now in the British Museum as Papyrus BM EA 10687, was published in Gardiner 1935: 55–65 (full translation), pls. 33–8 (full transcription, partial photographic record). Further images are available from the British Museum Collection Online, but a full published photographic record remains lacking. For the Chester Beatty papyri as coming originally from Deir el-Medina, see conveniently Pestman 1982. The text is a compendium of spells against scorpion stings.

parts along its way in order to be able to deliver its systemic impact reflected in the observable symptoms. It can be communicated with through the power of the spell, the aim being to get it to leave the body of the victim, for instance in a form of purging (e.g. spitting):[11]

> Papyrus Deir el-Medina 41:[12]
> Evacuate, venom (*mtwt*) (seven times) – Horus has conjured you, he has annihilated you, he has spat you out. You will not rise up, nor trample down. You will be weak, you will not be strong. You will be feeble, you will not be able to fight. You will be blind, you will not be able to see. You will fall, your face will not be lifted. You will be turned back and you will not find your way.

> Papyrus Chester Beatty VII, verso 6.1–2 and 6.5–6.6:
> I know you, I know your name. Come out from the right, come out from the left.
> Come out in [water (*mw*)], come out in vomit (*bš*), come out in urine (*wsš*). Come out at my word, just as I say … Make the venom (*mtwt*) come out which is in the body of A born of B in order to let him leave cured for his mother just as Horus left cured for his mother. The protection of Horus is protection enough.

The venom is thus treated as a force which needs to be combated, ultimately with the aim of forcing its ejection from the body. The actions of the practitioner are thus directed (including the spells and rites deployed) to this end. To engage directly with the venom inside the body he can utilise conjurative power, engaging the power of the gods (the forces of the cosmos) to attempt to weaken the venom and to attempt to compel it to be evacuated through an orifice of the body. The engagements come in various forms, but I would like to look at the following spell from Papyrus Chester Beatty VII, which deals with an attempt to repel the passage of the venom through the various parts of the body and which seeks to bring the power of the gods directly into the human body:[13]

---

11   This requires a concept of body in which the venom can move through the body from the site of injection, affecting various parts, through to being ejected from various orifices including the mouth. Because this body image is mostly taken for granted in these texts, with the focus being on ejecting the venom, I will not discuss this here. Compare Nyord 2009 for a discussion of the ancient Egyptian conception of the body which is commensurate with my work here.

12   An example of a prophylactic charm or amulet aimed at warding off the venom (*mtwt*). The text occurs in a number of variants. See Koenig 1982.

13   This type of text, associating the parts of the body with protective deities, is not restricted to such 'magical' texts. Similar listings can also be found in mortuary texts ranging from the Pyramid Texts through to the Book of the Dead. In these lists the primary focus is an association of the deity with each of the body parts of

Papyrus Chester Beatty VII, verso 2.3–5.9:

Then Isis the divine said, 'I am a Nubian. I have descended from the sky and I have come to reveal the venom (*mtwt*) which is in the body (*ḥꜥ*) of A born of B in order to allow him to emerge healthy for his mother just as Horus emerged healthy for his mother Isis …

You will not last (*ḥꜥ*) in his brow (*dhnt*);[14] [Hekayet? is against you, lady] of the brow,

You will not last in his eyes (*irty*); Horus-[Khent]enirti is against you, lord of the eyes.

You will not last in his ear (*msḏr*); Geb is against you, lord of the ear.

You will not last in his nostril (*šrt*); Khenemtjau-foremost-of-Hesret' is against you, lady of the nostril. Beware in case she extinguishes the north-breeze in the presence of the great ones.

You will not last in his lips (*spty*); Anubis is against you, lord of the lips.

You will not last in his tongue (*nst*), Sefekhabwy is against you, lady of the tongue.

You will not last in his neck (*nḥbt*); Wadjet is against you, lady of the neck.

You will not last in his throat (*šꜥš*); Meret is against you, lady of the throat. Beware in case her voice is hoarse in the presence of Ra.

You will not last in his breast-bone (*k3bt*); Nut is against you, mistress of the breast-bone, the lady who bore the gods and who gives suck […].

You will [not] last in his arm (*ḥpš*); Montu is against you, lord of the two arms.

You will not last in his spine (*i3t*); Ra is against you, lord of the vertebrae.

You will not last in his side (*drww*); Seth is against you, lord of the side.

You will not last in his liver (*mist*), in his lungs (*wf3*), in his heart (*ḥ3ty*), in his kidneys (*ggt*), in his spleen (*nnšm*), in his intestines (*mḫtw*), in his ribs (*spr*) or any of his internal organs (*iwf n ḥt*); Imseti, Hapy, Duamutef, Qebehsenuef, the gods in the torso (*imw ḥt*), are against you.

You will not last in his pelvic-region (*pḥwy*); Hathor is against you, lady of the pelvic-region.

You will not last in his penis (*ḥnn*); Horus is against you, lord of the penis.

You will not last in his testicles (*3st*); Reshpu is against you, lord of the testicles.

You will not last in his thighs (*mnty*); Horus is against you, lord of the thighs who went over the desert alone.

the deceased, rather than deployment of their antagonistic role. Chapter 42 of the Book of the Dead ends with a rubric which provides an overview of the notion at play here of the relationship between the body and protective divinity: 'There is no body-part of mine devoid of a god.'

14 While quite a few ancient Egyptian anatomical terms are well understood there are others which are not quite so secure. I follow here the presentation in Walker 1996: 265–79. Jim Walker was a practising GP who also gained a PhD in Egyptology. Walker 1996 is the posthumous publication of his PhD work.

You will not last in his knee (*pd̲*); Sia is against you, lord of the knee.
You will not last in his shin (*sd̲ḥ*); Nefertem is against you, lord of the shins.
You will not last in his feet (*t̲bty*); Nebet-debwet is against you, lady of the feet.
You will not last in his toenails (*ꜥnt*); Anuqet is against you, lady of
    the toenails.
You will not last in the sting (*psḥ*); Selqet is against you, lady of the sting.
You will not last, you will not get cool there, there is no place (*st*) to stay.

Come out down onto the ground. Look, I have charmed (*šnt.n=i*), I have spat
    out (*psg.n=i̓*) and I have drunk (*swr.n=i̓*) you. As Horus belongs to his
    mother, so A born of B belongs to his mother. As Horus lives, so does
    he live.

This antagonistic relationship can be analysed using the framework of force
dynamics,[15] the conceptual organisation (often by metaphorical transfer) of
various forms of interaction as between an agonist (the focal force entity) and an
antagonist (a resisting force). In this spell the ancient Egyptian conception of the
venom (*mtwt*) lends itself to being considered as an agonist, here an agentive
force whose presence within the body needs to be resisted and which needs to
be overcome and repelled. It is not the body itself which is conceived of here as
directly resisting (as antagonist) the venom; indeed the body, depicted through
its constituent parts, plays a passive or locative role (a site, as a series of containers, for the contest). Nor is the magical practitioner in this passage the direct
antagonist (though he is indirectly as the person conducting the rite). Rather the
antagonist force here comes from the divine invoked by the magical rites performed by the practitioner to engage the force of the venom with the power at
the disposal of the divine (as the stronger force) on the side of the victim within
the various parts of the victim's body. In the context of the spell, with no place
to go the venom is then forced out from the body.

References

Borghouts, J. F. (1978), *Ancient Egyptian Magical Texts* (Leiden: Brill).
The British Museum Collection Online (n.d.), www.britishmuseum.org/research/
    collection_online/search.aspx (last accessed 27 October 2014).
Černý, J. (1935), *Ostraca hiératiques: Nos 25501–25832*, Catalogue Général des Antiquités
    Égyptiennes du Musée du Caire (Cairo: Institut Français d'Archéologie Orientale).
Černý, J. and Gardiner, A. H. (1957), *Hieratic Ostraca* (Oxford: Griffith Institute).

15 More broadly I am presuming here a cognitive approach to 'magic', as for example
    in Sørensen 2007 (see e.g. Sørensen 2007: 42–3 on the utility of the framework
    of force dynamics). The framework of 'force dynamics' derives from the linguistic
    work of Leonard Talmy; see conveniently Talmy 2000.

Černý, J. (2001), *A Community of Workmen at Thebes in the Ramesside Period*, 2nd edn (Cairo: Institut Français d'Archéologie Orientale). First published 1973.

Collier, M. (2004), *Dating Late XIXth Dynasty Ostraca* (Leiden: Nederlands Instituut voor het Nabije Oosten).

Davies, B. G. (1999), *Who's Who at Deir el-Medina: A Prosopographic Study of the Royal Workmen's Community* (Leiden: Nederlands Instituut voor het Nabije Oosten).

The Deir el-Medina Database (n.d.), www.leidenuniv.nl/nino/dmd/dmd.html (last accessed 27 October 2014).

Demarée, R. J. (2002), *Ramesside Ostraca* (London: British Museum Press).

Gardiner, A. (1935), *Hieratic Papyri in the British Museum: Third Series, Chester Beatty Gift* (London: British Museum).

Grandet, P. (2000), *Catalogue des ostraca hiératiques non littéraires de Deîr el-Médînéh*, VIII: *Nos 706–830* (Cairo: Institut Français d'Archéologie Orientale).

Janssen, J. J. (1980), 'Absence from work by the necropolis workmen of Thebes', *Studien zur Altägyptischen Kultur* 8, 127–50.

Keenan, H. L. (1998), *Scorpions of Medical Importance*, reissue (London: Fitzgerald). First published 1980.

Koenig, Y. (1982), 'Deux amulettes de Deir el-Médineh', *Bulletin de l'Institut français d'archéologie orientale* 82, 283–93.

McDowell, A. G. (1999), *Village Life in Ancient Egypt: Laundry Lists and Love Songs* (Oxford: Oxford University Press).

Nyord, R. (2009), *Breathing Flesh: Conceptions of the Body in the Ancient Egyptian Coffin Texts* (Copenhagen: The Carsten Niebuhr Institute of Near Eastern Studies).

Pestman, P. W. (1982), 'Who were the owners, in the "community of workmen", of the Chester Beatty Papyri', in R. J. Demarée and J. J. Janssen (eds.), *Gleanings from Deir el-Medîna* (Leiden: Nederlands Instituut voor het Nabije Oosten), 155–72.

Salama, W. M. and Sharshar, K. M. (2013), 'Surveillance study on scorpion species in Egypt and comparison of their crude venom protein profiles', *Journal of Basic and Applied Zoology* 66, 76–86.

Shaw, I. (ed.) (2000), *The Oxford History of Ancient Egypt* (Oxford: Oxford University Press).

Sørensen, J. (2007), *A Cognitive Theory of Magic* (Lanham, MD: AltaMira Press).

Talmy, L. (2000), 'Force dynamics in language and cognition', in L. Talmy (ed.), *Towards a Cognitive Semantics*, I: *Concept Structuring Systems* (Cambridge, MA: MIT Press), 409–70. Minor revision of paper with this title originally published in 1988 in *Cognitive Science* 12, 49–100.

Walker, J. (1996), *Studies in Ancient Egyptian Anatomical Terminology* (Warminster: Aris and Phillips).

Wilfong, T. (1999), 'Menstrual synchrony and the "place of women" in Ancient Egypt (OIM 13512)', in E. Teeter and J. A. Larson (eds.), *Gold of Praise: Studies on Ancient Egypt in Honor of Edward F. Wente* (Chicago: The Oriental Institute of the University of Chicago), 419–65.

10

Magico-medical aspects of the mythology of Osiris

Essam El Saeed

The ancient Egyptian myth of Osiris can be reconstructed from various Pharaonic sources and includes some significant magico-medical aspects (Pinch 1994: 133–46; Koenig 2002; Campbell, El Saeed and David 2010; Győry 2011). It is likely that these had a special resonance for ancient Egyptian healing practitioners (Reeves 1992; David 2008, 2011). Several mythic episodes emphasise the transformative power of magic and healing, with special emphasis on the conception, birth and early life of Horus, the divine child and legitimate heir to Osiris (Wilkinson 2003: 118–23; Allen 2013; Leprohon 2008; Mathieu 2013). This concept of righteous succession by a healthy heir was the basis for the presentation of divine kingship in ancient Egypt (Baines 1995a, 1995b).

Horus as the legitimate heir to Osiris

Osiris was the rightful king of Egypt before his assassination by his brother, Seth, the god of confusion, who cut the dead god's body into several pieces (te Velde 1967; Turner 2013). Using her considerable magical powers (Pinch 1994; Teeter 2011: 161–81), Osiris's faithful sister and wife, Isis (Witt 1997), recited a spell to gather and restore the scattered pieces of the body of Osiris, and another spell to impregnate herself. She consequently gave birth to Horus, the legitimate heir to the throne of Egypt (Wilkinson 2003: 146). Through the effectiveness and strength of her magic (Koenig 2013) and the power of her words (Wilkinson 1994: 148–69), Isis was able to ensure her son's rule after the death of his father. Subsequently, the living king was the manifestation of Horus on the throne of Egypt (Nunn 1996: 218). The magical spells which Isis used to give birth to Horus refer to the will of Egyptian deities to confer legitimacy over the transfer of power from the father, Osiris, to their son, Horus

(Wilkinson 1992: 83). Thus Osiris was able to become the lord of the dead and of the underworld.

The divine conflict between Horus and Seth was a common theme in mortuary texts and literature (Tobin 1993; Baines 1996, 1999; Quack 2012), most notably featuring in 'The Contendings of Horus and Seth' preserved in the 20th Dynasty Chester Beatty Papyrus I (Broze 1996). The Ennead of Heliopolis (Wilkinson 2003: 78–9), among which Horus achieved a prominent place (Tillier 2013), expressed this in their judgement of Horus and Seth (Allam 1992) when Thoth said to Seth: 'Shall one give the office of Osiris to Seth while his son Horus is there?' (Lichtheim 1976: 215). Then the Ennead of Heliopolis (Griffiths 1960b) asked Thoth to write a letter to Neith the Great: 'What shall we do about these two people, who for eighty years now have been before the tribunal, and no one knows how to judge between the two? Write us what we should do!' (Lichtheim 1976: 215). Neith the Great sent a letter to the Ennead, saying: 'Give the office of Osiris to his son Horus, and don't do those big misdeeds that are out of place' (Lichtheim 1976: 215). Thus Horus became the legitimate king on the throne of Egypt deserving both the White Crown of Upper Egypt associated with Seth, as well as his own Red Crown of the Delta, his birthplace (Gardiner 1931; Wente 2003: 97). It was therefore possible in Egyptian art to see the king being crowned by a reconciled Horus and Seth, as seen in a rare three-dimensional rendering in a statue of Ramesses III in the Egyptian Museum, Cairo (Gardiner 1931; Figure 10.1).

Horus as a protective deity

When his mother, Isis, escaped to the Delta, Horus was protected by her and the deities of the Delta, including the cow-goddess Hathor, who breastfed and took care of him. These deities were thus considered sources of protection among the ancient Egyptians. Indeed, the name of Hathor means 'the House of Horus' (Wilkinson 2003: 140), which carries the implication of motherly protection. Protective deities associated with nurturing the child Horus provided the mythological scenario referenced in spells used in the context of magico-medical healing rituals. A transfer of power occurs between Horus the innocent son of Isis and Horus the child, who was considered to be a 'protector' or 'saviour' in his own right (Nunn 1996: 219). The concept of the saviour child Horus is also implicit in the presentation of divine kingship, where he is opposed to the god Seth, and by extension other chaotic forces (Wilkinson 2003: 64–9).

The Metternich Stela (Scott 1951), one of the category of objects known as 'Cippi of Horus' (Kákosy 2002; First 2013) with the motif of Horus standing on crocodiles (Altenmüller 1995; Sternberg-el-Hotabi 1999; Plate 3), carries a text

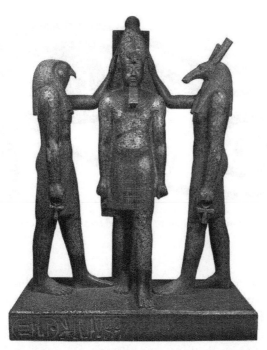

10.1 Ramesses III being crowned by Horus and Seth, Egyptian Museum, Cairo.
(www.globalegyptianmuseum.org/detail.aspx?id=14750)

stating that Seth had Horus poisoned by a scorpion. Isis was overcome with grief at the death of her child. She called out to Re and asked him for his aid. Re sent Thoth, who restored the child to life. On the cippi, Horus the child is depicted in the centre of the monument standing on crocodiles (Ritner 1989) and holding in each hand a serpent and scorpion, sometimes also with a lion and oryx in either hand (Sternberg-el-Hotabi 1987; Koemoth 2007). This motif inverts the concept of the powerless Horus in the myth of Osiris, and represents the innocent child god as the defeater against all evil forces (Sander-Hansen 1956: 2–76).

The struggle between Horus and Seth (Griffiths 1960a; Oden 1979) resulted in the destruction of the eye of Horus (Oestigaard 2011; Figure 10.2), restored by Isis as the Udjat eye, the 'complete', 'restored' and 'whole'. This hiero-glyphic symbol, with its different components, was used in recording quantities (Gardiner 1957: 197–200) especially in medicine (Allen 2005: 26–7). The Udjat eye could also represent the moon and its monthly destruction, which on a mythological level caused cosmic disorder until Thoth put the eye back and restored order (Koenig 2011). It is hardly surprisingly, therefore, that the Udjat

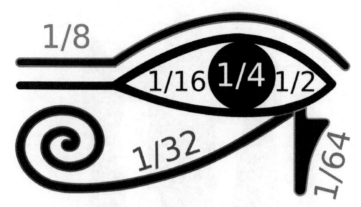

10.2 Mathematical values represented by the Udjat 'eye of Horus'.

eye represents one of the most important and well-attested amulets with heal-ing symbolism known from ancient Egypt (Andrews 1994: 43–4; see Andrews, Chapter 8, in this volume).

The violent destruction of the eye of Horus echoes Seth's murder and dis-memberment of Osiris, both events representing disorder in the cosmic cycle (Pinch 1994: 104–19). In 'The Contendings of Horus and Seth', we read that Seth removes both eyes of Horus:

> *iw.f rwy wd3.fy m st.w*
> *iw.f tmsw.w ḥr p3 dw r sḥd t3*
> *iw p3 bnrwy n irty.fy ḫprw m sḫrrty iw.sn rwd m sšnwy*

> He removed his two eyes from their sockets, and buried them on the moun-tain so as to illuminate the earth. His two eyeballs became two bulbs which grew into lotuses. (Gardiner 1932: 50, 11–13; Wente 2003: 98)

The injury to the eyes of Horus was in this case tended by the goddess Hathor, who is said to have applied milk:

> *wn.in.s mḥ m wʿ gḥst iw.s h3r.s iw.s ḥr dd n ḥr i.wn irt.k di.i n3y irtt im*
> *wn.in.f ḥr wn irt.f iw.s dit n3 irtt im iw.s dit r t3 imny iw.s dit r t3 smḥy*
> *iw.s ḥr dd n.f i.wn irt.k iw.f wn irt.f iw.s prt.f gm.(s) sw mnkw*

> She captured a gazelle and milked it. She said to Horus, 'Open your eyes that I may put this milk in'. So he opened his eyes and she put the milk in, putting (some) in the right one and putting (some) in the left one. She told him, 'Open your eyes!' He opened his eyes, and she looked at them; she found that they were healed. (Gardiner 1932: 51, 1–6; Wente 2003: 98–9)

In another episode, Seth attempts to have sexual intercourse with Horus (te Velde 1971; Borghouts 2008) and Horus takes revenge on him. Seth's favourite vegetable was lettuce, a symbol of the ithyphallic god Min that was considered to be an aphrodisiac (Pinch 1994: 120–32; Wente 2003: 97):

iw.s ḥr ḏd.n p3 k3ry n stḫ iḫ m smw p3 nty stḫ ḥr wnm.f di m-di.k ʿḥʿ.n p3 k3ry ḥr ḏd n.s bw ir.f wnm smw nb di m-di.i ḥr ʿbw

She (Isis) said to Seth's gardener, 'What sort of vegetable does Seth eat here in your company?' And the gardener answered her, 'He doesn't eat any vegetable here in my company except lettuce.' (Gardiner 1932: 52, 12–14; Wente 2003: 99)

Again, it is Isis who uses her magic to impregnate Seth with the semen of Horus, consumed after being applied to lettuce. This results in the creation of a sun-disk, 'born' from Seth's forehead. Although far-fetched to a modern (and perhaps an ancient) reader, the concept of cause and effect – application of a substance and subsequent action – had a powerful resonance with expected responses from ancient Egyptian healing practices. Use of a wide range of substances, including many plant products, was characteristic of the ancient Egyptian pharmacopoeia.

Conclusion

The magico-medical actions mentioned in the myth of Osiris were not intended simply to serve the narrative of the myth; rather their effectiveness relates to the problems that Horus faced for the completion of the process of his growth to ascend the throne of Egypt and occupy his hereditary seat. As a result, the magico-medical aspects of the myth were utilised as a divine model by the ancient Egyptians in blessings as well as curses, to heal diseases and especially to protect children by healing through magic by implication (Nordh 1996).

The primary purpose of the myth of Osiris, when pieced together from its varied sources, was to justify the accession of Horus to the throne of Egypt; indirectly, however, it also promoted psychological benefits in healing by placing magico-medical actions into the divine realm. The texts on many Horus cippi (Sternberg-el-Hotabi 1999) show the popularity of aspects of this universal myth in magico-medical actions (Abd El Razek 1995: 8).

Acknowledgements

I would like to dedicate this article as a token of love and gratitude to my teacher, Professor Rosalie David. Rosalie is a wonderful person and very gifted scholar. I have known her for many years and I have learned much from her. I thank Rosalie for her unique friendship and outstanding scholarship over many years, and wish her a long life full of health, happiness and prosperity. I am extremely grateful to Hussein Bassir, University of Arizona, for reading this article, making valuable comments and suggesting references. Finally, many thanks are due to Jacqueline Campbell.

References

Abd El Razek, E. M. (1995), 'A note on the difference between execration statues and prisoners' statues', *Göttinger Miszellen* 147, 7–8.

Allam, S. (1992), 'Legal aspects in the "Contendings of Horus and Seth"', in A. B. Lloyd (ed.), *Studies in Pharaonic Religion and Society in Honour of J. Gwyn Griffiths* (London: Egypt Exploration Society), 137–45.

Allen, J. P. (2005), *The Art of Medicine in Ancient Egypt* (New York and New Haven: Metropolitan Museum of Art and Yale University Press).

Allen, J. P. (2013), 'The name of Osiris (and Isis),' *Lingua Aegyptia* 21, 9–14.

Altenmüller, H. (1995), 'Der Sockel einer Horusstele des Vorstehers der Wab-Priester der Sachmet Benitehhor', *Studien zur Altägyptischen Kultur* 22, 1–20.

Andrews, C. (1994), *Amulets of Ancient Egypt* (London: British Museum Press).

Baines, J. (1995a), 'Kingship, definition of culture, and legitimation', in D. O'Connor and D. P. Silverman (eds.), *Ancient Egyptian Kingship* (Leiden: Brill), 3–47.

Baines, J. (1995b), 'Origins of Egyptian kingship', in D. O'Connor and D. P. Silverman (eds.), *Ancient Egyptian Kingship* (Leiden: Brill), 95–156.

Baines, J. (1996), 'Myth and literature,' in A. Loprieno (ed.), *Ancient Egyptian Literature: History and Forms* (Leiden: Brill), 361–77.

Baines, J. (1999). 'Prehistories of literature: performance, fiction, myth', in G. Moers (ed.), *Definitely: Egyptian Literature. Proceedings of the Symposium Ancient Egyptian Literature: History and Forms', Los Angeles, March 24–26, 1995* (Göttingen: Seminar für Ägyptologie und Koptologie), 17–41.

Borghouts, J. F. (2008), 'Trickster gods in the Egyptian pantheon', in S. E. Thompson and P. Der Manuelian (eds.), *Egypt and Beyond: Essays Presented to Leonard H. Lesko upon his Retirement from the Wilbour Chair of Egyptology at Brown University, June 2005* (Providence: Department of Egyptology and Ancient Western Asian Studies), 41–8.

Broze, M. (1996), *Mythe et roman en Égypte ancienne: les aventures d'Horus et Seth dans le papyrus Chester Beatty I* (Leuven: Peeters).

Campbell, J. M., El Saeed, E. and David, A. R. (2010), 'A reassessment of Warren Dawson's *'Studies in Ancient Egyptian Medical Texts'* 1926–1934, in the light of archaeobotanical and pharmacological evidence', in J. Cockitt and R. David (eds.), *Pharmacy and Medicine in Ancient Egypt: Proceedings of the Conferences Held in Cairo (2007) and Manchester (2008)* (Oxford: Archaeopress), 30–7.

David, A. R. (2008), 'Medical science and Egyptology', in R. H. Wilkinson (ed.), *Egyptology Today* (Cambridge and New York: Cambridge University Press), 36–54.

David, R. (2011), 'Ancient Egyptian medicine: an appraisal based on scientific methodology', in D. Aston, B. Bader, C. Gallorini, P. Nicholson and S. Buckingham (eds.), *Under the Potter's Tree: Studies on Ancient Egypt Presented to Janine Bourriau on the Occasion of her 70th Birthday* (Leuven: Peeters), 263–86.

First, G. (2013), 'The Horus cippus from National Museum in Poznań', *Folia orientalia* 50: 323–4.

Gardiner, A. H. (1931), *The Library of A. Chester Beatty: Description of a Hieratic Papyrus with a Mythological Story, Love-Songs, and Other Miscellaneous Texts; the Chester Beatty Papyri, No. 1* (London: Oxford University Press).

Gardiner, A. H. (1932), *Late-Egyptian Stories* (Brussels: Fondation Égyptologique Reine Élisabeth).

Gardiner, A. H. (1957), *Egyptian Grammar* (Oxford: Oxford University Press).

Golenischeff, W. S. (1877), *Die Metternichstele* (Leipzig: Engelmann).

Griffiths, J. G. (1960a), *The Conflict of Horus and Seth from Egyptian and Classical Sources: A Study in Ancient Mythology* (Liverpool: Liverpool University Press).

Griffiths, J. G. (1960b), 'The flight of the gods before Typhon: an unrecognized myth', *Hermes* 88, 374–6.

Győry, H. (2011), 'Some aspects of magic in ancient Egyptian medicine', in P. Kousoulis (ed.), *Ancient Egyptian Demonology: Studies on the Boundaries between the Demonic and the Divine in Egyptian Magic* (Leuven: Peeters), 151–66.

Kákosy, L. (2002), 'A late Horus cippus', in H. Győry (ed.), *Mélanges offerts à Edith Varga: 'le lotus qui sort de terre'* (Budapest: Musée Hongrois des Beaux-Arts), 217–20.

Koemoth, P. P. (2007), 'L'Atoum-serpent magicien de la stèle Metternich', *Studien zur Altägyptischen Kultur* 36, 137–46.

Koenig, Yvan (ed.) (2002), *La magie en Égypte: à la recherche d'une définition; actes du colloque organisé par le Musée du Louvre les 29 et 30 septembre 2000* (Paris: La Documentation Française).

Koenig, Y. (2011), 'Between order and disorder: a case of sacred philology', in P. Kousoulis (ed.), *Ancient Egyptian Demonology: Studies on the Boundaries between the Demonic and the Divine in Egyptian Magic* (Leuven: Peeters), 121–8.

Koenig, Yvan (2013), 'La magie égyptienne: de l'image à la ressemblance', in M. Tardieu, A. Van den Kerchove and M. Zago (eds.), *Noms barbares*, I: *Formes et contextes d'une pratique magique* (Turnhout: Brepols), 177–89.

Leprohon, R. J. (2008), 'Egyptian religious texts', in R. H. Wilkinson (ed.), *Egyptology Today* (Cambridge and New York: Cambridge University Press), 230–47.

Lichtheim, M. (1976), *Ancient Egyptian Literature. A Book of Readings*, II: *The New Kingdom* (Los Angeles: University of California Press).

Mathieu, B. (2013), 'Horus: polysémie et metamorphoses,' *Égypte Nilotique et Méditerranéenne* 6, 1–26.

Nordh, K. (1996), *Aspects of Ancient Egyptian Curses and Blessings: Conceptual Background and Transmission* (Uppsala: Acta Universitatis Upsaliensis).

Nunn, J. F. (1996), *Ancient Egyptian Medicine* (London: British Museum Press).

Oden Jr., R. A. (1979), '"The Contendings of Horus and Seth" (Chester Beatty Papyrus No. 1): a structural interpretation', *History of Religions* 18, 352–69.

Oestigaard, T. (2011), *Horus' Eye and Osiris' Efflux: The Egyptian Civilisation of Inundation c.3000–2000 BCE* (Oxford: Archaeopress).

Pinch, G. (1994), *Magic in Ancient Egypt* (London: British Museum Press).

Quack, J. F. (2012), 'Der Streit zwischen Horus und Seth in einer spätneuägyptischen Fassung', in C. Zivie-Coche and Guermeur (eds.), *'Parcourir l'éternité': hommages à Jean Yoyotte*, II (Turnhout: Brepols), 907–21.

Reeves, C. (1992), *Egyptian Medicine* (Princes Risborough: Shire).

Ritner, R. K. (1989), 'Horus on the crocodiles: a juncture of religion and magic in Late Dynastic Egypt', *Yale Egyptological Studies* 3: 103–16.

Sander-Hansen, C. E. (1956), *Die Texte der Metternichstele* (Copenhagen: Munksgaard).

Scott, N. E. (1951), 'The Metternich Stela', *The Metropolitan Museum of Art Bulletin* 9, 201–17.

Sternberg-el-Hotabi, H. (1987), 'Die Götterdarstellungen der Metternichstele: ein Neuansatz zu ihrer Interpretation als Elemente eines Kontinuitätsmodells', *Göttinger Miszellen* 97, 25–70.

Sternberg-el-Hotabi, H. (1999), *Untersuchungen zur Überlieferungsgeschichte der Horusstelen: ein Beitrag zur Religionsgeschichte Ägyptens im 1. Jahrtausend v. Chr* (Wiesbaden: Harassowitz).

Teeter, E. (2011), *Religion and Ritual in Ancient Egypt* (Cambridge: Cambridge University Press).

te Velde, H. (1967), *Seth, God of Confusion: A Study of his Role in Egyptian Mythology and Religion* (Leiden: Brill).

te Velde, H. (1971), 'The Egyptian god Seth as a trickster', in D. Sinor (ed.), *Proceedings of the Twenty-Seventh International Congress of Orientalists, Ann Arbor, Michigan, 13th–19th August, 1967* (Wiesbaden: Harassowitz), 50–1.

Tillier, A. (2013), 'Sur la place d'Horus dans l'ennéade héliopolitaine', *Zeitschrift für ägyptische Sprache und Altertumskunde* 140, 70–7.

Tobin, V. A. (1993), 'Divine conflict in the Pyramid Texts', *Journal of the American Research Center in Egypt* 30, 93–110.

Turner, P. J. (2013), *Seth. A Misrepresented God in the Ancient Egyptian Pantheon?* (Oxford: Archaeopress).

Wente, E. F. (2003), 'The Contendings of Horus and Seth', in W. K Simpson (ed.), *The Literature of Ancient Egypt: An Anthology of Stories, Instructions, Stelae, Autobiographies, and Poetry* (New Haven and London: Yale University Press), 91–103.

Wilkinson, R. H. (1992), *Reading Egyptian Art: A Hieroglyphic Guide to Ancient Egyptian Painting and Sculpture* (London: Thames and Hudson).

Wilkinson, R. H. (1994), *Symbol and Magic in Egyptian Art* (London: Thames and Hudson).

Wilkinson, R. H. (2003), *The Complete Gods and Goddesses of Ancient Egypt* (London: Thames and Hudson).

Witt, R. E. (1997), *Isis in the Ancient World* (Baltimore and London: Johns Hopkins University Press).

11

Trauma care, surgery and remedies in ancient Egypt: a reassessment

Roger Forshaw

I am pleased to be able to offer this new analysis of trauma care and surgery in ancient Egypt to Rosalie, as this is a topic of particular interest to her. Also I am grateful to Rosalie for inspiring me in my master's and doctoral studies in Egyptology and for inviting me to join her team at the KNH Centre for Biomedical Egyptology at the University of Manchester.

Trauma can be defined as any bodily injury or wound caused by an extrinsic agent. Evidence for trauma in a population may reflect many factors related to the lifestyles of individuals including culture, economy, living environment, occupation and interpersonal violence. The progress of healing of injuries in an ancient society is influenced by such factors as availability and quality of treatment, occurrence of complications and dietary status (Roberts and Manchester 2005: 84). A rich source of textual information relating to trauma care in ancient Egypt is provided by the Edwin Smith Papyrus, and there is some associated evidence in the Ebers Papyrus. In addition the palaeopathological record demonstrates further examples such as instances of splints used to immobilise fractures, described by Elliot Smith (1908: 732–4).

Trauma

The Edwin Smith Papyrus is referred to as a surgical papyrus in a number of publications such as those of Breasted (1930), Wilson (1952) and Chapman (1992) but in reality it is an ancient instructional text for the management of trauma to the head, the upper arms and the superior part of the thorax.[1] Other than

---

[1] For translations of the Edwin Smith Papyrus see Breasted (1930), von Deines, Grapow and Westendorf (1954–73), Allen (2005), Sanchez and Meltzer (2012).

simple procedures such as suturing of wounds there is little mention of surgical operative practices in the text. The papyrus lists forty-eight medical case descriptions, commencing at the top of the head and progressing downwards in a logical manner, terminating at the upper part of the thorax and arms, and not at waist level as Majno (1975: 91) suggests. The papyrus ends mid-sentence in Case 48; it would seem likely that at one time there would have been further parts to this treatise that would have related to cases of trauma in the lower parts of the body, but to date such texts have not been discovered.

That the ancient Egyptians understood the principles of trauma care is illustrated by many of the case descriptions recorded in the Edwin Smith Papyrus, reports which incorporate detailed anatomical, clinical and therapeutic information. Case 6 describes a severe head wound with a depressed skull fracture that has exposed the surface of the brain. [2] The explicit and detailed anatomical descriptions of the brain and the dura mater membrane enveloping the brain, while also recognising the existence of cerebrospinal fluid, are quite exceptional for this early date in history. The recommended treatment for Case 12, a depressed fracture of the nasal bone, involves reducing the fracture, intranasal cleansing, the insertion of a lubricated internal nasal packing and external splinting, followed by oil and honey dressings – treatment principles that are still employed today (Sanchez and Meltzer 2012: 69, 119).

There are a number of cases of trauma in the Edwin Smith Papyrus where either what may appear initially to be logical treatment is advised against or no treatment is prescribed. Case 4, a head injury with an open, elevated skull fracture, includes instructions that the wound is not to be bandaged. This advice appears logical as binding with a dressing would tend to restrict spontaneous intracranial decompression. Such decompression affords some relief from the build-up of intracranial pressure developing from brain swelling occurring with this type of serious injury. Case 44 is a description of fractures to the ribs for which no chest binding is advised, a not unreasonable treatment plan as cases of this nature often heal spontaneously. Today tight bindings in cases of rib fractures are considered counterproductive as they can result in reduced ventilation and associated lung collapse (Sanchez and Meltzer 2012: 58, 268).

The concept of infection was recognised in ancient Egypt as illustrated by Case 41, which describes a chest wound, although an understanding that bacteria were the cause of the problem was millennia away. Here the classical signs of superficial infection are described – swelling (*šf*), redness (*dšr*) and heat (*srf*) – signs that are still recognised as valid today. Cases 28 and 39 further

---

2 All case numbers refer to the notation system as established by Breasted (1930).

demonstrate this understanding, as here it is advised to carry out open drainage of an infective lesion. Such examples demonstrate that the ancient Egyptians understood and established sound clinical reasons for their treatment plans and recognised the existence and nature of possible complications.

Each of the forty-eight cases of the Edwin Smith Papyrus issues one of three verdicts related to the treatment potential in the circumstance: 'favourable', 'uncertain' or 'unfavourable'. The unfavourable verdict is translated by Breasted (1930: 46) as 'an ailment not to be treated' (*mr nn irw.ny*) with the implication that the case was hopeless and no treatment was to be provided. This translation has been followed in later publications (Majno 1975: 91; Ghalioungui 1980: 57; Nunn 1996: 28). However, each of the three verdicts can be interpreted as an expression of opinion and expectation of the individual's progress using the treatments that are available. A more recent translation of the unfavourable verdict is 'a medical condition that cannot be handled/dealt with', which is perhaps to be interpreted as not anticipating a successful outcome from the prescribed treatment (Sanchez and Meltzer 2012: 3).

This unfavourable prognosis was not a decision to withhold treatment, merely a recognition that the treatments available would be unlikely to help in this situation. This suggestion is supported by the fact that in the majority of these unfavourable cases, some form of care was provided. In Case 5, a head injury with an associated depressed skull fracture, the treatment was one of not bandaging the wound, which would have been contraindicated, but placing the patient on bed rest and observing progress. Similarly, in Case 6 the advice was not to bandage, but to gently apply oil to the wound and again monitor the progress of the condition. Further support for the provision of such palliative care is provided by a remedy in the Ebers Papyrus (200, 40, 5–10), where the advice for a stomach ailment is to provide treatment and not abandon the individual: 'Go against it, do not abandon' (*ʿk rf m bt sw*).

Such treatment advice and verdicts imply a hope of recovery in some of the cases, and in others, perhaps regarded as hopeless, the instructions provided are for observation associated with care and attention. This humanitarian concept is supported by a passage from a New Kingdom text, *The Instruction of Amenemope* (British Museum, Papyrus 10474, l. 24.9–10; translated in Simpson 2003: 241): 'Do not laugh at a blind man nor taunt a dwarf, neither interfere with the condition of a cripple.'

Surgery

The medical papyri, especially the Edwin Smith, demonstrate an understanding of anatomy and include a detailed vocabulary of Egyptian anatomical terms, particularly for the external and upper parts of the body. It can be

surmised that the same level of knowledge was attained for the lower parts of
the body not covered by the Edwin Smith Papyrus. This insight would suggest
that the ancient Egyptians studied anatomy and that at one time a treatise on
the subject may have existed. Clement of Alexandria (*Stromata* VI, 6: Roberts
and Donaldson n.d.) writing in the second century AD, stated that the ancient
Egyptians possessed six books of medical content, one of which related to
the structure of the body, although there is no evidence of such a text having
survived.

An appreciation of anatomy is essential to perform detailed surgical procedures. However, there is little evidence that human dissection was undertaken
in ancient Egypt to acquire this necessary anatomical skill until the Alexandrian
medical school was established during the Ptolemaic Period (Jackson 1988: 21,
27; von Staden 1989: 29). It is considered that traditions of respect for the dead
would have prohibited dissection, as such procedures would have been deemed
a desecration of the body (Baines and Lacovara 2002: 5–36). Battle casualties
and serious industrial accidents would have offered an opportunity to gain
some anatomical understanding although it is difficult to observe internal anatomical relationships *in vivo*. Evidence from mummified specimens indicates
that the embalmers possessed some technical expertise, and this knowledge
may have been passed onto the *swnw* (usually translated as 'doctors' or 'physicians') or other individuals involved with medical care (Nunn 1996: 42–3). Von
Staden (1989: 29) cautions that the level of anatomical familiarity required
for embalming is closer to that of a skilled butcher than to that of a surgeon.
Nevertheless, dressing animal carcasses would have provided a certain level
of anatomical knowledge, as is evident from the use of animal parts as hieroglyphic signs in references to parts of the human body. However, it is difficult
to comprehend that the detailed level of anatomical knowledge demonstrated
in the Edwin Smith Papyrus could be acquired without some form of dissection
experience.

A number of the medical papyri make reference to a 'knife treatment' (*dwꜥ*),
presumably some form of surgical procedure. Few details are provided about
such techniques except that at the conclusion of the procedure the advice is that
the wound should be treated 'like the treatment of a wound on any body-part of
man' (Ebers 868, 107, 5–9; translated in Ghalioungui 1987: 244).

The final section of the Ebers Papyrus (863–77) describes the surgical
removal and treatment of various swellings (*ꜥꜣwt*), some of which may refer
to tumours. For these procedures a number of separate knives are utilised,
the *ds*, *šꜣs*, *ḫpt* and *hmm* knife, and on two occasions the advice is to heat the
particular knife (Nunn 1996: 165–8). Ebers 875 introduces another term, the
hnw-instrument, a word which was determined by the sign for an animal hide
(Gardiner sign list F 28) and which could refer to a pair of forceps (Erman and

Grapow 1931: 494). All of these sixteen cases commence with an examination, diagnosis and prognosis which is then followed by treatment. This differentiation into logical component parts is also evident in cases 188–207, 831–3 and 857–62 of the Ebers Papyrus and is a characteristic again obvious in the trauma cases listed in the Edwin Smith Papyrus. In the remainder of the sections of the Ebers, the indication is that the diagnosis has already been made and the text is merely a remedy to eliminate a named disease. This obvious split between two styles of presenting cases reinforces the notion that the Ebers is a collection of medical texts from different sources that have been combined into a single document and arranged in a seemingly random order (Nunn 1996: 32; David 2008: 190).

Some of the sources of literature discussing surgery in ancient Egypt suggest that only the very simplest operative procedures were undertaken (Harris 1971: 125; Majno 1975: 86; Estes 1993: 51; Nunn 1996: 165). This perception appears to arise from the observation that the medical papyri do not usually provide extensive details of the surgical technique undertaken, as illustrated in the majority of cases 863–77 of the Ebers Papyrus, where there is merely reference to 'the knife treatment'. Certainly, there are no detailed descriptions of extensive surgery comparable to those portrayed by Celsus (*De medicina* VII, VIII: Spencer 1938: 295–587) in operations that were performed in ancient Rome.

However, a closer examination of some of the cases in the Ebers suggests that these procedures were carefully planned and executed, and while they are not examples of major surgery would, nevertheless, have required some anatomical knowledge as well as a degree of skill and experience. Ebers 871 (107,16 – 108,3) provides guidance for operating on a 'swelling of pain-matter' (ʿ*3 nt wḥdw*), which is considered by Nunn (1996: 167) to be an abscess. The instructions involve taking care to avoid one of the major vessels (*mtw*) and ensuring that no remnants of the swelling are retained. Ebers 875 (109, 2–11) refers to the possible removal of a guinea worm (Ghalioungui 1987: 251–2; Miller 1989: 249–54; Nunn 1996: 70, 168). The case describes the use of several different instruments during the procedure. A *ds* knife is used to make the initial incision, followed by a *ḥnw*-instrument (forceps?) to grasp the worm. A *š3s* knife is then utilised to extirpate the remnants, while taking care to avoid damaging the tissue boundaries and surrounding anatomical structures. Although this could be described as basic treatment, nevertheless the instructions provided in the papyrus follow a logical sequence and advise care in completing the various procedures, which is suggestive of a knowledge of anatomy and an awareness of possible complications, and is indicative of previous experience.

Until recently few cases of surgical procedures have been found from examinations of ancient Egyptian skeletal and mummified remains. Rowling (1989: 316) stated that of the estimated 30,000 mummies and skeletal remains of all periods of ancient Egyptian history that were investigated around the closing years of the nineteenth century and the first two decades of the twentieth century, no instance of a surgical scar was observed. However, Sullivan (1998: 113) indicated that it is extremely difficult if not impossible to identify a therapeutic incision in mummified specimens, particular in view of the previous use of embalming materials and the state of preservation of many of the mummified bodies.

In 2005 a multi-detector computed tomography (CT) scanner was used to take detailed tomograph images of the mummified head of Djehutynakht, a Middle Kingdom nomarch from Deir el-Bersha. Previous radiographic examinations of Djehutynakht had demonstrated systematic post-mortem facial mutilations, unrelated to the process of excerebration, practices which had not previously been observed in other mummified specimens (Gupta *et al.* 2008: 705–13). The 2005 investigation revealed a series of surgical procedures which seemed to be designed to remobilise the mandible, possibly following initial post-mortem rigor mortis. The technique involved a succession of soft tissue incisions and osteotomies which would appear to have been carried out with care and precision. Such a procedure could only have been performed by an operator who had a thorough knowledge of the anatomy and functional relationships of the jaw. The implementation of such a procedure on a mummified body could have ritual significance and may be related to the 'Opening of the Mouth' ritual, which conferred on the deceased the ability to speak and take nourishment in the afterlife.

No other similar examples have so far been identified, but this may relate to a lack of sufficiently preserved remains demonstrating this elaborate procedure. Additionally, this type of procedure may well have been restricted to royalty and the elite. Another problem relates to the quality of earlier computed tomography studies, which were generally not adequate to identify such procedures unless they were specifically sought (Chapman and Gupta 2007: 113–27). This demonstration of operative expertise and knowledge of detailed functional anatomy may have been repeated in the performance of other surgical procedures not yet identified in the palaeopathological record.

Another advanced surgical procedure, but one that was performed during life, is described for a mummified head unearthed in the Theban necropolis. The specimen is dated from between the Third Intermediate Period and the Late Period (Nerlich, Panzer and Lösch 2010: 117–21). This case displays severe blunt trauma to the left parietal bone, and on the basis of new bone deposition the individual is considered to have survived for some time following the episode. The trauma site shows an extensive osseous defect; however, the dura mater is undisturbed and is covered by an intact layer of skin and connective tissue. The bone fragment(s) are missing and because of the intact layer of skin,

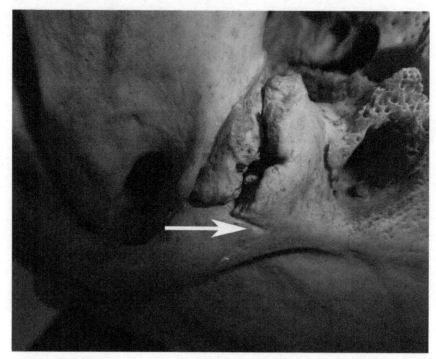

11.1 Skull NU 761 demonstrating ankylosis and possible incision. (Courtesy of Duckworth Laboratory, University of Cambridge. Image provided by M. Harris.)

these fragments are assumed to have been surgically removed from the defect. The procedure must have been carefully executed, as disturbing the dura mater would usually have fatal consequences.

A case displaying what appears to be surgical bony incisions in the region of the right temporomandibular joint has recently been described for an ancient Nubian skull (NU 761) excavated by the first Archaeological Survey of Nubia (1907–11) (Figure 11.1). The skull demonstrates a fracture of the right condylar head, part of which is separated from the mandible and ankylosed to the glenoid fossa, possibly as a result of a previous traumatic episode. The incisions appear to have been part of a procedure aimed at separating this fused joint and restoring normal joint movement. A micro-computed tomography scan of the area indicates that the sides of the incision are corticated, indicative of the procedure being performed ante-mortem. Additionally, the smooth-sided and tapering nature of the lesion suggests it was created by a double-sided sharp instrument (Harris, Lowe and Ahmed 2014: 41–50; Figure 11.2). If this hypothesis is correct then a procedure of this nature would indicate, as in the case of Djehutynakht, a thorough knowledge of the anatomy and functional relationships of the jaw, as

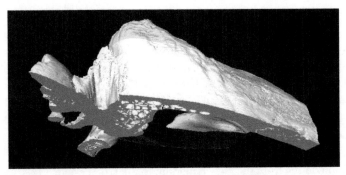

11.2 3D reconstruction of micro CT of section of skull NU 761 showing horizontal cut marks along the side of the lesion. (Courtesy of Duckworth Laboratory, University of Cambridge. Image provided by M. Harris.)

well as a high level of operative skill. While these cases are few in number, they do demonstrate a sophisticated level of surgical expertise.

Trepanation

Trepanation of the human skull, the removal of a piece of the calvarium without damage to the underlying anatomical structures, is a procedure well documented in antiquity. In ancient Egypt, while the medical papyri make no mention of trepanning there is some limited skeletal evidence of it being practised, although such evidence has been debated (Lisowski 1967: 651–72; Aufderheide and Rodríguez-Martín 1998: 31–4; Nerlich *et al.* 2003: 191–201; Martin 2013: 545–56). The purpose of trepanation in any ancient culture is difficult to identify but relief of intracranial disease processes, injuries, ritual significance and release of negative spiritual entities are among the motives suggested (Lisowski 1967: 651–72; Arnott *et al.* 2003).

Amputations

Amputations are often performed as treatment following a severe traumatic episode, and procedures of this nature may have been described in the 'missing' sections of the Edwin Smith Papyrus, which could have referred to the extremities of the body. However, there is a growing body of palaeopathological evidence that amputations were carried out in ancient Egypt, many of which appear to have been associated with traumatic incidents.

Amputations displaying successful healing patterns are recognised among the skeletal remains of the Old Kingdom pyramid builders excavated from the Giza necropolis (Zaki *et al.* 2010: 913–17). Brothwell and Møller-Christensen

(1963: 192–4) published details of an 11th Dynasty skeleton displaying an amputation of the forearm and subsequent distal fusion of the radius and ulna. Dupras *et al.* (2010: 405–23) describe four cases excavated from the necropolis of Deir el-Bersha, adjacent to an ancient quarry. This necropolis was in use from the late Old Kingdom to the New Kingdom. Three of these individuals display amputations with successful evidence of healing while the fourth died shortly after a traumatic incident and associated attempted amputations. Differential diagnoses indicated that these pathologies were probably due to trauma and not disease. Finally, Nerlich, Panzer and Lösch (2010: 117–21) describe two cases of amputation dating from the New Kingdom to the Late Period. These particular amputation sites are covered by layers of soft tissue and skin, indicating that the procedures were performed some time prior to death. However, Blomstedt (2014: 670–6), in a general review of original textual evidence and modern literature relating to surgery in ancient Egypt, considers that although fractures were treated, limb amputations were not routinely performed, although they may have been carried out under extraordinary circumstances.

There is evidence of amputations being carried out on the battlefield in ancient Egypt, where the victors would remove the right hands of their enemies to present to the king as evidence of their success.[3] A relief inscribed on the inner southern wall of the second courtyard of the temple of Ramesses III at Medinet Habu depicts amputated hands and penises being counted, and the biography of Ahmose son of Ebana (Lichtheim 1976: 12–14) describes how on a number of occasions Ahmose presented to the king an enemy hand as a trophy, for which he was rewarded with the gold of valour. Recently archaeological evidence of this practice has been discovered at Tell el-Daba (ancient Avaris), where sixteen skeletonised hands have been unearthed (Bietak 2012: 32–3).

Fractures

There is a considerable body of evidence revealing that the ancient Egyptians understood the principles involved in diagnosing and managing bone fractures (Nunn 1996: 174–7; Sanchez and Meltzer 2012). They used the method of 'closed treatment', a procedure which requires no surgical intervention. The technique consists of manipulation or 'reduction', followed by the application of a device such as a splint to maintain this reduction until healing occurs (Harkess, Ramsey and Harkess 1996: 29). The Edwin Smith Papyrus describes fractures and their treatment in some detail, and there is also widespread palaeopathological evidence of well-healed fractures. A study of 271 skeletons excavated

3   For a discussion of amputated hands in ancient Egypt see Abdalla 2005: 25–34.

from Old Kingdom cemeteries on the Giza plateau, probably to be identified as workers who built the pyramids, found a very high incidence of fractures. Nearly 44 per cent of the male skeletons and 26 per cent of the female skeletons displayed evidence of fractures, with 90 per cent of these fractures showing signs of complete healing with good alignment, an outcome which could be achieved only by the correct use of splints (Hussein *et al.* 2010: 85–9).

A study of long bones excavated from cemeteries at Saqqara dated to the Old Kingdom and Ptolemaic Periods, although showing a much reduced level of fractures (2.2 per cent), again found a high incidence displaying favourable healing patterns and good alignment, indicative of intervention and post-operative care (Kozieradzka-Ogunmakin 2013: 155). From a 26th Dynasty shaft tomb at Abusir a tibia and fibula were excavated which demonstrated well-healed fractures, again suggestive of treatment (Strouhal, Němečková and Kouba 2003: 334).

The archaeological record contains examples of splints that were used to immobilise these long bone fractures. Elliot Smith (1908: 732–4) describes two cases from Naga ed Deir, both dated to the 5th Dynasty. The first of these splints was applied to a compound fracture of the forearm involving both the radius and ulna. Elliot Smith considered that this type of splint, which consisted of rough bark, linen and coarse grass packing, would have supplied effective support. He based this conclusion on his study of many similar examples of fractures which displayed excellent healing patterns. The second example was a fracture of the right femur to which four wooden splints wrapped in linen had been fixed. The wood had been shaped in two of the splints, and they were all held in place on the leg by bandaging. Although Elliot Smith assessed that the splints had been carefully placed, he suggested that in this case they would have been of little value as the powerful leg muscles would have produced a tendency for the fragments to override and result in rotation and shortening of the healed limb.

However, Wood Jones (1908: 457) published illustrations of healed fractures of all six long bones of the limbs, which display good healing patterns and near perfect alignment, including a well-healed femur unlike the example described above. There is nothing in the surviving textual record, and no satisfactory explanation in more recent literature covering this topic, to suggest how the ancient Nubians could have arranged sustained traction to achieve this excellent result.

It is perhaps the works of the Hippocratic Corpus (*c.*440–340 BC) and in particular *De fracturis* III (I–XLIII) that we need to consult, as in these texts there are detailed accounts of fractures, displacements and instruments of reduction. The procedure that is described for reduction of this type of fracture involves, firstly, suspension of the patient and extension of the fractured femur either by weights or by the efforts of two assistants. Once alignment is achieved, linen bandages soaked in fat or oil mixed with wax or resins are applied to the fracture. These dressings are then changed daily, and at each bandage change, extension is reapplied and the position of the bone fragments adjusted. After approximately a week splints are applied, these being adjusted at intervals, with consolidation of the bones considered to have occurred after forty days. The detailed and careful manipulation, extension and splinting of fractures described in this source accords well with modern practice, and such a technique could well have resulted in near perfect bone union.

It is possible that a technique of this nature could have been utilised by the ancient Egyptians. Certainly, more complicated procedures than this were undertaken, as illustrated by the detailed descriptions of traumatic injuries and their treatment recorded in the Edwin Smith Papyrus. The 'missing' section of this text could have included a method to manage fractures of the long bones of the leg. It is not possible to say if such a technique originated in Egypt and influenced later Greek practices.[4]

Compounds utilised in ancient Egyptian remedies

The majority of the information relating to the medicaments used in the various ancient Egyptian remedies is based on the textual evidence of the medical papyri. These remedies have been variously described by Jonckheere (1947, 1958), Leake (1952), von Deines, Gravow and Westendorf (1954–73), Dawson (1967), Ghalioungui (1980, 1987), Estes (1993), Nunn (1996), Manniche (1989), Campbell and David (2005) and Campbell, Campbell and David (2010). Analysing the remedies in these papyri can be problematic because of the uncertainty in the translation of a number of the constituents, particularly in view of their unique vocabulary. Additionally, the Egyptians named these materials according to different criteria from those that are in use today. An important factor was appearance; thus chickpea was called (ḥr-bỉk) 'falcon-face', because the seeds resemble the face of a falcon complete with its beak. Other Egyptian names included šd-pnw 'mouse-tail' and šny-t3 'hair of the earth' (Germer 1998: 85).

Another difficulty is that a particular material used in ancient Egypt may not be the same material as we know today. ỉmrw, used in a number of the treatments listed in the medical papyri, has been the subject of considerable debate. Breasted (1930: 265) thought it might have a disinfectant function, and von Deines, Grapow and Westendorf (1959, VI: 33) consider it as an unknown

---

4 For the possible links between Egyptian and Greek medicine see Marganne 1993 and Jouanne 2012: 3–22.

material, while Nunn (1996: 176) suggests it may be equivalent to plaster of Paris as it is advised to be used with a bandage when treating a fractured bone. Allen (2005: 83), Sanchez and Meltzer (2012: 129) and Strouhal, Břetislav and Vymazalová (2014: 25) consider *imrw* to be alum, a view taken by this writer. However, the alum used by the ancients may have had a different chemical composition from the material we recognise as alum (hydrated potassium aluminium sulphate) today. Additionally, Pliny distinguished between different types of this material in his *Natural History* (35.183–90; Rackham 1952: 395–402).

Geographical and temporal influences need to be taken into consideration as it is quite possible that the names of some of the substances would not have remained the same throughout three thousand years of Pharaonic history. Germer (1998: 86) uses the example of the yellow dye fustic to illustrate this point. Fustic is obtained from the wig-tree (*Cotinus cogyggria*), which is native to Europe and Asia. However, when the New World was settled, Europeans transferred the name 'fustic' to the yellowwood tree (*Chlorophora tinctoria*), which resulted in fustic now being obtainable from a different plant.

Some of the materials used in the remedies have often been dismissed as being of little therapeutic value, and indeed in many cases this may be true. The choice of certain of the constituents may have been based on different crtiteria from those in use today. Compounds may have been added merely as a vehicle for the active constituent, some for taste and others because of their supposed magical properties. Papyrus Ramesseum V incorporates a number of animal products in the listed remedies, products derived from creatures such as the hippopotamus, crocodile, lion, mouse and donkey. Their inclusion may have been motivated by magical associations or based on the characteristics of the donor animal that were deemed to be desirable (Bardinet 1995: 472–5; Ritner 2001: 327).

More recent analyses of a number of these materials has revealed that, while they have previously been rejected as having no therapeutic value, there may be some rationale for their inclusion in a particular remedy. Case 9 of the Edwin Smith Papyrus describes a compound, comminuted fracture of the frontal bone of the skull. The treatment advised for this type of injury involves placing a mixture of ground ostrich shell and oil directly on the wound, followed by a coating of ground dry ostrich shell. During the application of these compounds a magical incantation was to be recited. Previous suggestions have been that the skull was equated to the shell of an egg and that this remedy was an example of sympathetic magic rather than rational medicine (Wilson 1952: 76; Westendorf 1992: 21–2; Nunn 1996: 138). However, recent studies indicate that the coarse granularity of the ground ostrich shell, mixed with oil, would have produced the consistency to plug bleeding cancellous bone. The additional application of powdered eggshell would have further sealed the wound (Sanchez and Meltzer

2012: 99–100). Ostrich shell, which is predominantly calcium carbonate, has been used both as an interpositional graft to fill a complete bone defect and as an onlay graft to fill partial defects (Dupoirieux, Pourquier and Souyris 1995: 187–94; Dupoirieux 1999: 467–71). Therefore, while the addition of powdered eggshell to a wound may give the appearance of a skull as well as looking similar to an ostrich shell, there is some practical benefit in the use of this material both to seal a wound and as a bone substitute to aid healing.

A remedy from the Middle Kingdom Kahun Papyrus may also warrant further investigation and again may have some basis for pharmaceutical use (col. 1, 15–20, translated in Quirke 2002): 'Examination of a woman aching in her teeth and gums (molars?) to the point that she cannot […] her mouth. You should say of it "it is toothache of the womb". You should treat it then fumigating her with incense and oil in 1 jar. Pour over her […] the urine of an ass that has created its like the day it passed it. …'

A woman who is unable to open her mouth may have muscle spasm caused by strong clenching, a severe gingival infection or possibly an acute attack of pericoronitis. These latter acute conditions often occur in an individual with a pre-existing condition of chronic periodontitis. A postmenopausal woman may have osteoporosis, which is a risk factor for the progression of periodontitis (Guers 2007: 36).

The first part of the treatment advised for this condition consists of fumigation with incense (*sntr*), a material which is mentioned in numerous texts from the Old Kingdom onwards and is believed to refer to resins or resinous products such as frankincense, myrrh and terebinth (Serpico 2000: 456). Myrrh is used today in aromatherapy; it is listed in the British Pharmacopoeia (2012: 3654–5), where one of its uses is for the treatment of gingivitis.

The other constituent in the remedy is the urine from an ass or a donkey that has 'created its like' (a donkey that has just given birth to offspring). The urine of such a donkey would contain a high concentration of oestrogens. Because of the presence of this high level of hormones, pregnant mare's urine has been utilised in hormone replacement therapy since the 1940s in the form of conjugated equine oestrogens, known as the drug premarin (Bhavnani 1998: 6–16). Premarin is available in tablet form or in a topical preparation for use in the vagina. In the Kahun remedy the urine is mixed with oil and then advised for internal use. One of the functions of hormone replacement therapy is as a treatment for osteoporosis. So again there may be some practical benefit in the use of this remedy.

However, few prescribing details are included for the urine used in this Kahun remedy, and so the link between premarin and unrefined donkey urine may be somewhat tenuous. Nevertheless, as with many other remedies listed in the papyri, selection was often based on experimentation and observation, and as these two examples demonstrate, some of the ancient Egyptian remedies may warrant further analysis.

Conclusion

Breasted's 1930 translation of the Edward Smith Papyrus was a landmark in understanding the treatment of trauma in ancient Egypt, and now Sanchez and Meltzer's 2012 translation and analysis of the original hieratic text has provided a new insight into one of the more important medical papyri from ancient Egypt. In the intervening years between these two translations major changes have occurred in the practice of medicine and in the understanding of ancient Egyptian texts, and so this new version is a welcome reinterpretation of a key work. Similarly, new studies into the constituents of the remedies listed in the papyri demonstrate that materials once thought to be of no therapeutic value may need to be reassessed.

Surgery and the treatment of trauma in ancient Egypt witnessed the development of an elaborate clinical methodology. Today a reassessment of this methodology in the light of more recent philological studies, modern medicine, palaeopathological studies and a reappraisal of pharmaceutical formulations can further our understanding of these two disciplines in this ancient culture.

References

Abdalla, M. A. (2005), 'The amputated hands in ancient Egypt', in K. Daoud, S. Bedier and S. 'Abd el-Fattāh (eds.), *Studies in Honor of Ali Radwan*, supplement to *Annales du Service des antiquités de l'Égypte* (Cairo: Supreme Council of Antiquities), 25–34.

Allen, J. P. (2005), *The Art of Medicine in Ancient Egypt* (New York and New Haven: Metropolitan Museum of Art and Yale University Press).

Arnott, R., Finger, S. and Smith, C. U. M. (eds.) (2003), *Trepanation: History, Discovery, Theory* (Lisse: Swets and Zeitlinger BV).

Aufderheide, A. C. and Rodríguez-Martín, C. (1998), *The Cambridge Encyclopedia of Human Paleopathology* (Cambridge: Cambridge University Press), 31–4.

Baines, J. and Lacovara, P. (2002), 'Burial and the dead in ancient Egyptian society: respect, formalism, neglect', *Journal of Social Archaeology* 2, 5–36.

Bardinet, T. (1995), *Les papyrus médicaux de l'Égypte Pharaonique* (Lyons: Fayard).

Bhavnani, B. R. (1998), 'Pharmacokinetics and pharmacodynamics of conjugated equine estrogens: chemistry and metabolism', *Proceedings of the Society of Experimental Biology and Medicine* 217, 6–16.

Bietak, M. (2012), 'The archaeology of the "Gold of Valour"', *Egyptian Archaeology* 42, 32–3.

Blomstedt, P. (2014), 'Orthopedic surgery in ancient Egypt', *Acta Orthopaedica* 85 (6), 670–6.

Breasted, J. H. (1930), *The Edwin Smith Surgical Papyrus: Hieroglyphic Transliteration, Translation and Commentary*, VI (Chicago: University of Chicago Press).

British Pharmacopoeia (2012), 'Myrrh', *British Pharmacopoeia*, IV (London: Stationery Office), 3654–5.

Brothwell, D. R. and Møller-Christensen, V. (1963), 'A possible case of amputation, dated to *c.*2000 BC', *Man* 63, 192–4.

Campbell, J. M., Campbell, J. R. and David, A. R. (2010), 'Do the formulations of ancient Egyptian prescriptions stand up to pharmaceutical scrutiny?' in J. Cockitt and R. David (eds.), *Pharmacy and Medicine in Ancient Egypt: Proceedings of the Conferences Held in Cairo (2007) and Manchester (2008)* (Oxford: Archaeopress), 15–19.

Campbell, J. M. and David, A. R. (2005), 'Some aspects of the practice of pharmacy in ancient Egypt 1850 BC to 1300 BC', *Journal of Biological Research* 80, 331–4.

Chapman, P. H. (1992) 'Case 7 of the Smith Surgical Papyrus: the meaning of *tp3w*, *Journal of the American Research Center in Egypt* 29, 35–42.

Chapman, P. H. and Gupta, R. A. (2007), 'Reinvestigation of a Middle Kingdom head provides new insights concerning mummification and its relationship to contemporary anatomic knowledge and funerary ritual', *Journal of the American Research Center in Egypt* 43, 113–27.

David, R. (2008), 'The ancient Egyptian medical system', in R. David (ed.), *Egyptian Mummies and Modern Science* (Cambridge and New York: Cambridge University Press), 181–94.

Dawson, W. R. (1967), 'The Egyptian medical papyri', in D. Brothwell and A. T. Sandison (eds.), *Diseases in Antiquity: A Survey of the Diseases, Injuries and Surgery of Early Populations* (Springfield, IL: Charles C. Thomas), 98–111.

Dupoirieux, L. (1999), 'Ostrich eggshell as a bone substitute: a preliminary report of its biological behaviour in animals – a possibility in facial reconstructive surgery', *British Journal of Oral and Maxillofacial Surgery* 37, 467–71.

Dupoirieux, L., Pourquier, D. and Souyris, F. (1995), 'Powdered eggshell: a pilot study on a new bone substitute for use in maxillofacial surgery', *Journal of Cranio-Maxillo-Facial Surgery* 23, 187–94.

Dupras, T. L., Williams, L. J., De Meyer, M., Peeters, C., Depraetere, D., Vanthuyne, B. and Willems, H. (2010), 'Evidence of amputation as medical treatment in ancient Egypt', *International Journal of Osteoarchaeology* 20, 405–23.

Erman, A. and Grapow, H. (1931), *Wörterbuch der ägyptischen Sprache*, III (Berlin and Leipzig: J. C. Hinrichs).

Estes, J. Worth. (1989), *The Medical Skills of Ancient Egypt* (Canton, MA: Science History Publications).

Germer, R. (1998), 'The plant remains found by Petrie at Lahun and some remarks on the problems of identifying Egyptian plant names', in S. Quirke (ed.), *Lahun Studies* (New Malden, Surrey: SIA Publishing), 84–91.

Ghalioungui, P. (1980), 'Medicine in ancient Egypt', in J. E. Harris and E. F. Wente (eds.), *An X-ray Atlas of the Royal Mummies* (Chicago and London: University of Chicago Press), 52–98.

Ghalioungui, P. (1987), *The Ebers Papyrus: A New English Translation, Commentaries and Glossaries* (Cairo: Academy of Scientific Research and Technology).

Guers, N. C. (2007), 'Osteoporosis and periodontal disease', *Periodontology 2000* 44, 29–43.

Gupta, R., Markowitz, Y., Berman, L. and Chapman, P. (2009), 'High-resolution imaging of an ancient Egyptian mummified head: new insights into the mummification process', *American Journal of Neuroradiology* 29, 705–13.

Harkess, J. W., Ramsey, W. C. and Harkess, J. W. (1996), 'Principles of fractures and dislocations', in D. P. Green, C. A. Rockwood, R. W. Bucholz and J. D. Heckman (eds.), *Rockwood and Green's Fractures in Adults* (Philadelphia and New York: Lippincott Raven), 1–120.

Harris, J. R. (1971), 'Medicine', in J. R. Harris (ed.), *The Legacy of Egypt* (Oxford: Clarendon Press), 112–37.

Harris, M., Lowe, T. and Ahmed, F. (2014), 'An interesting example of a condylar fracture from ancient Nubia suggesting the possibility of early surgical intervention', in R. Metcalfe, J. Cockitt and R. David (eds.), *Palaeopathology in Egypt and Nubia: A Century in Review* (Oxford: Archaeopress), 41–50.

Hussein, F., El Banna, R., Kandeel, W. and Sarry El Din, A. (2010), 'Similarity of fracture treatment of workers and high officials of the pyramid builders', in J. Cockitt and R. David (eds.), *Pharmacy and Medicine in Ancient Egypt: Proceedings of the Conferences Held in Cairo (2007) and Manchester (2008)* (Oxford: Archaeopress), 85–9.

Jackson, R. (1988), *Doctors and Diseases in the Roman Empire* (London: British Museum Press).

Jonckheere, F. (1947), *Le papyrus médical Chester Beatty* (Brussels: Fondation Égyptologique Reine Élisabeth).

Jonckheere, F. (1958), *Les médecins de l'Égypte pharaonique: essai de prosopographie* (Brussels: Fondation Égyptologique Reine Élisabeth).

Jones, F. Wood (1908), 'Some lessons from ancient fractures', *British Medical Journal* 2 (2486), 455–8.

Jouanne, J. (2012), *Greek Medicine from Hippocrates to Galen: Selected Papers* (Leiden: Brill).

Kozieradzka-Ogunmakin, I. (2013), 'Patterns and management of fractures of long bones: a study of the ancient population of Saqqara, Egypt', in R. David (ed.), *Ancient Medical and Healing Systems: Their Legacy to Western Medicine*, supplement to *Bulletin of the John Rylands University Library of Manchester* 89 (Manchester: Manchester University Press), 133–56.

Leake, C. (1952), *The Old Egyptian Medical Papyri* (Lawrence: University of Kansas Press).

Lichtheim, M. (1976), *Ancient Egyptian Literature*, II: *The New Kingdom* (Berkeley, CA: University of California Press).

Lisowski, F. P. (1967), 'Prehistoric and early historic trepanation', in D. Brothwell and E. T. Sandison (eds.), *Diseases in Antiquity: A Survey of the Diseases, Injuries, and Surgery of Early Populations* (Springfield, IL: Charles C. Thomas), 651–72.

Majno, G. (1975), *The Healing Hand. Man and Wound in the Ancient World* (Cambridge, MA: Harvard University Press).

Manniche, L. (1989), *An Ancient Egyptian Herbal* (London: British Museum Press).

Marganne, M.-H. (1993), 'Links between Egyptian and Greek medicine', *Forum* 3 (5), 35–43.

Martin, D. C. (2013), 'Like you need a hole in the head: tool innovation a possible cause of trepanation. A case from Kerma, Nubia', *International Journal of Osteoarchaeology* 23, 545–56.

Miller, R. L. (1989), '*Dqr*, spinning and treatment of guinea worm in P. Ebers 875', *Journal of Egyptian Archaeology* 75, 249–54.

Nerlich, A. G., Panzer, S. and Lösch, S. (2010), 'Surgery in ancient Egypt – palaeopathological evidence for successful medical treatment by surgery', in J. Cockitt and R. David (eds.), *Pharmacy and Medicine in Ancient Egypt: Proceedings of the Conferences Held in Cairo (2007) and Manchester (2008)* (Oxford: Archaeopress), 117–21.

Nerlich, A. G., Zink, A., Szeimies, U., Hagedorn, H. G. and Rösing, F. W. (2003), 'Perforating skull trauma in ancient Egypt and evidence for early neurosurgical therapy', in R. Arnott, S. Finger and C. U. M. Smith (eds.), *Trepanation, History, Discovery, Theory* (Lisse: Swets and Zeitlinger BV), 191–201.

Nunn, J. F. (1996), *Ancient Egyptian Medicine* (London: British Museum Press).

Quirke, S. (2002), Digital Egypt for Universities, *Kahun Medical Papyrus*, www.digital-egypt.ucl.ac.uk/med/birthpapyrus.html (last accessed 20 February 2014).

Rackham, H. (trans.) (1952), Pliny the Elder, *Natural History IX* (London: William Heinemann).

Ritner, R. K. (2001), 'Magic in medicine', in D. B. Redford (ed.), *The Oxford Encyclopedia of Ancient Egypt*, II (Oxford: Oxford University Press), 326–9.

Roberts, A. and Donaldson, J. (trans.) (n.d.) Clement of Alexandria, 'Stromata part VI', in P. Kirby, *Early Christian Writings*, www.earlychristianwritings.com/text/clement-stromata-book6.html (last accessed 11 February 2014).

Roberts, C. and Manchester, K. (2005), *The Archaeology of Disease* (Stroud: Sutton Publishing).

Rowling, J. T. (1989), 'The rise and decline of surgery in dynastic Egypt', *Antiquity* 63, 312–19.

Sanchez, G. M. and Meltzer, E. S. (2012), *The Edwin Smith Papyrus: Updated Translation of the Trauma. Treatise and Modern Medical Commentaries* (Atlanta, GA: Lockwood Press).

Serpico, M. (2000), 'Resins, amber and bitumen', in P. T. Nicholson and I. Shaw (eds.), *Ancient Egyptian Materials and Technology* (Cambridge: Cambridge University Press), 430–74.

Simpson, W. K. (2003), 'The instruction of Amenemope', in W. K. Simpson (ed.), *The Literature of Ancient Egypt* (New Haven and London: Yale University Press), 223–44.

Smith, G. E. (1908), 'The most ancient splints', *British Medical Journal* 1 (2465), 732–4.

Spencer, W. G. (trans,) (1938), Celsus, *De Medicina* (Cambridge, MA: Harvard University Press).

Strouhal, E., Břetislav, V. and Vymazalová, H. (2014), *The Medicine of the Ancient Egyptians* (Cairo and New York: The American University in Cairo Press).

Strouhal, E., Němečková, A. and Kouba, M. (2003), 'Palaeopathology of Iufaa and other persons found beside his shaft tomb at Abusir (Egypt)', *International Journal of Osteoarchaeology* 13, 331–8.

Sullivan, R. (1998), 'Proto-surgery in ancient Egypt', *Acta Medica* (Hradec Králové) 41, 109–20.

von Deines, H., Grapow, H. and Westendorf, W. (1954–73) *Grundriss der Medizin der alten Ägypter*, 11 vols. (Berlin: Akademie-Verlag).

von Staden, H. (1989), *Herophilus: The Art of Medicine in Early Alexandria* (Cambridge: Cambridge University Press).

Westendorf, W. (1992), *Erwachen der Heilkunst: Die Medizin im alten Ägypten* (Zurich: Artemis and Winkler).

Wilson, J. A. (1952), 'A note on the Edwin Smith Surgical Papyrus', *Journal of Near Eastern Studies* 11, 76–80.

Zaki, M. E., Sarry El-Din, A. M., Al-Tohamy Soliman, M., Mahmoud, N. H. and Abu Baker Basha, W. (2010), 'Limb amputation in ancient Egypt from Old Kingdom', *Journal of Applied Sciences Research* 6, 913–17.

12

One and the same? An investigation into the connection between veterinary and medical practice in ancient Egypt

Conni Lord

During the last one hundred years, there has been an increase in scholarly interest in ancient Egyptian health, disease and management of medical conditions (Filer 1995: 40–4; David 2008: 237). Fortunately, the environmental conditions of Egypt have assisted the investigation of these topics through the preservation of papyri, artistic representations and the remains of the ancient Egyptian themselves. An area of research that, until recently, has lagged behind the study of human health and disease is that of the ancient Egyptian animal population. This is a significant omission in view of the importance that the ancient Egyptians placed on animals in both the economic and religious spheres (Houlihan 1996: 10). Once domestication of animals took place,[1] man became responsible for their care, in health and in sickness (Wilkinson 2005: 2). It seems reasonable to assume that the origins of medicine and veterinary care are intertwined; however, this raises a question concerning the evidence from ancient Egypt and its ability to validate this idea. This chapter will look at human and animal diseases in ancient Egypt, what evidence scholars can utilise to confirm these, as well as evidence of human intervention in animal care. Special attention will be given to the unique Veterinary Papyrus of Kahun, in order to ascertain whether it is possible to determine whether human and animal care in ancient Egypt were one and the same.

[1]   The earliest undisputed evidence for domestication in ancient Egypt comes from Merimde at approximately 5000 BC. However, it is possible that some form of domestication was established as early as 8000 BC (MacDonald 2000: 5–9).

Disease in ancient Egypt

As an agricultural society, humans and animals in ancient Egypt would have regularly shared the same space, often to the detriment of each other. While disease would have been present in the prehistoric population, its incidence increased when people began to remain in one location. Before the change to a more sedentary lifestyle of farming communities, Egyptian hunter-gatherers moved from place to place, leaving their waste behind. Once fixed communities were established, this waste built up and, despite the ancient Egyptians' desire for cleanliness (Herodotus, *Histories*, II, 37; Waterfield 1998: 109–10), the lack of an effective method of human waste disposal perpetuated the constant threat of disease being transmitted by insects and parasites (Peck 2013: 110). While Juliet Clutton-Brock (2006: 74) argues that, despite images showing the closeness and even affection between man and beast, there is little reason to believe that the ancient Egyptians 'lived in any closer communion with their animals than pastoral peoples of the rest of the world over the past millennium', it cannot be in doubt that the contact between man and animal increased significantly after domestication and that with this, a sometimes fatal pattern of disease transmission between them was established (Porter 2003: 4; see Figure 12.1).

Threats to health and wellbeing were present through all stages of life in ancient Egypt. Dangers such as snake and scorpion bites, infectious and parasitic diseases such as tuberculosis and schistosomiasis, and ophthalmic complaints through environmental conditions, as well as trauma such as fractures

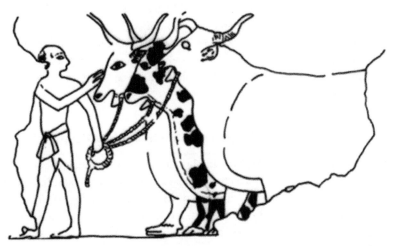

12.1 A herdsman shows his affection for his charges, Tomb of Kenamun, New Kingdom. (Created by Mary Hartley after Scanlan 2004: 95.)

and dislocations, were constant problems for the ancient Egyptians (Halioua and Ziskind 2005: 82–7; Allen 2005: 9; Forshaw 2013: 201). Tooth wear caused by the gritty nature of the diet caused problems at a relatively early age, and if one was fortunate enough to live into middle and old age, arthritis and cardio-vascular disease could well develop (Halioua and Ziskind 2005: 96–103). Egypt's hot dry climate and the funerary customs practised during the Pharaonic Period have allowed scholars to investigate not only medical complaints but also how such debilitating conditions were managed (David 2013: 162).

Like humans, domesticated animals had their own disease vulnerabilities (Dunlop and Williams 1996: 73). The fertile strip of land running along the banks of the Nile river and its delta would have been capable of supporting a heavy concentration of stock. However, such crowded conditions would have rendered them susceptible to imported respiratory and enteric plagues such as those introduced by the Egyptian military fighting outside Egypt or by invading forces such as the Hyksos during the Second Intermediate Period. Epidemics of environmental origin, such as rinderpest and anthrax, must have also been common and recurrent (Dunlop and Williams 1996: 73). The fifth plague of the ten plagues of Egypt in the Bible is said to have devastated herds of livestock belonging to the Egyptians (Exodus 9: 1–7). Some scholars have attempted to identify this plague from the symptoms described, with four possibilities suggested – rinderpest, foot and mouth disease, Rift Valley fever and anthrax (Halioua and Ziskind 2005: 201; Ehrenkranz and Sampson 2008: 32). Of the four, the most feasible is anthrax, which would fit the types of animals affected, the enzootic nature and the ominous prognosis given (Halioua and Ziskind 2005: 201).

Animals, like their human carers, would have displayed a high incidence of parasitic disease while the harsh glare of the Egyptian sun and frequent dust storms must have led to a high occurrence of both human and animal eye disease (Dunlop and Williams: 1996: 73). The environmental conditions of ancient Egypt would have facilitated animal and human disease patterns, the evidence for which is discussed below.

Evidence for human healing in ancient Egypt

The information available for studying human disease and healing comes from a range of sources, none of which are persuasive enough to stand alone. For example, the artistic representations from the tombs of the higher echelons of society are incomplete and open to different interpretations. However, while aiming to represent the deceased as young and healthy, a state in which they wished to spend eternity, the scenes occasionally depict servants of the tomb owner with signs of ageing or physical incapacity as well as medical disorders

(David 2013: 168). Examples of these include a possible case of Potts disease found in the 19th Dynasty tomb of Ipwy (Theban tomb 217) and images of blind musicians such as that in the 18th Dynasty tomb of Nakht (Theban tomb 52) (Filer 1995: 32–3; Halioua and Ziskind 2005: 111).

From the Old Kingdom onwards, there are a series of medical titles based on the ancient Egyptian word *swnw*, commonly translated as 'physician'. Approximately 150 such titles have been discovered which relate to the entire the Pharaonic Period (Nunn 1996: 115–18); however, the actual roles and responsibilities of their owners remain unclear. If we consider the evidence from the false door of Irenakhty (First Intermediate Period) that was set up in his tomb, discovered in Giza (tomb G4760), we see that he possessed a number of leadership roles as well as various specialist medical titles. These include palace *swnw*, inspector of palace *swnw* and *swnw* of the eyes, belly and gastro-intestinal tract, as well as non-*swnw* titles such as the delightfully named shepherd of the anus[2] and keeper of the secrets (Ghalioungui 1983: 17).

One of the most significant sources of evidence comes from the twelve major medical papyri, dating from the Middle Kingdom to the Ptolemaic Period.[3] Like the artistic representations and medical titles, the medical papyri should be viewed with caution; while they provide important information concerning the Egyptian understanding of disease, the workings of the human body and healing, they are open to interpretation (Shaw 2012: 40). It has been all too easy to ascribe modern insight to the ancient texts, assigning the ancient Egyptian healers a scientific and technological understanding that was simply not available in their time. An example of this is Ebbell's (1937: 35) over-enthusiastic translation of the Ebers Papyrus, particularly his translation of the *aaa* disease, which is mentioned close to fifty times in the treatments as haematuria, in which he went well beyond what could be judged as probable. However, Ebbell's explanations have been regularly referred to by many non-Egyptologists such as Aboelsoud (2010: 83) and Salem *et al.* (2010: 207).

---

2   'Shepherd of the anus' has been interpreted either as the world's first recorded proctologist or as one who was responsible for the king's enemas.

3   The best-known medical papyri that have been discovered so far are: Kahun Gynaecological (currently housed in the Petrie Museum of Egyptian Archaeology, University College London), Ramesseum (III, IV, V) (Ashmlolean Museum, Oxford), Edwin Smith (New York Academy of Medicine), Ebers (Leipzig University Library), Hearst (University of California), London (British Museum), Carlsberg VIII (University of Copenhagen), Berlin (Ägyptisches Museum und Papyrussammlung), Chester Beatty VI (British Museum), Brooklyn snake (Brooklyn Museum), London and Leiden (British Museum and Rijksmuseum van Oudheden), Crocodilopolis (Kunsthistorisches Museum, Vienna).

Ancient Egyptian remains provide the most important evidence for disease in this culture (Filer 1995: 27; Dunand and Lichtenberg 2006: 2; David 2013: 168–9). While definite disease identification can be contentious, mainly owing to post-mortem conditions that can mimic disease signs, the scientific study of mummies and skeletal material has uncovered congenital diseases, acquired disorders, dental disease and trauma (Filer 1995: 53–102; Forshaw 2013: 195–8).

While human remains have revealed a large amount of information concerning the diseases of the past, they are limited in what they can disclose about the medical treatments used by the ancient Egyptians. Studies of skeletal material have demonstrated the management of long bone fractures by traction, bandaging and splinting, information which is also recorded in the Edwin Smith Papyrus (Kozieradzka-Ogunmakin 2013: 154–5). However, despite a section in the Ebers Papyrus dedicated to the treatment of tooth and gum disorders and the record of a title corresponding to 'dentist',[4] extensive analysis of Egyptian skulls has provided little to no evidence of dental intervention. Even simple procedures such as extractions of mobile teeth or the draining of abscesses, which would have been relatively easy to perform and would have provided considerable pain relief, are not attested in the palaeopathological record (Forshaw 2013: 188). Also it is currently not possible to fully understand the ancient Egyptian usage of remedies, such as those recorded in the Ebers Papyrus. As scientific analytical techniques continue to advance, identification of more of the constituents used in these remedies may become possible, providing another layer of understanding of health, disease and healing in ancient Egypt.

Evidence for animal healing in ancient Egypt

While the above evidence for human healing in ancient Egypt is limited and often difficult to interpret, it is far more comprehensive than that available for the Egyptians' animal counterparts. A rich relationship between man and beast in ancient Egypt is clear to see in the numerous artistic representations of domestic and wild animals throughout the Pharaonic Period. The depiction of animals and people in tomb reliefs covers a variety of animal husbandry pursuits including the branding of cattle, assistance with the birthing of calves and the feeding

---

4   Until recently, the title *ibḥ* (dentist) had been attested five times in the Old Kingdom and once in the Late Period (Nunn 1996: 119). In 2006, it was announced by the Supreme Council of Antiquities that excavations near the Step Pyramid at Saqqara had uncovered inscriptions of a further three dentists, all from the same Old Kingdom tomb (Mathieson and Dittmer 2007: 90).

and watering of a number of animal species (Houlihan 1996: 10; Scanlan 2004: 85). Examples of such activities include fattened cattle being force-fed, probably for sacrifice, from the tomb of Khnumhotep at Beni Hasan (BH3) and a milking scene from the tomb of Kagemni at Saqqara (LS10) (Houlihan 1996: 12; Scanlan 2004: 94). These tomb scenes go some way to helping with the reconstruction of ancient Egyptian agricultural and pastoral practices, as well as demonstrating what appears to be a genuine affection that the agricultural workers had for their animal charges. Unfortunately, there are no such scenes of ailing animals or veterinary practice. While it is obvious from archaeological remains and tomb reliefs that animals were essential for ancient Egyptian agriculture, it is likely that the experienced herdsmen attended to most animal needs. As these herdsmen would have mostly been illiterate, any skills and knowledge they possessed would not have been written down but may well have been passed on orally or learned anew by trial and error. In many scenes involving herdsmen and their stock, the men can be seen making magical gestures of protection towards the animals. Captions to these scenes include simple charms aimed at protecting both the animals and the people on the land. Such incantations were also carried out by priests or magicians as well as the herdsmen, and like the practical knowledge of the herdsmen regarding animal husbandry, the basic magic involved in the protection spells would have been passed down orally from generation to generation (Ritner 1993: 227–33; Pinch 1994: 59).

Very early in the history of ancient Egypt, the priests of Sekhmet were associated with the medical profession. Sekhmet, the lion-headed goddess, could inflict death and disease, and her priests were charged with the responsibility of intervening in the favour of those whom she punished. In addition, as mentioned previously, the *swnw* were involved in the treatment of human medical problems (Nunn 1996: 120; Halioua and Ziskind 2005: 7–8; Shaw 2012: 47–9). If we turn to the healing of animals, the titles and responsibilities of the personnel involved become less clear. No title relating to 'veterinary surgeon' has been identified, and although Gordon (2007: 131) believes the absence of the word implies that the *swnw* were responsible for both human and animal healing, there is little evidence to support this claim. From the Old Kingdom, three Sekhmet priests are pictured supervising the sacrificial butchery of offering cattle. One such scene is that of Wenen-nefer, who was both a *wab* priest of Sekhmet and an inspector of *swnw* (Ghalioungui 1963: 113). Also involved in cattle sacrifice are holders of the title *sš swnw* (the scribe of the physicians). An example occurs in the Middle Kingdom tomb of Khnumhotep at Beni Hasan, in which a *sš swnw* called Nakht is pictured with a reed and papyrus sheet talking to herdsmen. An interpretation offered by Chassinat (1905: 3–8) is that Nakht was an inspector that travelled to farms in order to catalogue cattle suitable for sacrifice (Ghalioungui 1983: 3).

A graffito from the calcite quarries at Hatnub, dated to the 12th Dynasty, contains the biographical detail of two men. The main figure is Heryshef-nakht, who claims to be chief of the king's *swnw* and a *wab* priest of Sekhmet, confirming the sometime dual roles of the priests of Sekhmet and the *swnw*[5] (Ghalioungui 1983: 9). Next to his graffito, and of a much inferior size, is the information regarding one of Heryshef-nakht's colleagues, Aha-nakht, another priest of Sekhmet, who describes his duties in similar terms to his colleague. Both are skilled in examining a sick man using their hands,[6] however, Aha-nakht is also a *rḫ k3w* 'one who knows oxen' (Nunn 1996: 129); this phrase has been interpreted as 'veterinary surgeon' (Sauneroun 1960: 161; Ghalioungui 1963: 113; Nunn 1996: 129; Gordon 2007: 137). However, to refer back to the duties related to the titles *sš swnw* and *w'b swnw*, it is far more likely, in this writer's opinion, that this title is again connected to proclaiming cattle suitable for sacrifice, not the healing of ailing animals.

From a much later date, there is one inscription that could support the idea of the *wab* priests of Sekhmet being involved in some form of veterinary practice or at least animal care. This comes from the early Ptolemaic tomb of Petosiris at Tuna el-Gebel, where there is a text in which Petosiris's daughter says: 'Your herds are numerous in the stable, thanks to the science [lit. 'secrets'] of the priest of Sekhmet' (Lefebvre 1924, II: 30; Ghalioungui 1983: 12). This single text unfortunately is too brief and unique to offer any conclusions.

Mummified and skeletal remains of ancient Egyptian animals have been discovered in considerable numbers (Ikram *et al.* 2014: 48–66). Many of these finds are in extremely poor condition, impeding pathological analysis. However, while not yet on the scale of human mummy studies, research has been conducted on animal remains that provides information on some of the medical conditions animals suffered in ancient Egypt. In addition these studies suggest that some form of animal healing by human intervention was provided from at least the Predynastic Period onwards (Hierakonpolis Online 2014).

Within an elite Predynastic cemetery, HK6, at Hierakonpolis a number of interesting animal remains have been discovered, including an elephant, wild cats, aurochs and a hippopotamus (Hierakonpolis Online 2014). In a semi-intact burial (Tomb 12), remains of seven baboons were excavated, some of which displayed fractures of the jaw as well as of the hand and foot bones, probably resulting from capture or conditions experienced during captivity. However, the healing patterns of these fractures suggest that the animals were in a protected

---

5 Five individuals from the Old Kingdom have been discovered holding the dual titles of *wab*-priest of Sekhmet and *swnw*.

6 The phrases used by Heryshef-nakht and Aha-nakht mirror the Ebers Papyrus 854a and the Edwin Smith Surgical Papyrus, Case 1.

environment which included some form of human care (Hierakonpolis Online 2014).

An early study, based at the British Museum, of fifty-three mummified cats found that all but one were healthy at the time of their death (Armitage and Clutton-Brock 1981: 195). The exception was a kitten that had abnormally thin limb bones and unusually small vertebrae, both signs of juvenile osteoporosis. The researchers believed this not to be a case of neglect and rather to be associated with a meat-only diet. This condition today is seen in only the most pampered of house cats (Armitage and Clutton-Brock 1981: 195).

In 1996, Goudsmit and Brandon-Jones investigated a number of baboons and Barbary macaques from the baboon catacombs at Saqqara, which demonstrated a number of healed skull and long bone injuries (Goudsmit and Brandon-Jones 1999). Also found were a significant number of animals displaying dental and skull development abnormalities, indicative of a vitamin D deficiency. The study found three possible cases of rickets in the baboon skeletons, which would strengthen the diagnosis of vitamin D deficiency in the other material (Goudsmit and Brandon-Jones 1999: 51). As primates obtain their vitamin D from the reaction of ultraviolet light on the skin and not through diet, it appears that the Saqqara baboons and monkeys were kept indoors out of the sunlight, at least during the period of their physical development (Goudsmit and Brandon-Jones 1999: 53).

More recently, a study using high-magnification macrophotographs has been conducted in order to examine mummified dogs from the site of el-Deir and dated to the Roman Period (Huchet *et al.* 2013: 165). The examination of one young mummified dog revealed what is believed to be the first report of canine ectoparasitosis in ancient Egypt (Huchet *et al.* 2013: 173).

As much as the study of human mummies and skeletal material has provided valuable insights into human medical problems and their treatment, the potential is present for the study of the animal mummies of ancient Egypt to do the same. The limited but informative research that has been undertaken so far has demonstrated that such investigations can provide evidence for the types of conditions suffered by animals of the past, as well as human intervention into the healing process.

The Veterinary Papyrus

The Veterinary Papyrus of Kahun (UC 32036, lot LV.2; Plate 4) bears the first, and only, recorded rational approach to animal healing in ancient Egypt. Egyptologists have largely ignored it, presumably because of the severe fragmentation of the original document. All that remains is a main section outlining three treatments probably relating to the treatment of bovines, and some smaller fragments for which their positioning in the overall papyrus is unknown. The text follows the standard formula of medical treatises: title, symptoms, treatment, prognosis, re-examination and further symptoms and finally further treatment. The clinical signs described are somewhat general, making disease identification speculative at best; however, some of the symptoms and the treatment thereof are both understandable and rational to a modern reader. The content and layout attest to the papyrus's practical use, rather than simply being an object of historical curiosity. The text of the first and third case studies is extremely damaged, and in the few interpretations of the papyrus, scholars are in disagreement as to the type of diseases that are being recorded.

The first few lines of the first preserved case study, entitled '[Eye examination of a bull with] nest of a worm', are so badly damaged as to make meaningful translation impossible, although it is assumed by the context that the sufferer is a bovine. An interpretation by Professor Peter Windsor (University of Sydney, Australia, personal communication, 2010) suggests that 'nest of a worm' could be a literal translation for an external parasite such as Old World screw-worm fly.

The third case study is also badly damaged, possibly documenting a case of bovine photosensitisation causing lethargy and severe eye problems (Windsor, personal communication). Unfortunately, because of the damage to the text, it is impossible to interpret the clinical signs or the treatment.

Case study 2, entitled 'Eye examination of a bull with an airborne disease', is the longest and the best preserved and therefore the soundest of the three case studies to examine in terms of clinical signs and treatment:

> If I see a bull with an airborne disease, its eyes running, its tears heavy, the roots of its teeth reddened, and its neck taut, it should be read as follows:
>
> It should be lain on its side, and sprinkled with fresh/cool water
> And its eyes should be rubbed, along with its flanks and all its limbs
>
> With *khenesh*-plants or *shu*-plants, and fumigated by (?)
> It is saved from damp … to be kept away from water
> It is rubbed with *khenesh* parts of *qadet*-plants
> Then you should cut it at its nostrils and its tail and say of it:
> It is under treatment – it will die from it or it will live from it
> If it does not recover, and is heavy under your fingers and its eyes are blocked
> You should wrap its eyes with fine linen, heated at a fire, for the bleariness.
> (UC 32036; Collier and Quirke 2004: 55)

There is no doubt that the patient is bovine as the hieroglyph for k_3 or 'bull' can be seen in the title (Collier and Quirke 2004: 54). Despite the limited and non-specific clinical signs, there is general agreement on the diagnosis of this case study. Most scholars believe the condition to be the viral infection malignant catarrh fever (MCF), which is characterised by high fever, profuse discharge from the eyes and nose, bilateral corneal opacity, necrosis of the muzzle and erosion of the buccal epithelium (Walker 1964: 200; Dunlop and Williams 1996: 68; Windsor, personal communication).

From the initial description – eyes running, discharge thick, reddened gums and swollen neck – it appears that the bull is suffering from a fever, and therefore the aim of its ancient Egyptian carer is to cool the animal down, as it would be for a veterinary surgeon of today. In order to do so, the bull is forcefully placed on its side and cooled with water. It is then rubbed all over with *khenesh* and *shu* plants; later in the case study, another plant (*qadet*) is also employed in the treatment. None of the plants have been identified; however, from their context, it appears likely that they are being utilised for believed cooling properties, in much the same way as aloe vera is utilised today. The next stage of the treatment involves bloodletting, a common ancient treatment for fever.

Once this initial treatment is complete, the prognosis is stated: 'it [the bull] will live from it or it will die from it'. Finally, the bull is examined for further signs, for which additional treatment is suggested. The bull now appears to be suffering from lethargy and its eyes are blocked. Its ancient Egyptian carer attempts to lessen the ocular concerns by covering its eyes with fine warm linen; heating the linen would enable the cloth to be as sterile as the ancient environment would allow, although the concept of sterility would not have been understood by the Egyptian healers. The warmth of the linen would also encourage blood supply to the eye, which may have aided healing depending on the condition (Windsor, personal communication). At this point the second study ends.

Comparison of texts

Unfortunately, a comparison of the few treatments in the Veterinary Papyrus with those in the medical corpus does little to answer the question of whether animal and human healing was connected during the Pharaonic Period. The Edwin Smith Papyrus is probably the medical document most comparable to the Veterinary Papyrus in that both have a logical approach rather than being a collection of remedies and both seem to concentrate on case studies. According to Nunn (1996: 29), a medical doctor himself, the Edwin Smith Papyrus 'has an instant appeal to the doctor of today' as its approach relates to current surgical practice. This appeal was also obvious when the Veterinary Papyrus was shown to a veterinary surgeon of today. Professor Peter Windsor (personal communication) had no trouble in recognising certain modern veterinary techniques, in spite of the language difficulties.

While the Veterinary Papyrus has some treatment and disease commonalities with the other medical documents (mainly the Ebers and Hearst Papyri: see below), there is little else that can be used as evidence to connect the two

types of texts. While the Veterinary Papyrus was found in Kahun with the
Kahun Gynaecological Papyrus, there are no similarities in format or subject
matter between these two papyri. The Veterinary Papyrus is written in hieroglyphic script,[7] as is one of the other known medical papyri, the Ramesseum
V. However, as with the Kahun Gynaecological Papyrus, there are no other
similarities of content or form.

Case study 2 is the most straightforward text to compare with that of the
medical papyri as its language is most understandable to the modern reader.
The bovine patient is evidently suffering a fever and the healer must cool the
animal down. A number of plants are rubbed over the bull's limbs, but none of
them can be identified with any certainty. The *qadet* plant is seen in the Ebers
and Hearst Papyri (Ebers 278 and 294, Hearst 35 and 64); however, in these
cases it is being used for very different purposes including the elimination of
excessive urine and letting out of mucus (Ghalioungui 1987: 91, 93). The *shu*
plant is not seen in this form in any of the medical papyri, but a similar word is
found in Ebers 484 as part of a treatment for a burn, and it is tempting to think
that in both cases this plant was utilised for its cooling properties (Ghalioungui
1987: 134). The *kenesh* plant is not recorded in any of the medical papyri.

The bull is then fumigated, a common treatment for a number of conditions
in the medical papyri, none of which match the clinical signs exhibited by the
bull patient in case study 2. Many of them are concerned with gynaecological
complaints, for example Ebers 793, where it is used to return the uterus to its
place. Ebers 852 and 853 recommend fumigation treatments to sweeten the
smell of the house and clothes (Ghalioungui 1987: 202, 216). Fumigation is also
prescribed on several occasions to treat snake bites in the Brooklyn Papyrus
(Nunn 1996: 189). Unfortunately, the last part of the treatment in the Veterinary
Papyrus is damaged and it is not possible to ascertain with what material the
bull was fumigated (Collier and Quirke 2004: 55).

The animal is then bled from the nose and the tail. Bloodletting was used
as a way to reduce fever in many ancient cultures but is not mentioned in any
of the Egyptian medical papyri. The Greek physician Hippocrates noted the
use of therapeutic bloodletting for human patients in the fifth century BC, and
its use on animal patients has been recorded as early as 1000 BC in China; it
became the cornerstone of Roman veterinary treatment (Hosgood 1991: 238;
Dunlop and Williams 1996: 93, 166). It was believed to reduce fever by the
removal of toxins (Hosgood 1991: 234), and was still used for that purpose in
the 1940s. While the context fits here, the writer of this chapter does not believe
this is a case of veterinary bloodletting as the tail and the nose do not allow

---

7   All the medical papyri, with the exception of the Ramesseum V, are in the hieratic
    script.

the blood flow required; it is more likely to be ritualistic in nature rather than medical.

Finally in case study 2, fine linen, which is heated by fire, is used to treat the bull's bleary eyes (Collier and Quirke 2004: 55). The condition of 'bleary' or 'veiled' eyes is seen in four Ebers prescriptions (339, 340, 385 and 415), and in one (339) the eyes are bandaged (Ghalioungui 1987: 103). It is difficult to tell in the Ebers case if the bandaging is a treatment in itself or is used to hold the accompanying poultice in place. All eye treatments in this long but disorganised section of the Ebers Papyrus involve medication applied externally to the eye (Nunn 1996: 199). In contrast, the linen in the Veterinary Papyrus appears to be the treatment.

There are very few parallels between the treatments and remedies of the medical texts and the Veterinary Papyrus. As they stand today, it is very difficult to use the written documents to see any connection between animal and human healing.

Conclusion

It is tempting to think that animal and human healing in ancient Egypt were allied together. From the time of domestication, man had responsibility for the health and welfare of his animals as well as that of his human kin. However, the evidence for the formation of comparative medicine in ancient Egypt is currently lacking conviction. What evidence we do have, especially for the area of animal healing, is limited and open to insupportable interpretations. The titles utilised in human healing, specifically *swnw* and/or the priests of Sekhmet, certainly seem also to be involved in animal matters; however, it would appear that this is more focused on the suitability of cattle for sacrifice. A comparison of the medical papyri with the solitary veterinary text demonstrates some commonalities in language, but in general there appear to be few similarities in form or content; one exception is the Edwin Smith Papyrus, which follows the same logical progression of treatments. Data in the form of human and animal mummies and skeletal material cannot be effectively compared because of the limited number of studies focusing on the diseases of ancient Egyptian animals and the healing methods employed by their human carers. This may change in time and with the advancement of scientific analytical techniques. However, until more evidence is available, only educated guesses can be made. In the opinion of this author, human and animal medicine did develop at the same time soon after animal domestication was established. However, as Egyptian bureaucracy and technology advanced, the two areas branched apart and the few similarities witnessed in the papyri are possibly a relic of this once-close association. Additional evidence and research are needed to either advance this argument further or disprove it.

References

Aboelsoud, N. H. (2010), 'Herbal medicine in ancient Egypt', *Journal of Medicinal Plants Research* 4 (2), 82–6.

Allen, J. P. (2005), *The Art of Medicine in Ancient Egypt* (New York and New Haven: Metropolitan Museum of Art and Yale University Press).

Armitage, P. L. and Clutton-Brock, J. (1981), 'A radiological and histological investigation into the mummification of cats from ancient Egypt', *Journal of Archaeological Science* 8, 185–96.

Chassinat, E. (1905), 'Note sur le titre [...]', *Bulletin de l'Institut français d'archéologie orientale* 4, 223–28.

Clutton-Brock, J. (2007), 'How domestic animals have shaped the development of the human species', in L. Kalof (ed.), *A Cultural History of Animals in Antiquity* (Oxford and New York: Berg), 71–96.

Collier, M. and Quirke, S. (2004), *The UCL Lahun Papyri: Religious, Literary, Legal, Mathematical and Medical* (Oxford: Archaeopress).

David, R. (2008), 'The International Ancient Egyptian Mummy Tissue Bank', in R. David (ed.), *Egyptian Mummies and Modern Science* (Cambridge and New York: Cambridge University Press), 237–46.

David, R. (2013), 'Ancient Egyptian medicine: the contribution of twenty-first century science', in R. David (ed.), *Ancient Medical and Healing Systems: Their Legacy to Western Medicine*, supplement to *Bulletin of the John Rylands University Library of Manchester* 89 (Manchester: Manchester University Press), 157–80.

Dunand, F. and Lictenberg, R. (2006), *Mummies and Death in Egypt* (Ithaca and London: Cornell University Press).

Dunlop, R. H. and Williams, D. J. (1996), *Veterinary Medicine: An illustrated History* (St Louis, Baltimore and Boston: Mosby).

Ebbell, B. (1937), *The Papyrus Ebers: The Greatest Egyptian Medical Document* (London: Oxford University Press).

Ehrenkranz, N. J. and Sampson, D. A. (2008), 'Origin of the Old Testament plagues: explications and implications', *Yale Journal of Biology and Medicine* 81, 31–42.

Filer, J. (1995), *Disease* (London: British Museum Press).

Forshaw, R. (2013), 'Hesyre: the first recorded physician and dental surgeon in history', in R. David (ed.), *Ancient Medical and Healing Systems: Their Legacy to Western Medicine*, supplement to *Bulletin of the John Rylands University Library of Manchester* 89 (Manchester: Manchester University Press), 181–202.

Ghalioungui, P. (1963), *Magic and Medical Science in Ancient Egypt* (London: Hodder and Stoughton).

Ghalioungui, P. (1983), *The Physicians of Ancient Egypt* (Cairo: Al-Ahram Center for Scientific Translation).

Ghalioungui, P. (1987), *The Ebers Papyrus* (Cairo: Academy of Scientific Research and Technology).

Gordon, A. H. (2007), 'The observation and use of animals in the development of scientific thought in the ancient world with especial reference to Egypt', in L. Kalof (ed.), *A Cultural History of Animals in Antiquity* (Oxford and New York: Berg) 127–50.

Goudsmit, J. and Brandon-Jones, D. (1999), 'Mummies of olive baboons and Barbary macaques in the Baboon Catacomb of the Sacred Animal Necropolis at North Saqqara', *Journal of Egyptian Archaeology* 85, 45–53.

Griffith, F. Ll. (1898), *Hieratic Papyri from Kahun and Gurob* (London: Bernard Quaritch).

Halioua, B. and Ziskind, B. (2005), *Medicine in the Days of the Pharaohs* (Cambridge, MA, and London: Belknap Press).

Hierakonpolis Online (2014), 'HK6 – elite cemetery', www.hierakonpolis-online.org/index.php/explore-the-predynastic-cemeteries/hk6-elite-cemetery (last accessed 23 October 2014).

Hosgood, G. (1991), 'Bloodletting: the old and the new', *Journal of the American Veterinary Medical Association* 198 (2), 238–4.

Houlihan, P. F. (1996), *The Animal World of the Pharaohs* (London: Thames and Hudson).

Huchet, J. B., Callou, C., Lichtenberg, R. and Dunand, F. (2013), 'The dog mummy, the ticks and the louse fly: archaeological report of severe ectoparasitosis in ancient Egypt', *International Journal of Paleopathology* 3, 165–75.

Ikram, S., Nicholson, P., Bertini, L. and Hurley, D. (2014), 'Killing man's best friend?', *Archaeological Review from Cambridge* 28 (2), 48–66.

Kozieradzka-Ogunmakin, I. (2013), 'Patterns and management of fractures of long bones: a study of the ancient population of Saqqara, Egypt', in R. David (ed.), *Ancient Medical and Healing Systems: Their Legacy to Western Medicine*, supplement to *Bulletin of the John Rylands University Library of Manchester* 89 (Manchester: Manchester University Press), 133–56.

Lefebvre, G. (1924), *Le tombeau de Petosiris*, 3 vols (Cairo: Institut Français d'Archéologie Orientale).

MacDonald, K. (2000), 'The origin of African livestock: indigenous or imported?', *Origins and Development of African Livestock: Archaeology, Genetics, Linguistics and Ethnography* (Abingdon and New York: Routledge), 2–17.

Mathieson, I. and Dittmer, J. (2007), 'The geophysical survey of North Saqqara 2001–7', *Journal of Egyptian Archaeology* 93, 79–93.

Morgan, L. W. and McGovern-Huffman, S. (2008), 'Non-invasive radiographic analysis of an Egyptian falcon mummy from the Late Period 664–332 BC', *Journal of Avian Biology* 39, 584–7.

Nunn, J. F. (1996), *Ancient Egyptian Medicine* (London: British Museum Press).

Peck, W. (2013), *The Material World of Ancient Egypt* (Cambridge: Cambridge University Press).

Pinch, G. (1994), *Magic in Ancient Egypt* (London: British Museum Press).

Porter, R. (2003), *Blood and Guts: A Short History of Medicine* (London: Penguin).

Ritner, R. K. (1993), *The Mechanics of Ancient Egyptian Magical Practice* (Chicago: The Oriental Institute of the University of Chicago).

Salem, S., Mitchell, R. E., El-Dorey, A. E., Smith, J. A. and Barocas, D. A. (2011), 'Successful control of schistosomiasis and the changing epidemiology of bladder cancer in Egypt', *British Journal of Urology International* 107 (2), 206–11.

Sauneron, S. (1960), *The Priests of Ancient Egypt* (London: Evergreen Books).

Scanlan, B. (2004), 'Animals: the hunted and the domestic', in L. Donovan and K. McCorquodale (eds.), *Egyptian Art: Principles and Themes in Wall Scenes* (Sydney: Macquarie University Press), 83–100.

Shaw, I. (2012), *Ancient Egyptian Technology and Innovation* (London: Bristol Classical Press)

Walker, R. E. (1964), 'The Veterinary Papyrus of Kahun: a revised translation and interpretation of the ancient Egyptian treatise known as the Veterinary Papyrus of Kahun', *Veterinary Record* 75, 198–200.

Waterfield, R. (trans.) (1998), Herodotus, *The Histories* (Oxford: Oxford University Press).

Wilkinson, L. (2005), *Animals and Disease: An Introduction to the History of Comparative Medicine* (Cambridge and New York: Cambridge University Press).

13

Bread and beer in ancient
Egyptian medicine

Ryan Metcalfe

The environment of ancient Egypt was ideally suited to the cultivation of cereal crops. Nile floods brought fertile sediments from upstream to reinvigorate the soil, and the water itself could be diverted and stored in a series of channels and basins to irrigate the plants (Butzer 1976: 17). The importance of these crops to the ancient Egyptians can be seen in their incorporation into many different parts of life other than just the diet. Grain in the form of bread and beer formed the basis of remuneration (e.g. Kemp 1991: 125). Offerings of bread and beer were made to the gods and left with the dead to nourish them in the afterlife, and there are surviving depictions of agriculture that show people at all levels of society, from the pharaoh down to the lowliest peasant, working on the land (Emery 1961: 42–3; Brewer, Redford and Redford 1994: 14). The presence of the ruler working the land, albeit in a ceremonial role, underlines the importance of agriculture to the Egyptian state.

In good years, the bounty of the fields was more than sufficient to feed the population, and vast granaries, like those still visible at the Ramesseum, would provide substantial reserves against poor yields in the future (Kemp 1991: 195). However, the floods were not always reliable, and a series of floods that varied substantially from the norm could be disastrous. Too little, and there would not be enough water for irrigation or silt to provide fertile land. Too much, and irrigation systems and food stores could be damaged (Butzer 1976: 51). Food shortages are known from history, for example from the depiction of starving people on the causeway of the pyramid of Unas, and it has been suggested that such shortages may well have been factors in social upheaval (Butzer 1976: 54–6).

The amount of water the floods brought with them allowed the Egyptians to grow crops that would otherwise be almost impossible to cultivate in a North African environment. Emmer and barley were the most common cereal crops, despite requiring large amounts of water to grow successfully. More drought-tolerant crops, such as millet and sorghum, were widely cultivated in Nubia but appear not to have been a significant part of the ancient Egyptian diet (Touzeau *et al.* 2014).

Grain in its raw state is not particularly palatable, and it needs to be processed to make it more suitable for consumption. The nature of this processing can have a significant effect on the nutritional content, taste and texture of the end result (Samuel 2000). Two of the more common products made from cereal crops are bread and beer, both of which formed a significant part of the ancient Egyptian diet.

Baking and brewing in ancient Egypt

The importance of bread and beer to the ancient Egyptians has led to substantial interest in the methods used in their production. Originally, it was assumed not only that the two had ingredients in common, particularly grain and a leavening agent, but that the manufacturing processes showed many similarities and were carried out together. Tomb scenes and models provide further evidence, as the two processes are often shown side by side (Kemp 1991: 120–2).

Brewing

Modern brewing is, in essence, a very simple procedure (see, for example, Koch, Wagner and Clemens 2011: 17–19). Numerous variations exist, but all revolve around the conversion of starch from grains into sugars which are then fermented. Generally, grain is first malted through a controlled germination to increase the amount of amylase enzymes, which can digest starch into soluble, fermentable sugars. The malted grain is mixed with warm water at or near to the optimum temperature for these enzymes to work (around 60–65°C). The sugars and the remnants of the grains are then separated, and the sugar solution (wort) is boiled with hops for flavour and aroma and to increase the longevity of the beer by inhibiting bacterial growth. Yeast is then added to convert the sugar into alcohol. Boiling helps to keep the brew clean by killing any bacteria or fungi that may have contaminated the wort, but is not required from a functional viewpoint. The other stages must be present in one form or another, however, as yeast cannot ferment starch.

Ancient Egyptian brewing techniques have attracted a great deal of attention. Early ethnographic work suggested that the methods were similar to those used for the production of *bouza*, a traditional fermented drink from Egypt (Lucas and Harris 1962: 13–14). This process involves converting the majority of the grain into a coarse, lightly baked bread, with the remainder being allowed to germinate for a few more days. These two batches are mixed together with water and a small amount of old *bouza* (Morcos, Hegazi and El-Damhougy 1973). In this case, baking part of the grain would change some of the starch into a form that is easier for enzymes to convert into sugar. The enzymes would be supplied by the smaller, germinated portion of grain, and the old *bouza* would provide yeast. This would mean that conversion of starch to sugar and the conversion of sugar into alcohol would happen simultaneously, in contrast to modern brewing, where the two happen sequentially. This is a simpler process, and would also have the benefit of protecting the beer from spoilage organisms during brewing. Wort is vulnerable to contamination by bacteria and fungi from the environment. Fermenting the sugars as they are produced, as in *bouza*, reduces this risk as the production of alcohol at an early stage helps to keep the brew free of contaminating micro-organisms. Ethanol is highly toxic, and presents what has been referred to as a 'fermentation wall' – a barrier to the growth of other organisms (Ishida 2005).

It has also been suggested that the ancient Egyptians used a method similar to but less complicated than that used in the manufacture of *bouza* (Samuel 2000: 538–9). This method used heavily yeasted but lightly baked bread, which was then crumbled into water and allowed to ferment. However, according to Samuel (2000: 555), analysis of the physical evidence argues against this method as it would not be possible to both convert the starch into the form seen in beer residues and leave yeast viable. The evidence also precludes the use of a method identical to that of *bouza* production (Samuel 2000: 557), but has allowed Samuel to suggest an alternative but somewhat similar method.

Samuel's method is based on the mixing of two batches of grain, but in this case one is not baked into bread but is instead turned into something more like porridge or gruel. The other is malted, ground and mixed with cold water (Samuel 2000: 540). The two batches are then mixed, allowing the enzymes from the malt to digest the cooked starch quickly. Combining a hot and a cold fraction would result in a warm mixture, near to the optimum temperature for amylases (Samuel 2000: 554).

It is important to note that Samuel's method reflects just one method used in the New Kingdom, and there may have been much variation across time. There will also have been a number of different styles of beer available, either fundamental alterations to the process or more minor variations in the ingredients used. Numerous different beers are recorded in texts, such as strong beer, beer of Nubia and sweet beer (see, for example, Utterances 90 and 151 of the Pyramid Texts (Faulkner 1969) and Papyrus Ebers 6 (Ghalioungui 1987) respectively). How these differed from 'standard' beer is not currently known: sweet beer may have been flavoured with honey, for example, or fermentation may have been stopped before all of the sugars were converted to alcohol. The artistic record, despite presenting many scenes of brewers going about their work, does not provide details of specific brewing processes as it was intended to represent brewing as a concept rather than being a true record of the methods used (Samuel 1999). However, Ishida (2005) attempted to determine detailed brewing methods from two tomb scenes of the Old and New Kingdoms. Although these methods are capable of producing alcoholic beverages from grain, they are extremely complicated and based on an incomplete understanding of ancient Egyptian artistic conventions. For example, Ishida suggested that the number of red and yellow pots on a stand indicated the ratio of water to wort in a dilution step, when the different colours may more plausibly have been used to make each pot easier to distinguish from its neighbours.

Baking

Much of the discussion of ancient Egyptian bread revolves not around the recipe or the baking, but around the grinding of grain into flour. Leek (1972: 131) examined several ancient bread samples and found that they contained large quantities of inorganic material. Some of this he attributed to sand or grit that may have been intentionally added to the grain during grinding to enable a finer flour to be produced, a theory that was supported by experimental reproduction carried out at the Manchester Museum. Later experiments by Samuel, however, showed that it was possible to produce fine flour on a saddle quern without the need for any such additives (Samuel 1994: 237). As the loaves investigated by Leek were from funerary contexts, it is quite possible given the quantity of inorganic material seen in some samples that they were not prepared as carefully as those intended for human consumption (Samuel 2000: 564).

Although there is some evidence for the use of yeast in bread making, it is difficult to say what proportion of loaves included yeast or whether other leavening agents (such as lactic acid bacteria) were used (Samuel 2000: 558). However, it is difficult to imagine that yeast was the sole leavening agent employed by Egyptian bakers, since there are several naturally occurring yeasts and bacteria that can be used in baking, such as those responsible for making sourdough (De Vuyst and Neysens 2005). In addition to the choice of grain and which leavening agent, if any, to use, a baker may produce different breads by adding other ingredients, altering the shape by hand or with a mould or varying the baking time. Such adjustments would help to make a basic staple food a more interesting and enjoyable part of the diet.

Medical uses of bread and beer

The ancient Egyptians had a sophisticated and well-developed system of medical care. We are fortunate that so much literary, artistic and physical evidence has survived, as this has allowed the medical traditions to be studied in far greater detail than would otherwise have been the case. The techniques used included surgical interventions, magical spells and entreaties to various gods for their intercession on behalf of the patient. This apparent lack of distinction between magic and medicine may be surprising to those familiar with the evidence-based approaches used in modern Western medicine. However, an ancient culture without knowledge of germ theory would have had no 'rational' basis for understanding the onset or transmission of diseases caused by pathogenic organisms. While a heavy blow or awkward fall would be an obvious cause for a broken bone, diseases such as tuberculosis would appear to have no obvious cause other than, perhaps, divine displeasure or a rival's curse.

On the spectrum between surgery and spell lie many of the herbal and other remedies recorded in the medical papyri. These have attracted considerable interest as many of the ingredients can still be found in traditional, alternative or even mainstream medicine today (e.g. Manniche 1989: 139–40). It is unfortunate that many of the components cannot be identified (Nunn 1996: 145, for example, states that 80 per cent of the names of botanical species cannot be translated), but in several recipes there is sufficient evidence to form at least a plausible hypothesis regarding the efficacy of the treatment. Some certainly appear to be implausible, such as the cure for impotence (Papyrus Ebers 663; Ghalioungui 1987: 173–4), which contains thirty-seven ingredients including six types of sawdust, four different types of leaf, goose fat and ox fat.

In addition to the herbs, minerals and animal products that make up the majority of the remedies, beer and, to a lesser extent, bread are also common ingredients. The Ebers Papyrus features fourteen remedies that include bread, and 106 that include one or more types of beer. Sweet beer is the most common type used, being mentioned sixty-eight times; the second most common (simple 'beer' with no adjective) is mentioned only twenty-one times. Without being able to determine which constituent made beer 'sweet' it is difficult to understand why it was so commonly used. Beer could be made sweet using honey or fruit juice, for example, and the extra sugars thus provided could have prolonged fermentation and produced a stronger beer. Alternatively, sweet beer may have only had a short, incomplete fermentation, with unconverted sugars providing the sweetness and producing a weaker beer. Honey is a very common ingredient in the medical papyri, being used in over 200 remedies in the Ebers Papyrus (Ghalioungui 1987), so it is possible that if honey was used to produce sweet beer then the resulting beverage would also be seen as beneficial. Unfortunately, as both honey and sweet beer are used together in fifteen remedies in the Ebers Papyrus with no clear pattern in ailment or administrative route, and as there is, at best, scant physical evidence regarding additional ingredients used in ancient Egyptian brewing (Samuel 2000: 548–50), the nature of sweet beer remains obscure.

It is possible to develop some hypotheses regarding the practical uses of beer without fully understanding its composition. Perhaps the most obvious is that it was used to disguise unpleasant flavours from other ingredients. For some of the remedies, the patient would be certain to appreciate such concern. Papyrus Ebers 333 has, for example: 'Another [remedy to kill the *ghw* disease]: *t3-msh* (crocodile dung?) 5 ro; ... of dates 5 ro; sweet beer 5 ro; ground; made into a mass; eaten on 4 days' (Ghalioungui 1987: 101). Similarly, Papyrus Ebers 326, prescribed for the same disease, also features excrement, this time from a bird, and sweet beer. The strongest argument against sweet beer being used solely for flavour is that some of the remedies featuring it are not administered orally. The majority are, with fifty-five being swallowed and two more being spat out after rinsing the mouth, but sweet beer is also used in nine poultices and two enemas. Other types of beer are used non-orally as well, including remedies that are placed or poured into the vagina.

There are numerous other reasons why beer may have been used in these remedies besides hiding the taste of unpleasant ingredients, one of which is simply availability. Beer formed a standard part of the diet, and so would be easy to obtain. Conversely using a more unusual or special type of beer, such as the 'excellent' beer mentioned in three of the Ebers remedies (772, 791 and 812) (Ghalioungui 1987), may have added to any placebo effect by making the patient feel well treated during their convalescence. In either case, the alcohol in the beer may also have had a slight euphoric and/or sedative effect on the patient, if it was consumed in sufficient quantities or was sufficiently strong.

Another possible, and practical, reason for using beer is related to one of the reasons why it was so common in the diet of the ancient Egyptians and many other cultures throughout history. As discussed above, the ethanol produced during fermentation is highly toxic to many organisms, including micro-organisms such as fungi and bacteria. The comparatively low number of harmful micro-organisms would make beer a relatively clean source of fluid in comparison to the most commonly available source of water, the river Nile. It is known that the river was home to the schistosome parasite (see Rutherford in Chapter 16 below), and would certainly have included many other bacteria and parasites both naturally and from the use of the river as a sewer. Using this water in remedies that would be swallowed, inserted into the body as an enema or a vaginal douche, or placed in contact with open wounds or sores would have provided a serious infection risk. Although the ancient Egyptians would not have understood the cause of secondary infections from using Nile water, it is possible that they observed better results from those remedies that used beer.

As well as being microbiologically safer than Nile water, ancient styles of beer are likely to have been highly nutritious, with large amounts of protein and soluble fibre, along with vitamins from the yeast and carbohydrates from any unfermented sugars or starch. It is quite probable that beer was used not just for fluid but also for calories and nutrition. This certainly appears to be the case in two remedies from Papyrus Ebers (291 and 293) which are used 'to cause the stomach to receive food' (Ghalioungui 1987: 92–3). Both of these appear to be recipes for broth based mainly on sweet beer, with several other ingredients cooked in them and strained out. Fat meat and figs feature in both, with other fruit and vegetables included. If the patient was ill and refusing food, these recipes may have provided the nutrition they needed to recover in a form that was easily consumed.

Next to beer, which is nutritious, clean and slightly alcoholic, bread seems to hold little promise as a pharmaceutical ingredient. It would certainly be commonly available, and it could help to add body and thickness to remedies, which appear to be the main rationale for its use in many of the prescriptions in the Ebers Papyrus in which it features. It also appears in a remedy (289) for either stimulating the appetite or allowing food to be kept down (Ghalioungui 1987: 92). As with remedies 291 and 293 mentioned above, this does not appear to be a treatment for the cause so much as for the symptoms. Dried bread is mixed with water, a legume, a little honey and an unidentified mineral, then strained and drunk. A similar but simpler recipe for invalids can be found from a far more recent source. The mid-nineteenth-century *Mrs Beeton's Everyday Cookery* (Beeton n.d.: 673) includes a number of recipes for invalids, one of which calls for a crust of bread to be toasted until hard before being added to water, soaked for an hour and then strained. The ancient Egyptian version sounds more palatable, and more nutritious, but the parallels are striking.

One remedy, however, may indicate that bread could have a practical effect under certain circumstances. Papyrus Ebers 522 describes a complicated, multi-step process for healing a wound. The first step is applying ox fat or ox flesh to the wound so that it 'fouls'. If the wound becomes very foul, the papyrus instructs that the wound is dressed with sour bread so that it dries up (Ghalioungui 1987: 141–2). The adjective 'sour' may indicate that the bread contains lactic acid, which is produced naturally by the lactic acid bacteria. As it is produced, the local environment becomes increasingly acidic to the point where other bacteria cannot survive, and so sufficiently sour bread may be able to kill putrefying bacteria within a wound and make it less 'foul'.

As with many aspects of ancient Egyptian medicine, several assumptions need to be made before the ability of sour bread to clean wounds can be made confidently. Some certainty over the translation is required. The description of the bread as sour, with all the connotations that it carries in modern English, may not adequately convey what the ancient scribes intended. A modern cook may sour cream by adding lemon juice, for example. Similar issues can be found with many remedies, making specific insights difficult to gather. There is also some suggestion that metaphor and punning may play a part in naming the ingredients, possibly to restrict the ability to perform medicine to those who had received the appropriate training. 'Crocodile dung' for example may actually refer to Ethiopian clay, which would change the character of some remedies significantly, including remedy 333 mentioned above (Dieleman 2005: 190–1). Ebers remedy 344 would become far more pleasant to apply around the eyes if this were the case (Ghalioungui 1987: 104).

Beer and medicine in ancient Nubia

In comparison to the abundant evidence provided by the medical papyri from ancient Egypt, the evidence of a medical tradition in ancient Nubia is extremely poor. However, the celebrated discovery of traces of tetracycline (an antibiotic) in skeletal remains from the area has been the cause of considerable interest and debate (Basset *et al.* 1980; Hummert and Van Gerven 1982; Nelson *et al.* 2010). This represents an interesting problem, as the physical evidence of this chemical is convincing but how it was ingested and why are less certain.

As we have already seen with brewer's yeast and lactic acid bacteria, many micro-organisms produce substances that help to secure their position within the environment at the cost of other species. The question of how tetracycline was produced in an ancient civilisation has the same answer: it is made naturally by certain species of *Streptomyces* bacteria. These bacteria live naturally in soil, and as they can produce spores they can survive in harsh environments for a considerable period of time (Madigan *et al.* 2014: 525). Contamination of food stuffs by these bacteria is easy to imagine, especially for stored grains that may come into contact with earthen floors of granaries.

It would appear that the most probable route by which tetracycline entered the body was through drinking beer that had been made with contaminated grain. Beer in its unfermented state is certainly an ideal medium for bacterial growth, full as it is with sugars and protein. Ancient Nubian beer was, however, probably very different in character from that of ancient Egypt as the Nubians had a far greater reliance on drought-tolerant crops than the Egyptians (e.g. Iacumin *et al.* 1998). These crops, such as millet and sorghum, are less well suited to making bread and so the Nubian diet would have been based on foods more similar to porridge or dumplings than to bread (Edwards 2003: 143), but they are a suitable base for making beer.

It has been assumed that Nubian beer would be similar to a traditional Sudanese beverage called *merissa*, which is made from sorghum (see, for example, Edwards 2003: 143). This requires a fairly complex, multi-step and multi-batch process, with some malting, some cooking and some lactic acid fermentation

(Dirar 1978). Crucially, a small amount of a previously brewed batch of *merissa* is also added, which according to Nelson *et al.* (2010) would be vital for the production of tetracycline in sufficient quantities to leave a detectable trace in the bones. It appears that this antibiotic-laced beer was consumed by all sections of society, including children, and that it was consumed with some regularity (Nelson *et al.* 2010). This has led to the assumption, mainly expressed in the popular media, that it was brewed purposefully for medical use (see, for example, McNally 2010). The proportion of skeletons that have tested positive for tetracycline is high but with some variation between populations, ranging from 100 per cent in an X-group population (fifteen individuals: Basset *et al.* 1980) to 63 per cent in a Christian population (110 individuals: Hummert and Van Gerven 1982). This widespread consumption would indicate that, if the beer was being consumed primarily for medical reasons, it was not being used to cure a specific illness. Rather, it would point towards use as a prophylactic against ill health more generally.

Consumption by a large proportion of the population would make any beneficial effects, specifically those due to this beer, difficult to recognise, especially if it was a common part of the diet alongside other staple foodstuffs. Instead, it is possible that the health benefits were, at least originally, an unrecognised positive side effect rather than an intentional aim. Rather, the presence of antibacterial substances in the beer would help to prevent contamination without affecting the ability of yeast to thrive. As grains would most probably be infected with *Streptomyces* during storage in granaries, it may have been noted that old grain was more reliable for brewing, whereas beer made with fresh grain might be more likely to become contaminated and fail. If this was the case, the lactic acid fermentation in modern *merissa* production may have been supplemented with or even replaced by a tetracycline fermentation stage. The latter may have had an effect on the taste and texture of the resulting beer, but an experimental reproduction was described as 'sour' (McNally 2010) and so the difference may have been only slight.

Antibiotic beer in Egypt

Nubian beer is referred to in the Pyramid Texts (e.g. Utterance 151 from the Pyramid Text of Unas; Faulkner 1969), but it does not appear likely that the Egyptians were importing it for medical reasons. The bones that have tested positive for tetracycline from Nubia date to between AD 350 and AD 550 or later (Hummert and Van Gerven 1982; Nelson *et al.* 2010), whereas the earliest evidence of the Pyramid Texts is from the pyramid of Unas of *c.*2375–2345 BC (Malek 2000: 112–13). It is possible that tetracycline beer was brewed significantly earlier in Nubia, but as yet no evidence for this has been found. There are also logistical reasons to doubt that this beer was exported to Egypt. *Merissa* is drunk while still actively fermenting (Dirar 1978), and so must be consumed within a very short space of time after production. Transporting it in time from Nubia to Egypt would be difficult if not impossible.

It is possible that 'Nubian beer' was, rather than being made in Nubia, simply beer in a Nubian style, either brewed by Nubians living in Egypt or brewed to a traditional recipe. However, the diet of the ancient Egyptians was based on wheat and barley almost to the exclusion of sorghum and millet. Indeed, the latter appear to have been restricted to use as animal feed (Dupras, Schwarcz and Fairgrieve 2001). This would make consumption of beer made from one of these grains unlikely, and particularly so if it was considered an important enough beverage to have been mentioned specifically in the Pyramid Texts. Recipes can of course be adjusted to suit local tastes, so it is possible that wheat and/or barley were used instead of millet or sorghum for the version consumed in Egypt, but the end result may have been similar enough in texture and flavour to be recognisable as essentially Nubian in character. Unfortunately, as with several of the named beers of Egypt, in the absence of further evidence we are limited to speculation as to what made each drink different.

There is, however, evidence for the consumption of tetracycline in ancient Egypt (Cook, Molto and Anderson 1989). This is, so far, isolated to the Dakhleh Oasis at around AD 400–500, though the concurrence with Nubian evidence may be coincidental. Rather, the location may be the key to explaining the lack of evidence from the Nile valley. *Streptomyces* grow in dry soils (Madigan *et al.* 2014: 527), so while the valley may have been relatively inhospitable to these bacteria because of the regular flooding and irrigation, the harsh conditions of the Dakhleh Oasis may have allowed them to survive and infect grain stores there. It is possible that populations from other isolated oases in Egypt may also show evidence of tetracycline-labelled bones, but no confirmation of this has yet been reported.

Conclusion

The fertile silt and water provided by the inundation of the Nile allowed the ancient Egyptians to base their agriculture, and thereby their economy, on wheat and barley. These crops are ideally suited to the production of bread and beer, which became the staple components of their diet. These same foodstuffs also became incorporated into their medical traditions, and although their use is sometimes obscure or difficult to rationalise, some of their applications indicate an effective treatment. In some circumstances, bread may have offered real benefit, being able to clean up infected wounds. While the use of beer seems mainly to revolve around its cleanliness and nutritional content, a truly pharmaceutical brew appears to have been used to the south in Nubia and in the Dakhleh Oasis, but there is as yet no evidence for its consumption in the population centres of the Egyptian Nile valley.

References

Basset E. J., Keith, M. S., Armelagos, G. J., Martin, D. L. and Villanueva, A. R. (1980), 'Tetracycline-labelled human bone from ancient Sudanese Nubia (AD 350)', *Science* 209, 1532–4.

Beeton, I. (n.d.), *Mrs Beeton's Everyday Cookery* (London: Ward, Lock & Co.).

Brewer, D. J., Redford, D. B. and Redford, S. (1994), *Domestic Plants and Animals: The Ancient Egyptian Origins* (Warminster: Aris and Phillips).

Butzer, K. (1976), *Early Hydraulic Civilization in Egypt* (Chicago: University of Chicago Press).

Cook, M., Molto, E. L. and Anderson, C. (1989), 'Fluorochrome labelling in Roman Period skeletons from Dakhleh Oasis, Egypt', *American Journal of Physical Anthropology* 80, 137–43.

De Vuyst, L. and Neysens, P. (2005), 'The sourdough microflora: biodiversity and metabolic interactions', *Trends in Food Science and Technology* 16, 43–56.

Dieleman, J. (2005), *Priests, Tongues, and Rites: The London—Leiden Magical Manuscripts and Translation in Egyptian Ritual (100–300CE)* (Leiden: Brill).

Dirar, H. A. (1978), 'A microbiological study of Sudanese merissa brewing', *Journal of Food Science* 43, 1683–6.

Dupras, T. L., Schwarcz, H. P. and Fairgrieve, S. I. (2001), 'Infant feeding and weaning practices in Roman Egypt', *American Journal of Physical Anthropology* 115, 204–12.

Edwards, D. N. (2003), 'Ancient Egypt in the Sudanese Middle Nile: a case of mistaken identity?', in D. O'Connor and A. Reid (eds.), *Ancient Egypt in Africa* (London: UCL Press), 137–50.

Emery, W. (1961), *Archaic Egypt* (Harmondsworth: Penguin Books).

Faulkner, R. O. (1969), *The Ancient Egyptian Pyramid Texts* (Oxford: Oxford University Press).

Ghalioungui, P. (1987), *The Ebers Papyrus* (Cairo: Academy of Scientific Research and Technology).

Hummert, J. R. and Van Gerven, D. P. (1982), 'Tetracycline-labelled human bone from a medieval population in Nubia's Batn El Hajar (550–1450 AD)', *Human Biology* 54, 355–71.

Iacumin, P., Bocherens, H., Chaix, L. and Mariothe, A. (1998), 'Stable carbon and nitrogen isotopes as dietary indicators of ancient Nubian populations (northern Sudan)', *Journal of Archaeological Science* 25, 293–301.

Ishida, H. (2005), 'Two different brewing processes revealed from two ancient Egyptian mural paintings', *Master Brewers Association of America Technical Quarterly* 42, 273–82.

Kemp, B. (1991), *Ancient Egypt: Anatomy of a Civilisation* (London: Routledge).

Koch, G., Wagner, S. and Clemens, R. (2011), *The Craft of Stone Brewing Co.* (New York: Ten Speed Press).

Leek, F. F. (1972), 'Teeth and bread in ancient Egypt', *Journal of Egyptian Archaeology* 58, 126–32.

Lucas, A. and Harris, J. R. (1962), *Ancient Egyptian Materials and Industries*, 4th edn (London: Edward Arnold).

Madigan, M., Martinko, J., Bender, K., Buckley, D. H., Stahl, D. A. and Brock, T. (2014), *Brock Biology of Microorganisms*, 14th edn (Harlow: Pearson).

Malek, J. (2000), 'The Old Kingdom', in I. Shaw (ed.), *The Oxford History of Ancient Egypt* (Oxford: Oxford University Press), 89–117.

Manniche, L. (1989), *An Ancient Egyptian Herbal* (London: British Museum Press).

McNally, J. (2010), 'Ancient Nubians made antibiotic beer', www.wired.com/2010/09/ antibiotic-beer/ (last accessed 4 October 2014).

Morcos, S. R., Hegazi, S. M. and El-Damhougy, S. T. (1973), 'Fermented foods of common use in Egypt, II: The chemical composition of *bouza* and its ingredients', *Journal of the Science of Food and Agriculture* 24, 1157–61.

Nelson, M. L., Dinardo, A., Hochberg, J. and Armelagos, G. J. (2010), 'Mass spectrometric characterization of tetracycline in the skeletal remains of an ancient population from Sudanese Nubia 350–550 CE', *American Journal of Physical Anthropology* 143, 151–4.

Nunn, J. F. (1996), *Ancient Egyptian Medicine* (London: British Museum Press).

Samuel, D. (1994), 'An Archaeological Study of Baking and Bread in New Kingdom Egypt' (PhD thesis, University of Cambridge).

Samuel, D. (1999), 'Brewing and baking in ancient Egyptian art', in H. Walker (ed.), *Food in the Arts* (Totnes: Prospect Books), 173–81.

Samuel, D. (2000), 'Brewing and baking', in P. T. Nicholson and I. Shaw (eds.), *Ancient Egyptian Materials and Technology* (Cambridge: Cambridge University Press), 537–76.

Touzeau, A., Amiot, R., Blichert-Toft, J., Flandroisc, J.-P., Fourela, F., Grossia, V., Martineau, F., Richardin, P. and Lécuyera, C. (2014), 'Diet of ancient Egyptians inferred from stable isotope systematics', *Journal of Archaeological Sciences* 46, 114–24.

14

On the function of 'healing' statues

Campbell Price

I first encountered the work of Rosalie David when, aged five or six, I borrowed a book entitled *Mysteries of the Mummies* from my local library. The book drew largely on work done by the Manchester Museum Mummy Project, and proved instrumental in confirming my nascent interest in ancient Egypt. Little did I realise then that one day I would inherit from Rosalie, a fellow Liverpool University alumnus, the stewardship of the Manchester Museum's exceptional Egyptology collections. It is therefore a special pleasure to offer this study to someone who has done so much to promote the museum and attempts to understand its contents.[1]

The so-called 'healing' statues form a relatively small but well-studied category of monuments attested chiefly from between the 26th Dynasty and early Ptolemaic Period. They represent men of elite status and generally derive from Delta sites (Kákosy 1999; Sternberg el-Hotabi 1999: 99–112).[2] Although the statues are widely cited in discussions of Egyptian religion (e.g. David 2002: 313),

---

1 This is a revised version of a paper presented during a session chaired by Rosalie David at the 'Pharmacy and Medicine in Ancient Egypt' conference held in Manchester in September 2008. It draws upon some aspects of my doctoral dissertation (Price 2011), currently being revised for publication.

2 It is valid to draw a distinction between those statues of private individuals, covered in magical texts, and those of goddesses, where such texts are confined to back pillars, seats and bases – although their functions are likely to have been similar. For the distinction, and list of examples, see Kákosy 1987: 171–6, to which should be added the seated statue of Isis recently auctioned by Christie's in October 2012 (sale 7207, lot 37). No healing statues representing mortal women are known for certain, although texts voiced by a female donor do occur on at least one statue base (Louvre 2540; Ritner 1992: 499–501). Compare Bernard Bothmer's assertion (1969:

most scholarly attention has been focused on the magico-medical spells they carry, rather than the function and perception of the statues in their original contexts. These are the aspects of the statues I attempt to address here.

Medicine and materiality

Perhaps the best-known example of a 'healing' statue is that depicting a man named Djedhor, of very early Ptolemaic date (Cairo JE 46341; Jelínková-Reymond 1956; Sherman 1981: 82–102; Plate 4). The form of this sculpture – a block statue with Horus cippus in front of the shins – is, however, unusual within the genre, which more commonly depicts standing figures. The means by which Djedhor's statue functioned in context seems self-evident: it sits upon a socle with a depression forming a basin, apparently worn from repeated use, which collected the run-off from liquids poured over the heavily inscribed statue. Water, or other liquid, that came into contact with the statue absorbed and was therefore able to transfer the power of the healing spells to those who drank or applied it. This principle of contagion is well attested in many ancient and modern societies (Frankfurter 1998: 48; cf., for example, Finneran 2009 on Christian Ethiopia) and has been the focus of a number of studies of Egyptian magico-medical practice (e.g. Lacau 1922: 189–209; Satzinger 1987: 189–204). Discussion of the healing statues thus tends to proceed on the assumption that each of the statues must regularly have been *used* in the same way.

The efficacy of the written word in magico-medical healing is well known (e.g. Ritner 1993),[3] although the resulting implication that such literate responses to affliction were an elite product is relatively little explored. Bearing in mind that elite context, it is worth emphasising the latent power of the inscribed text itself. The curative potential of a divine name is neatly expressed on a stelophorus statue of the 25th–26th Dynasty potentate Montuemhat from the Karnak Cachette.[4] In the inscriptions, Montuemhat addresses the god Amun:

> I trust (ḥnw) in your name: it is my physician (swnw),[5]
> it drives out suffering (mnt) from my flesh (ḥʿw), it expels disease (ḫ3)

xxxvii) that there was a prohibition against representations of the female form in temple statuary between the 26th Dynasty and the Ptolemaic Period.

3 Frankfurter (1994: 179–221) helpfully contrasts the uses of hieroglyphic and Greek scripts. I maintain that the distinction between medical and magical approaches would have been an artificial one for the ancient Egyptians.

4 Cairo, CG 42237, front of stela, lines 5–7; Leclant 1961: 33; see now the Karnak Cachette Database no. 522.

5 For a convenient collection of references for 'swnw' as a practitioner of healing (= 'physician'), see Nunn 1996: 115–18.

Inscribing the very names of gods on a monument invoked and assured divine presence. In a text on the back pillar of a late Ptolemaic statue from Dendera occurs the following appeal:

> O, these gods and goddesses upon this statue (ḥr snn pn); come to establish his [the deceased's] name and the names of his children for ever and eternity[6]

This statue does not carry any purely figural decoration (Abdalla 1994: 6, pl. IV), so the invocations of the divine names in the statue's inscriptions are apparently sufficient to secure the desired effect. Extensive listings of gods' names (e.g. Sternberg el-Hotabi 1994) and their characteristic images (Spencer 2006: 26) fulfilled apotropaic functions, especially on cosmically vulnerable areas such as temple walls and naos shrines. Contemporary healing statues, with their dense textual and pictorial imagery, echo these trends and reflect a broader shift in the rules of decorum governing the application of hieroglyphic texts to monumental surfaces in the second half of the first millennium BC. It should be borne in mind that this period witnessed the decreasing use of hieroglyphic script, with the result that monuments bearing hieroglyphs carried a heightened cultural premium (Houston, Baines and Cooper 2003: 445).

Encountering the statues

As with the great majority of non-royal temple sculpture to survive from Pharaonic Egypt, the precise original context of the healing statues is archaeologically inaccessible.[7] Yet the statues' forms and inscriptions give important insights into their intended encounters with the living, and their possible settings. It is notable that most of the healing statues – which are generally less than life-size in scale – take theophorus form (one might coin the term 'cippophorous'): that is, in a standing position, holding, supporting or proffering a Horus cippus (Plate 5). This choice is unsurprising; in contrast to the passive block statue form – which was, in fact, more suited to the application and collection of liquids – the standing statues appear more active, and more easily engage the attention of the passer-by.

The visual impact of a densely inscribed statue is likely to have been significant. A steady increase in the amount of text on non-royal statues can be traced from the early Old Kingdom, where inscriptions are sparse (Eaton-Krauss 2009:

---

6   JE 46320, back pillar, col. 3: Abdalla 1994: 7–8, fig. 2.
7   On the problems of interpretation caused by this lack of context, see Price 2011: 173–213. The suggestion of Daumas (1957: 47–9) that healing statues were installed in sanatoria at Dendera, in order for water from channels to run over them, is difficult to substantiate.

129–53) and through the Middle Kingdom, with ever more dense hieroglyphic texts and figural motifs in the New Kingdom, Third Intermediate and Late Periods. Some block statues of the 25th–26th Dynasties are particularly heavily inscribed, and it is notable that this practice is revived during the fourth century BC (Perdu 2012: 90, 93 n. 42). The healing statues, however, go a step further.

Choices in the arrangement of texts were constrained by the fact that at no point was it common for Egyptian sculpture to bear extensive inscriptions on the unclothed skin of a statue, with text instead being focused on a clothed or shrouded surface. This is in contrast to, for example, Mesopotamian sculpture, in which continuous text frequently extends onto the upper body and face (e.g. Marchesi and Marchetti 2011: pls. 35–7). In Pharaonic sculpture, display of the royal name on the bare upper arms or chest of some elite male sculpture is a special case; here the cartouche is employed for its conspicuous amuletic properties, combined with a more prosaic concern to assert loyalty.

An important development, related to the amuletic use of royal and divine names, is the increasing use of figural surface decorations on non-royal statues of stone and metal during the Third Intermediate Period. These predominantly consist of images of gods and have been plausibly interpreted as a means of connecting an individual with the gods depicted in order to harness their divine protection (Taylor 2007: 65–81); parallel increases in divine iconography occur in contemporary Third Intermediate Period coffin decoration. Such changes have been recognised as the precursors of the distinctive iconography of healing statues (Taylor 2007: 80).

A notable detail of the healing statues is that texts and images extend onto the wig area. This innovation seems to be restricted to the healing statues themselves and some contemporary stone sarcophagi (e.g. Buhl 1959: 153–4, fig. 61), although the tomb context of the latter reduced their visual impact among the living. In temples, even if dimly lit, the eye is normally drawn to the face of an anthropomorphic sculpture. The appearance of a healing statue, with dense text extending onto the wig, would have made an obvious departure from traditional elite sculpture. The surviving wigged head of at least one example shows markedly realistic indications of age on the face, which would have heightened this striking effect.[8]

8   The 'Nadler Head' in New York (Allen 2005: 68–9; Bothmer 2004: 425, with the assumption that the statue was 'seen by a great many pilgrims'). On the likelihood of a more restricted intended audience, see below. Compare the reaction of the third-century AD Philostratus, in his *Heroikos*, to the lifelike appearance of a healing statue of Hektor in Greece: 'The statue of Hektor in Ilion resembles a semi-divine human being and reveals many delineations of his character to one inspecting it with the right perspective. In fact, he appears high-spirited, fierce, radiant, and with the splendour of full health and strength, and he is beautiful despite his short hair. The statue is something so alive that the viewer is drawn to touch it' (Gorrini 2012: 121).

A hierarchy of text arrangement is recognisable on some naophorus statues. Most notable is the 27th Dynasty example belonging to a man named
Udjahorresnet (Vatican 196; Baines 1996: 83–92), with sacred content in texts
(such as direct appeals to gods) concentrated around the naos element and
more 'secular' biographical content in visually subordinate positions (Baines
1996: 90–2). More generally, Late Period statue owners – in either naophorus or
theophorus stances – were able to assert not only the talisman-like quality of the
divine image itself (Baines 2004: 52) but also the authority to display and protect it (Price 2011: 190–3). This interpretation accords with the observation by
Kákosy (e.g. 1987: 180) that the hands of the healing statues – which came into
contact with the cippus element – were conceptualised as especially effective.

In attempting to gauge the visual impact of the healing statues in context,
we must recognise the competitive nature of temple spaces in which the statues
are likely to have been set up. Assuming the healing statues to have shared
space with other elite sculpture – and there seems no good reason to doubt
this – the main aim was to achieve sufficient prominence to receive offerings
and the verbalising of prayers (or at least a name) from those with access to the
temple. Conspicuously archaising forms were one means to achieve the same
result: to stand out from other, more common statue types in order to attract the
attention of passers-by (Price 2011: 219–20; Price in press). A targeted audience
among those with privileged access to temple space is made clear in the healing
statues' inscriptions.

Expected interactions

The concept of reciprocity underscores the relationship between deceased
individuals and the living. This is formulated in the text of episode 71 of the
'Opening of the Mouth' ritual

> He (= the deceased) hears the call of those among his relatives, he protects the
> limbs (*mki=f ḥ'w*) of the one who pours water for him (*sti n=f mw*). (Otto
> 1960, I: 194; II: 159)

The pouring of water was a normal ritual gesture in Pharaonic Egypt (e.g.
Gardiner 1902: 146; Sweeney 1985: 214), and in the Late and Graeco-Roman
Periods came to designate a priestly occupation, the *choachytes* (Donker van Heel
1992: 19–30). The precise contexts of rituals which included the pouring of water
– or other liquids – are not made clear in texts, simply because no need is felt to
explain norms of behaviour in explicit ways that answer questions from a different cultural perspective (Eyre 2013: 109). This general interpretational problem
highlights our lack of firm knowledge about how people would normally have
interacted with objects like the healing statues. Texts on monuments like statues

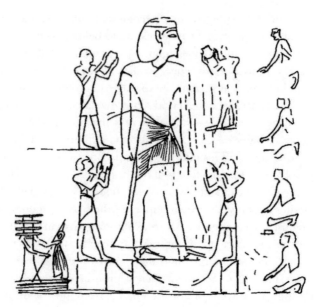

14.1 Scene of lustration from the tomb of Amenemopet, Theban Tomb 41.
(Created by the author after Spieser 1997: fig. 4.)

are a guide to practice, but they are in an important sense prospective – for eternity – and idealised, reifying their expressed wishes for offerings.

Although the stipulation to pour water 'on the ground' occurs in texts (Clère 1995: 120–1; Gardiner 1902: 146), the drenching of entire statues may be implied in some New Kingdom tomb chapel scenes showing the lustration of the deceased (plausibly to be interpreted in the form of a statue in some contexts)[9] (Figure 14.1). This may suggest an otherwise ephemeral practice that is given material expression in the form of the healing statues.

A small group of statues that embody, more than any other, the desire to *drink* liquid offerings are the New Kingdom 'begging' statues, the so-called *chauves d'Hathor*. These bald-headed statues assert their ability to intercede with the divine, in return for interactions with passers-by. In a typical example, a *chauve* proclaims:

> I am a bald one of the goddess, the mediator for his mistress. Anyone with petitions, speak [them to] my ear so that I may repeat them to my mistress in return for offerings (*ḥtpw*).[10] Give me beer upon my hand, *sermet*-beer for my

9   For a list of relevant scenes, see Buzov 2005: 274. The lustration of a statue may be interpreted as part of the 'Opening of the Mouth' ritual (Spieser 1997: 224–8).

10   I follow the interpretation by Pinch (1993: 334) of the hieroglyphs here.

mouth, sweet ointment for my bald head ... if there is no beer give me cool water because the mistress wants a bald one who is satisfied. [11]

The begging statues are unusual because they represent the elite statue owner in an apparently abject attitude, with a hair-style normally associated with the unkempt agricultural worker (Clère 1995); it is as if the bounds of artistic decorum have been pushed to permit this strikingly undignified pose in a special attempt to catch the attention of passers-by. That this should be necessary is perhaps a reflection of the competitive nature of the sacred spaces where such statues were set up. The 'begging' type was an innovative but relatively short-lived means of engaging the living; although an intermediary function is asserted in texts on the statues of other notable individuals, such as Amenhotep son of Hapu (Galán 2003: 221–9), the form of the *chauve* statues makes the expectation of reciprocity – *do ut des* – unusually explicit.

By the Late Period, statue forms became generally more conservative,[12] but their inscriptions contain a number of statements promising reciprocal action for those who act positively for the statue owner (e.g. Jansen-Winkeln 1999: 54–61; Perdu 2000: 185–91; Price 2011: 229–38). A typical example of such a rhetorical appeal to passers-by emphasises the expected pious attitude of temple staff:

> You shall adore He-whose-name-is-hidden [= Amun] for the Ka of the possessor of this statue (*nb snn pn*) because I was one of you ... I spent my lifetime praying (*dw3-ntr*) for every statue I passed by. He who does good, good is done for him double, he who does bad, bad is done to him likewise.[13]

A number of the healing statues carry similar statements focusing on the reciprocal encounter between the statue and the living (Ritner 1992: 499; Vernus 1985: 71–9). But who are the living people who are expected to benefit from such interactions? Are the healing statues and monumental cippi evidence of a reduction in priestly mediation of ritual and a corresponding rise of independent access to healing cults, as David Frankfurter (1998: 49) suggests?

Who were the healing statues for?

Commentators tend to emphasise the supposed accessibility of the healing statues and cippi (e.g. Kákosy 1995: 91–8; Allen 2005: 68–9), imagining them to

---

11   Luxor Museum J 131, left side, l. 4–9: Kitchen 1987, 128, 7–11; Frood 2007: 189–91.
12   At least one *chauve* statue is attested for Montuemhat, of the 25–26th Dynasties: JE 31884 (Leclant 1961: 97–104, pls. 25–8). Most Late Period elite sculpture was of block, naophorus or theophorus form, but exceptions existed and may have been a special means of attracting attention (Price 2011: 214–64).
13   JE 37843 = JE 38696, front, l. 7–10 (Price 2011: 230).

have been placed in areas 'frequented by the general public' (Sherman 1981: 84), as the result of 'public gift' (Ritner 1992: 501) or 'public benefactions' (Ritner 1993: 107). This impression of the statues being set up *for the common good* arises, in part, from modern assumptions about the broad appeal of the healing statues.[14] Comparison with the public accessibility of the roughly contemporary 'healing' statues of athletes in Greece and Rome (Gorrini 2012: 107–30) does not seem justified. The Egyptian context is a significantly different one, at least on the basis of the inscriptions of Late Period non-royal temple sculpture. Despite a clear concern to maximise potential contact through interactions with the living and articulating a more general fear of neglect, Late Period statue inscriptions also state an abhorrence of deliberate damage (Price 2011: 254–5) or contact with the impure and unclean (Rizzo 2004: 511–21; cf. Price 2011: 250–4). Desired interactions were between the statue and a properly purified temple staff (e.g. Gee 1998), those with sanctioned (and sanctified) access to sacred space: the same sort of people who set up the (healing) statues.

Another reason for the perceived popular appeal of the healing statues lies in an over-literal interpretation of universalising claims in their inscriptions. These texts emphasise the effectiveness of their spells by asserting them to be of benefit to people. Yet righteous boasting about having helped the afflicted is a standard cliché dating back to the Old Kingdom (Lichtheim 1992; cf. Coulon 1997: 109–38); are we to believe these all represent genuine records of such charitable actions?

Putting aside modern, egalitarian assumptions about access to healthcare, a much more restricted use of the statues seems probable. The healing statues, like much Late Period elite sculpture, carry inscriptions targeting a specific audience among knowledgeable, literate temple staff. Thus, the famous statue of Djedhor carries an appeal on its base (Jelínková-Reymond 1956: 122–3) to a restricted, literate group concerned to keep control over the powerful magical content of inscriptions:

> O, every pure-priest, every scribe, every knower-of-things who sees this 'saviour'-statue (*šd*): read out its writings (*sd sšw=f*), know its magical formulae (*rḫ=sn s3ḫw=f*), keep its texts safe (*swd3=tn sš=f*), protect its (ritual) recitations(?) (*mk=tn sḫ3w(?)=f*). Say the offering-formula ... !

On the base of another healing statue representing Djedhor, speech ascribed to him states that he 'put [spells] in writing on this statue in order to save[15]

14   There is evidence of later, Greek graffiti marking the appreciation of the healing qualities of Pharaonic monuments – such as New Kingdom statues at Deir el-Bahri (Metawi 2013: 110–14) – but these are obviously secondary and were written when access to the statues was apparently unmediated.

15   *s͗nḫ* means 'to cause to live' (Erman and Grapow 1953, 46 (line 4) –47 (line 13)) and

everyone (*r sᶜnḫ s nb*) thereby from the poison of every male and female viper and all snakes' (Sherman 1981: 91 and n. ee). In fact, the same phrase for 'everyone' (lit.: 'every man') appears in a number of contemporary 'appeals to the living' in statue inscriptions; the context of these suggests a restricted, priestly group of 'men' (Price in press: text note j) and not the 'general public' that Sherman (1981: 84) and others seem to envisage.

Self-interest is more characteristic of the motivations behind the healing statues than the public-spiritedness that is often used to explain their creation. Thus, while a priest called Nesatum claims to have commissioned the carving of the Metternich Stela (Plate 3) (an elite monument comparable to the healing statues) for the benefit of his mother,[16] he also makes clear that he acted for the gods, in expectation of divine reciprocation. Nesatum claims to have:

> renewed this writing after he found it absent from the house of Osiris Mnevis, for the sake of making his mother's name live (*sᶜnḫ rn=s*), forestalling for her death and every divine pain, giving air to the suffocating, and for the sake of making live the families of all the gods. Then his lord Osiris Mnevis was heightening his lifetime with sweetness of mind and a final burial after old age because of this which he has done for the house of Osiris Mnevis. (Allen 2005: 63)

The Metternich Stela is one of a few 30th Dynasty non-royal monuments that employ particularly perplexing cryptographic writings. Indeed, it seems that the small group that commissioned and fully understood these inscriptions did so for literary and aesthetic delight (Klotz 2012: 144). The very selective removal of one of the royal names on the stela's base (Allen 2005: 53) shows the potential scrutiny of the monument's texts that might be carried out by a sufficiently interested party.

The stela, in common with the few surviving healing statues, are finely executed works for the use of ritual specialists – and not the hoi polloi. An awareness of the restricted access to such texts on statues is echoed by a Demotic papyrus, Leiden I 384, of around the second century AD. It closes with a Greek section which lists thirty-seven entries which claim to provide a translation key for a proper understanding of the ingredients prescribed in magico-medicinal recipes. This is preceded by a short introduction that explains the function of the list:

---

is well attested in dedication inscriptions on Late Period statues (e.g. Price 2011: 100–2); the rendering 'save' conflates this with a modern understanding of '*šdᵓ*' as 'saviour', the Judaeo-Christian overtones of which are inappropriate in this context.

16 Such an assertion of filial piety is especially fashionable at this period (Price in press).

Interpretations translated from the holy (writings), of which the temple scribes made use. Because of the nosiness of the masses, they (the temple scribes) wrote the (names of the) herbs and other things that they made use of on statues of gods in order that they (the masses) … do not meddle … due to the inevitable result of their mistake. (Papyri Graecae Magicae XII.401–7; Dieleman 2005: 185–6)

The impression of wilfully concealed temple wisdom is, of course, part of a much broader perception of Pharaonic culture (Baines 1990: 1–23). Yet the idea of deliberate secrecy by the temple staff and required initiation to understand statue inscriptions strikes a significant chord with the restricted physical and intellectual access to the healing statues.

Summary

Often of extremely fine workmanship, the healing statues are an embodiment of material practices that are likely to have been both long-lived and widespread among social groups, but which leave little archaeological trace. The statues stand, however, at the most privileged end of the spectrum of responses to affliction; they are a reflection of the concerns of a small group of literate temple staff and are likely to have been designed principally to serve their interests. The statues vaunt access to ancient magico-medical knowledge, inviting passers-by to stop awhile and consider their powerful inscriptions. Yet it seems likely that such interactions took place within the closed, and increasingly rarefied, world of the Egyptian temple during the fourth and fifth centuries BC.

Interaction with sculpture in any Pharaonic temple is likely to have been far more 'hands-on' than the clinical settings of most of the statues' modern museum contexts would imply. Yet the power of the healing statues did not, perhaps, lie so much in their actual use as in their potential to be used; their presence reified the magico-medical texts written on them and stood out among other, less visually intriguing sculpture. The healing statues are a forceful expression of a much wider concern for reciprocal action: they not only promise the role of intercessor with the gods and the dead, but vaunt quick-fix material solutions to real problems. The statues conspicuously – perhaps cynically, given knowledge of how temple spaces operated – exploited human vulnerability, attracting those in need of a remedy as a means to increase interactions and enhance the perpetual presence (and not merely the 'reputation') of the person(s) depicted and named on the statue. As the work of Rosalie David herself has helped to show, the health problems which resulted from a privileged priestly diet and lifestyle were significant (David 2010: 105–18), creating a host of ailments for which relief might be sought from within the temple.

The power of objects comes from ability to restrict access to and knowledge of them; had the healing statues been as widely accessible as so many claim then it is unlikely that their cultural prestige and perceived effectiveness would have been so pronounced. This interpretation of the function of the healing statues acknowledges both the unequal access to aesthetic and sacred materials in Pharaonic Egypt (Baines 2013: esp. 6–14) and the misleading effects of a sentimental vision of Pharaonic healing practices.

Acknowledgements

I am grateful to Simon Connor of the Museo Egizo Turin for generous assistance with photography.

References

Abdalla, A. (1994). 'Graeco-Roman Statues Found in the Sebbakh at Dendera', in C. Eyre, A. Leahy and L. Montagno Leahy (eds.), *The Unbroken Reed: Studies in the Culture and Heritage of Ancient Egypt in Honour of A. F. Shore* (London: Egypt Exploration Society), 1–24.

Allen, J. P. (2005), *The Art of Medicine in Ancient Egypt* (New York and New Haven: Metropolitan Museum of Art and Yale University Press).

Baines, J. (1990), 'Restricted knowledge, hierarchy, and decorum: modern perceptions and ancient institutions', *Journal of the American Research Center in Egypt* 27, 1–23.

Baines, J. (1996), 'On the composition and inscriptions of the Vatican statue of Udjahorresne', in P. der Manuelian and R. Freed (eds.), *Studies in Honor of William Kelly Simpson*, I (Boston: Museum of Fine Arts), 83–92.

Baines, J. (2004), 'Egyptian elite self-presentation in the context of Ptolemaic rule', in W. V. Harris and G. Ruffini (eds.), *Alexandria: Between Egypt and Greece* (Leiden: Brill), 33–61.

Baines, J. (2013). *High Culture and Experience in Ancient Egypt* (Sheffield: Equinox)

Bothmer, B. V. (1969), *Egyptian Sculpture of the Late Period, 700 B.C. – A.D. 100*, 2nd edn (New York: Brooklyn Museum).

Bothmer, B. V. (2004), 'Egyptian Antecedents of Roman Republican Verism', in M. Cody (ed.), *Egyptian Art: Selected Writings of Bernard V. Bothmer* (Oxford: Oxford University Press), 408–31.

Buhl, M.-L. (1959), *The Late Egyptian Anthropoid Stone Sarcophagi* (Copenhagen: Nationalmuseet).

Buzov, E. (2005), 'The Role of the Heart in the Purification', in *L'acqua nell'antico Egitto: Proceedings of the First International Conference for Young Egyptologists* (Rome: L'Erma di Bretschneider), 273–81.

Clère, J.-J. (1995), *Les chauves d'Hathor* (Leuven: Peeters).

Coulon, L. (1997). 'Véracité et rhétorique dans les autobiographies égyptiennes de la Première Période Intermédiaire', *Bulletin de l'Institut français d'archéologie orientale* 97, 109–38.

Daumas, F. (1957), 'Le sanatorium de Dendara', *Bulletin de l'Institut français d'archéologie orientale* 56, 35–57.

David, R. (2002), *Religion and Magic in Ancient Egypt* (London: Penguin).

David, R. (2010), 'Cardiovascular disease and diet in ancient Egypt', in A. Woods, A MacFarlane and S. Binder (eds.), *Egyptian Culture and Society: Studies in Honor of Naguib Kanawati*, I (Cairo: Supreme Council of Antiquities), 105–18.

Dieleman, J. (2005). *Priests, Tongues, and Rites: The London–Leiden Magical Manuscripts and Translation in Egyptian Ritual (100–300 CE)* (Leiden: Brill).

Donker van Heel, K. (1992), 'Use and meaning of the Egyptian term *wꜥb mw*', in R. J. Demarée (ed.), *Village Voices: Proceedings of the Symposium 'Texts from Deir el-Medina and their Interpretation', Leiden, May 31 – June 1, 1991* (Leiden: Centre of Non-Western Studies), 19–30.

Eaton-Krauss, M. (2009), 'The location of inscriptions on statues of the Old Kingdom', in D. Magee, J. Bourriau and S. Quirke (eds.), *Sitting beside Lepsius: Studies in Honour of Jaromir Malek at the Griffith Institute* (Leuven: Peeters), 129–53.

Erman, A. and Grapow, H. (1953), *Wörterbuch der ägyptischen Sprache*, IV (Berlin and Leipzig: J. C. Hinrichs).

Eyre, C. (2013), 'Women and prayer in Pharaonic Egypt', in E. Frood and A. McDonald (eds.), *Decorum and Experience: Essays in Ancient Culture for John Baines* (Oxford: Oxford University Press), 109–16.

Finneran, N. (2009) 'Holy waters: pre-Christian and Christian water association in Ethiopia: an archaeological landscape perspective', in T. Ostegaard (ed.) *Water, Culture and Identity in the Nile Basin* (Bergen: University of Bergen Press), 165–87.

Frankfurter, D. (1994), 'The magic of writing and the writing of magic,' *Helios* 21, 179–221.

Frankfurter, D. (1998), *Religion in Roman Egypt: Assimilation and Resistance* (Princeton: Princeton University Press).

Frood, E. (2007) *Biographical Texts from Ramessid Egypt* (Atlanta: Society of Biblical Literature).

Galán, J. (2003), 'Amenhotep son of Hapu as intermediary between the people and God', in Z. Hawass and L. Pinch Brock (eds.), *Egyptology at the Dawn of the Twenty-First Century*, II (Cairo: American University in Cairo Press), 221–9.

Gardiner, A. (1902), 'Imhotep and the scribe's libation', *Zeitschrift für ägyptische Sprache und Altertumskunde* 40, 146.

Gee, J. (1998), 'The Requirements of Ritual Purity in Ancient Egypt' (PhD dissertation, Yale University).

Gorrini, M.E. (2012), 'Healing statues in the Greek and Roman world', in I. Csepregi and C. Burnett (eds.), *Ritual Healing: Magic, Ritual and Medical Therapy from Antiquity until the Early Modern Period* (Florence: Sismel Edizioni del Galluzzo), 107–30.

Houston, S., Baines, J. and Cooper, J. (2003), 'Last writing: script obsolescence in Egypt, Mesopotamia, and Mesoamerica', *Comparative Studies in Society and History* 45 (3), 430–79.

Jansen-Winkeln, K. (1999), *Sentenzen und Maximen in den Privatinschriften der ägyptischen Spätzeit* (Berlin: Achet).

Jelínková-Reymond, E. (1956) *Les inscriptions de la statue quérisseuse de Djedher-le-sauveur* (Cairo: Institut Français d'Archéologie Orientale).

Kákosy, L. (1987), 'Some problems of the magical healing statues', in A. Roccati and A. Siliotti (eds.), *La Magia in Egitto ai tempi dei Faraoni* (Milan: Rassegna Internazionale di Cinematografia Archeologica Arte e Natura Libri), 171–86.

Kákosy, L. (1995), 'Heilstatuen in den Tempeln', in *Systeme und Programme der ägyptischen Tempeldekoration: 3. ägyptologische Tempeltagung, Hamburg 1. – 5. Juni 1994* (Wiesbaden: Harrassowitz), 91–8.

Kákosy, L. (1999), *Egyptian Healing Statues in Three Museums in Italy: Turin, Florence, Naples* (Turin: Museo Egizio).

Karnak Cachette Database (n.d.), www.ifao.egnet.net/bases/cachette/ (last accessed 6 February 2015).

Kitchen, K. A. (1987). *Ramesside Inscriptions: Historical and Biographical*, VII (Oxford: Blackwell).

Klotz, D. (2012), 'The peculiar naophorous statuette of a Heliopolitan priest: Hannover, Museum August Kestner 1935.200.510', *Zeitschrift für ägyptische Sprache und Altertumskunde* 139, 136–44.

Lacau, P. (1922), 'Les statues guérisseuses dans l'ancienne Égypte', *Monuments et mémoires de la Fondation Eugène Piot* 25, 189–209.

Leclant, J. (1961), *Montouemhat quatrième prophète d'Amon, prince de la ville* (Cairo: Institut Français d'Archéologie Orientale).

Lichtheim, M. (1992), *Maat in Egyptian Autobiographies and Related Studies* (Freiburg and Göttingen: Vandenhoeck and Ruprecht).

Marchesi, G. and Marchetti, N. (2011), *Royal Statuary of Early Dynastic Mesopotamia* (Winona Lake, IN: Eisenbrauns).

Metawi, D. (2013), 'A brother for Tuthmose III (Cairo Museum BN 104)', *Journal of Egyptian Archaeology* 99, 101–16.

Nunn, J. F. (1996), *Ancient Egyptian Medicine* (London: British Museum Press).

Otto, E. (1960), *Das ägyptische Mundöffnungsritual*, 2 vols. (Wiesbaden: Harrasowitz).

Perdu, O. (2000), 'Florilège d'incitations à agir', *Revue d'Égyptologie* 51, 175–193.

Perdu, O. (2012), *Les statues privées de la fin de l'Égypte pharaonique*, I: *Hommes* (Paris: Khéops).

Pinch, G. (1993) *Votive Offerings to Hathor* (Oxford: Griffith Institute).

Price, C. (2011), 'Materiality, Archaism and Reciprocity: The Conceptualisation of the Non-Royal Statue at Karnak during the Late Period (c. 750–30 BC)' (PhD dissertation, University of Liverpool).

Price, C. (in press), 'Archaism and filial piety: an unusual pair statue from the cachette (JE 37136)', in L. Coulon (ed.), *La cachette de Karnak: nouvelles perspectives sur les découvertes de G. Legrain* (Cairo: Institut Français d'Archéologie Orientale and Supreme Council of Antiquities).

Ritner, R. (1992), 'Religion vs. magic: the evidence of the magical statue bases', in U. Luft (ed.), *The Intellectual Heritage of Egypt. Studies presented to Laszlo Kákosy* (Budapest: Eötvös Loránd University), 495–501.

Ritner, R. K. (1993), *The Mechanics of Ancient Egyptian Magical Practice* (Chicago: The Oriental Institute of the University of Chicago).

Rizzo, J. (2004), 'Une mesure d'hygiène relative à quelques statues-cubes déposées dans le temple d'Amon à Karnak', *Bulletin de l'institut français d'archéologie orientale* 104, 511–21.

Satzinger, H. (1987), 'Acqua guaritrice: le statue e le stele magiche ed il loro uso magico-medico nell'Egitto faraonico', in A. Roccati and A. Siliotti (eds.), *La magia in Egitto ai tempi dei faraoni: atti, convegno internazionale di studi, Milano, 29–31 ottobre 1985* (Milan: Rassegna Internazionale di Cinematografia Archeologica Arte e Natura Libri), 189–204.

Sherman, E. J. (1981), 'Djedhor the saviour: statue base OI 10589', *Journal of Egyptian Archaeology* 67, 82–102.

Spencer, N. (2006), *A Naos of Nakhthorheb from Bubastis: Religious Iconography and Temple Building in the 30th Dynasty* (London: British Museum Press).

Spieser, C. (1997), '*L'eau* et la régénération des morts d'après les représentations tombes thébaines du Nouvel Empire', *Chronique d'Égypte* 72, 211–28.

Sternberg-el-Hotabi, H. (1994), 'Der Untergang der Hieroglyphenschrift', *Chronique d'Égypte* 69, 218–48.

Sternberg-el-Hotabi, H. (1999), *Untersuchungen zur Überlieferungsgeschichte der Horusstelen: ein Beitrag zur Religionsgeschichte Ägyptens im 1. Jahrtausend v. Chr.* (Wiesbaden: Harrassowitz).

Sweeney, D. (1985), 'Intercessory Prayer in Ancient Egypt and the Bible', in S. Israelit-Groll (ed.), *Pharaonic Egypt, the Bible and Christianity* (Jerusalem: Magnes Press), 213–30.

Taylor, J. (2007), 'Figural surface decoration on bronze statuary of the Third Intermediate Period', in M. Hill (ed.), *Gifts for the Gods: Images from Egyptian Temples* (New York and London: Yale University Press), 65–81.

Vernus, P. (1985), 'La retribution des actions: à propos d'une maxime', *Göttinger Miszellen* 84, 71–9.

15

Writings for good health in social context: Middle and New Kingdom comparisons

Stephen Quirke

Among writings for good health from ancient Egypt, two substantial groups are the Ramesseum Papyri, from the late Middle Kingdom, and the Deir el-Medina and Chester Beatty Papyri from the Ramesside Period. The former were found with other writings in a box, at the bottom of a tomb shaft, beside figurines, clappers, worked tusks, beads and writing tools. None of the finds bears a title with a personal name, leaving the identities of the owner(s) and user(s) uncertain; Egyptologists have interpreted the materials as equipment of a magician, a lector at rituals or a nurse. The Deir el-Medina and Chester Beatty Papyri also include other writings along with those for good health, and here the archaeological context is secure: the owner was principal accountant managing the primary project of any reign, the creation of the tomb of the king. Comparison of the contents, and of the Egyptological reception of the two groups, offers an opportunity to reconsider the social location of writings for good health in Egypt in the second millennium BC.

The late Middle Kingdom finds in a three-chamber shaft tomb under the Ramesseum store-rooms

In 1895–96, Flinders Petrie continued the apprenticeship of James Quibell, an Oxford classics and chemistry student, in supervising part of the work on New Kingdom king-cult temple sites along the edge of the fields on the West Bank at Thebes. Petrie summarised the division of responsibility in his brief report:

> the ruins behind the Kom el Hettan were attributed to Amenhotep III. The result of my work was to fix the last-named ruin as the temple of Merenptah, and to discover the sites of the temples of Amenhotep II, Tausert, and Siptah; at the same time the sites of Tahutmes IV and of Uazmes were fully cleared and planned. Meanwhile Mr. Quibell cleared the Ramesseum and the great

buildings around that, working for the Egyptian Research Account. (Petrie 1897: 1)

In his publication of work on the Ramesseum, Quibell provided the following description of architecture of one tomb, which yielded material from the Middle Kingdom, Third Intermediate Period and Roman Period:[1]

> The most important tomb of the XIIth dynasty period consisted of a long, oblong shaft, skew to the wall of one of the chambers (No. 5, pl. I) and running under it. ... At the bottom of the shaft, 13 feet down, two small chambers opened. ... There was a third chamber pierced in the long S. side of the well, half way down. (Quibell 1898: 3–4)

The triple chamber tomb is well attested for the late Middle Kingdom, though its interpretation is uncertain (Miniaci and Quirke 2009). The original number of burials intended for three-chamber tombs may vary; there is no guarantee that architects were working to a concept of one chamber for one individual. Two other possibilities must be considered: (a) that a single individual might be buried in a tomb with multiple chambers; and (b) that a single chamber was intended to contain more than one burial. The best-documented burial of the period, that of Senebtysy at Lisht, demonstrates how burial equipment for a single person might be distributed across two spaces on one level (Mace and Winlock 1916). At least in theory, a single individual may have been provided with one chamber for the body, a second chamber at the same level for one set of offerings or burial equipment, and a third chamber midway down the shaft for another set (as speculated in Miniaci and Quirke 2009). Conversely, the Middle Kingdom cemetery at Lisht North, around the pyramid of Amenemhat I, shows a range of population density in triple-chamber tombs: remains of four individuals were found in the upper chamber of shaft tomb 466; the lower chambers of shaft tomb 391 contained remains of at least seven individuals (Quirke 2015). Original intentions may be obscured by re-use of existing space by kin or associates of the deceased, or by later unconnected generations. Whatever the initial plan for the three-chamber tomb published by Quibell, the record from cemeteries for the period indicates a trend to multiple burials (Grajetzki 2007). Quibell did not refer to human remains in his report on the tomb, and therefore the number of burials in each phase of its use is unknown.

At the bottom of the shaft, the Qurna and Qift excavators working for Petrie and Quibell unearthed a group of finds:

---

1   In Quibell's citation, his 'No. 5' refers not to a tomb, as some previous commentators have inferred, but to the Ramesseum store-room chamber built over the tomb-shaft, as is clear from the sequence of numbers on his plate I.

Lastly, the heap left in the middle of the shaft was removed, and in it, in a space about 2 feet square, was found a group of objects, some of which are shown in PL. III.

First was a wooden box about 18 × 12 × 12 inches. It was covered with white plaster, and on the lid was roughly drawn in black ink the figure of a jackal. The box was about one third full of papyri which were in extremely bad condition, three quarters of their substance having decayed away...

In the box was also a bundle of reed pens, 16 inches long and a tenth of an inch in diameter, and scattered round it were a lot of small objects. (Quibell 1898: 3)

Quibell added confidently that 'the position can leave no doubt that all these objects are from one interment and of one date'; in the absence of any sketch-plan of the find, or more precise documentation of the object scatter, the attribution to a single burial is difficult to confirm, but the handwriting of the papyri and the parallels for the objects confirm a broad dating for the group to the late Middle Kingdom (Gardiner 1955; Kemp and Merrillees 1980: 166; Bourriau 1991: 20).

A combination of papyri and other objects is a rare find in Egyptian archae-ology. In this find-group, both the artefacts and the majority of the separable manuscripts have been ascribed to the performative aspect of healing (I avoid here the English term 'magical', on account of its specific associations, mainly negative, in definition against supposedly more advanced practices; cf. Gutekunst 1986: cols. 1320–6). Accordingly, the find stimulated speculation over the identity of the person (assumed to be singular) buried. In his introduction to the papyri, Alan Gardiner interpreted the entire group as 'the professional outfit of a magi-cian and medical practitioner', citing specifically the papyri and 'castanets, ape in blue glaze, dd-sign of ivory, and above all the figure of a masked girl holding a serpent in each hand' (Gardiner 1955: 1). In my doctoral dissertation, I also assumed a single burial, and I followed Gardiner in connecting a list of seventy days on Papyrus Ramesseum 13 with the seventy days cited in other sources as the duration of embalming: 'this could be taken to imply that the owner of the box held the profession of wtw "embalmer", in accordance with the predomi-nant ritual and magical tone of the papyri and the other objects in the burial' (Quirke 1990: 187–8). Against such interpretations, Janine Bourriau drew atten-tion to the regular inclusion of female figurines, faience animals and plants, and objects with related imagery in late Middle Kingdom tombs, and argued that the Ramesseum find was 'unremarkable within the general context of burial groups of the late XII to XIII Dynasties' (Bourriau 1991: 20). As such items are found on settlement sites and in votive deposits, they were presumably used on earth; Bourriau distinguished the burials containing them from burials of the same date but equipped with regalia made for embalming rites and burial.

Andrea Gnirs has discussed the range of objects in the Ramesseum find-group most recently and systematically, and acknowledged the point made by Bourriau on the wider distribution of the figurines and the figured tusks and rod-segments (Gnirs 2009). Nevertheless, within that context of late Middle Kingdom burial equipment, Gnirs emphasised as exceptional items the papyri and the leonine-faced or masked naked snake-holder, as did Gardiner, adding the hair-tangled snake staff as a third item that removes the find from the burial customs of the day (Gnirs 2009: 143).[2] Another distinguishing feature, according to Gnirs, may be the presence of multiple female figurines and worked tusks; certainly, whether with single or multiple burials, no other late Middle Kingdom tomb is known to have contained four tusks. Further, in an important break from previous assumptions, Gnirs pointed out that, in the absence of any direct evidence from human remains or inscription with name, the sex of any individual buried in the tomb is unknown. From a review of Middle Kingdom sources for nurses and midwives, Gnirs concluded that the objects 'als das Berufsgerät einer Amme und Hebamme angesehen werden dürfen' (Gnirs 2009: 153–4). As indicated in a footnote to that sentence, her hypothesis, along with all the other interpretations of the find, would contradict the analysis by Stephan Seidlmayer of burial equipment at Beni Hasan and other sites; Seidlmayer had found that Old and Middle Kingdom burial equipment related to age, gender and above all status, and not to a 'profession', that is, a dominant activity in life (Seidlmayer 2006). Gnirs cited as counter-example the burial equipment of the overseer of works Kha, which included measuring devices (Gnirs 2009: 154, n. 165). However, again, measuring equipment is typical for burials of a group of men not with the same title but of the same status, high-ranking officials of the late 18th Dynasty. Commenting on new finds of cubit rods in the tomb of the vizier Aperel, Alain Zivie noted that another is inscribed for the treasurer Maya, and that the official titles on the measuring-rod inscribed for Aperel concern his status as, for example, 'child of the inner palace', rather than any role in overseeing works (Zivie 1990: 136–7). If items were placed in a tomb primarily to secure the social status of an individual, then the equipment can reveal the status that is claimed for her or him for eternity, but not the sphere of activity where the individual spent most of her or his life on earth. For both the objects and the papyri, the quest for the professional owner turns out to be a misconception at its starting point. An analogy may be drawn with the tendency to identify model tools in burials as medical equipment, and, by extension, as the work kit ('Berufsgerät') of an ancient surgeon or other healer. Fifty years ago, Khalil and Hishmet Messiha compared the forms

2   From its relatively short length, 16 cm, Gnirs considers that the snake staff may be a metal figurine, rather than a functional staff, or may be a metal figurine in itself.

of such models with other items identified as anatomical instruments, and with depictions of artists at work, and concluded that 'these implements are engraving tools and not surgical tools' (Messiha and Messiha 1964: 209). Yet the idea of such prestigious ancestry seems to have eclipsed their study, and the 'professional' interpretation still circulates.

Leaving aside the objects found around the box, and the uncertainties over association and number of burials, the 'professional' identity of any ancient owner of the papyri proves more elusive than even the contents might suggest. As all the papyri were deposited in the same box and in a burial-place, they have, reasonably enough, been taken to constitute an intentional collection, rather than, for example, an accidental accumulation or waste-paper; for the latter possibility, the baskets found containing papyri in second- to-third-century AD contexts at Tanis and Tebtunis (Cuvigny 2009: 50) seem suggestive to a modern user of waste-paper baskets, though they too may have been regular book-roll containers. The interpretation of the deposit has not been methodically theorised, in the manner undertaken in other archaeologies for the ways in which materials enter the archaeological record, that is, enter and emerge from the ground (Sommer 1991). Instead, much as the find-group has been equated implicitly with a single burial, the papyri in the box have implicitly provided modern investigators with an individual book-owner, book-collector or reader, on the basis that some person or persons did at some point place these particular papyri into that one box. Therefore, one ancient identity, singular or collective, ought to materialise out of the writings on the papyri. A single property-owner has tended to be the focus of researchers. The papyri have resisted this reduction to the singular, because their contents and even their script types are diverse, as the summary in Table 15.1 indicates (letters and numbers of separate manuscripts following Gardiner 1955, but noting possible joins between his items; see also the more detailed list in Table 15.4 below)

Reviewing the Gardiner book on the papyri, Jean Yoyotte argued that

Table 15.1   Summary of the Ramesseum Papyri by content type (after Gardiner 1955)

Cursive hieroglyphic manuscripts	Hieratic manuscripts
Senusret I statue ritual (B)	one: onomasticon (D)
Funerary rites at a mastaba (E)	Tale of Sanehat, Tale of Khuninpu, Teachings (A, 1, 2)
Prescriptions, ointments to relax body (5)	one: (?) prescriptions and incantations at birth (3, 4)
Hymns to Sobek (6)	five: (?) incantations, longer books (C, 8, 9, 10, 16, 17)
Incantations (7: possibly part of 6)	six: (?) incantations, shorter MSS (11–15, 19)

'la presence de ces livres ne denote, à proprement parler, ni le sorcier, ni le guérisseur, ni le conteur, ni le maître d'école; ils sont le bien propre d'un prêtre-officiant (ẖry-ḥbt)' (Yoyotte 1957: 175). In order to govern correct procedure and pronouncement in rituals, a lector would need competence in reading the cursive hieroglyphic script used for ritual manuscripts at this period, on the evidence of this group and of rare contemporary finds (Berger-el Naggar 2004). However, the crucial position of lector, and its status as 'profession' and 'role', remain to be researched from the dataset of attestations within each period; for the present, the extent and social profile of hieroglyphic literacy remain even more difficult to assess than hieratic literacy, though at least the two scripts can be distinguished in the process (Vernus 1986). The administrative jottings and accounts on the back of several papyri provide some clues to the socio-economic status of the person(s) using, and perhaps writing or acquiring, these (papyri D, E, 1, 3 and 4, and the seventy-day check-list on 13). The reference to *pr.i* 'my house/estate' on the back of no. 3 seems to place at least that item in the domain of an individual, rather than an institution such as a bureau or temple at regional or national level (Quirke 1990: 189). Further research into quantities of items and seasonality of entries might produce additional information on the scale of activity and, in comparison with accounts of the same and other periods, size of the estate. However, the fragmented entries on the different manuscripts yield no clear connections (Quirke 1990: 187–94), and no singular or professional identity seems to emerge. Here, to complicate and enrich our reading of the ancient society, a second group of manuscripts miraculously preserved from the second millennium BC is at hand to guide us.

The papyri of Qenherkhepshef

Twenty years before he presented his summary of the papyri in the box found under the Ramesseum, Alan Gardiner produced a fuller edition of a substantial group of hieratic manuscripts and fragments, provisionally identified as eighteen separate items, in addition to the largest and best-preserved book-roll, which he had published separately and is today preserved in the Chester Beatty Library and Gallery in Dublin:

> They were one and all presented to the British Museum by Mr. and Mrs. Chester Beatty, and emanate from a single find which included, besides a number of fragments of letters, inventories, etc., another magnificent papyrus (No. I) retained by Mr. Chester Beatty for his own collection (Gardiner 1935: vii)

The remarkable contents include the earliest book of dream interpretations apparently to be consulted in practice, rather than solely for reading in the

Table 15.2   Summary of the papyri of Qenherkhepshef (after Gardiner 1935)

Ritual manuals	Literary manuscripts (including hymns)	Manuscripts for good health
Dream Book (ChB 3)	Horus and Seth Tale, love songs (ChB 1)	prescriptions (ChB 6)
Offering Ritual (ChB 9)	Tale of Truth and Falsehood (ChB 2)	incantations (ChB 6–8, 9, 11–18)
	Battle of Qadesh (ChB 3 verso)	aphrodisiacs (ChB 10)
	Teaching of Khety (ChB 19)	
	hymns to the creator, to Amun (ChB 4, 11)	
	hymn to the Nile flood	
	hymn to Amun (ChB 11)	
	excerpts from Satirical Letter (ChB 17)	
	Didactic excerpts (ChB 5, 18)	

Abbreviation
ChB – Chester Beatty

manner of a literary manuscript, and one papyrus that may have been used as a practical manual for someone guiding the performance of an offering ritual. The other manuscripts contain literary compositions, prescriptions for medicaments and the words to be spoken in healing rites. In Table 15.2, the group can be compared with the late Middle Kingdom papyri from the Ramesseum site (see Table 15.5 for a fuller list).

As on the Ramesseum Papyri, accounts and notes were added to some manuscripts, along with a copy of a letter to Panehesy, vizier of king Merenptah, from the *sš n p3 ḥr* 'Accountant of the Project' Qenherkhepshef (Gardiner 1935: 24–6, on Papyrus Chester Beatty 3). The title of Qenherkhepshef identifies him as the person responsible for keeping the accounts for one focal project of any 19th or 20th Dynasty reign, to decorate the tomb of the king at Thebes; this task was accomplished by a force of varying size, including higher status artists and their support teams, residing at a purpose-built village on the desert-cliff foot-hills, a site now known as Deir el-Medina (Černý 1973). As Gardiner noted, Jaroslav Černý identified the handwriting of the Qadesh Battle narrative on the same Papyrus Chester Beatty 3 as that of Qenherkhepshef; Černý could also cite other sources for men named in another note there, attesting to their activity as members of Project teams into the reign of Ramesses IV, one to two generations later than Qenherkhepshef himself (Gardiner 1935: 8, 26–7).

The full extent of the group and the find-place were revealed by Georges Posener, in completing the publication by Černý of a series of letters and separate list of tools, with part of a related legal document and one further literary manuscript from excavations at Deir el-Medina:

> Il est permis de dire à present que la découverte dépassa en importance les papyrus recueillis par le fouilleur le 20 février 1928. Le lendemain de cette découverte, Bernard Bruyère note dans son Journal de fouilles avoir entendu que "trois ouvriers du chantier le volaient" et il decide de les congédier. On saura plus tard que les papyrus Chester Beatty proviennent de la même trouvaille. Cinquante ans se sont écoulés depuis ces événements et il n'y a plus lieu d'entourer d'un voile pudique l'origine de la grande collection. (Posener 1978: viii)

Posener pin-pointed the location of the find as a deposit in a tomb courtyard south from chapel no. 1166, 'dans l'angle inférieur droit du plan du site publié dans *FIFAO* 6, II, pl. I' (Posener 1978: vii). Černý himself had earlier published the legal documents from the group; by the dispersal of the find, these are now divided between the French Institute in Cairo and the Ashmolean Museum, Oxford (Černý 1945). Their contents may be added to those of the Chester Beatty Papyri in Table 15.2 above.

Table 15.3   Further Deir el-Medina papyri assigned to the Qenherkhepshef group (after Posener 1978)

Contents	Location
Teaching of Any, incantations for good health	Institut Français d'Archéologie Orientale, DeM 1
Will of a woman named Niutnakht	Institut Français d'Archéologie Orientale DeM 2; Ashmolean Museum, Oxford
Letters	Institut Français d'Archéologie Orientale, DeM 3–16, 21–2
List of bronze tools	Institut Français d'Archéologie Orientale, DeM 17

From the observations by Gardiner on the condition of the manuscripts, from the personal names in notes added to the main contents and from the associated legal documents and letters, Pieter Pestman (1982) proposed to reconstruct an ancient life of the group, focusing on the Dream Book, Papyrus Chester Beatty 3:

> 1270s–1250s BC, early reign of Ramesses II: Dream Book is written down on the *recto*

1230s–1200s BC, late reign of Ramesses II or later later: Qenherkhepshef copies Qadesh Battle narrative on the verso
1213–1203 BC, reign of Merenptah: Qenherkhepshef adds to the verso a copy of his letter to vizier Panehesy
1170s–1130s BC, mid-20th Dynasty: note added to recto 'made by the writer Amennakht son of Khamnun, brother of the carpenter Neferhotep, of the carpenter Qenherkhepshef, and of the writer Pama ...'

In a final stage, a now presumably brittle papyrus suffered from being 'torn', according to Gardiner; this is interpreted as a destructive act by a later custodian or owner of the books, perhaps Maanakhtef, another son of Khamnun, known from other sources including letters and letter drafts concerning furniture-making (Pestman 1982: 159–61, noting that letter IFAO (Institut Français d'Archéologie Orientale) DeM (Deir el-Medina) 10 was written over an erased literary composition). Letter DeM 13 is the latest dated item, from the reign of Ramesses IX, *c*.1125–1107 BC. The legal documents include the transfer of property from Niutnakht in favour of the children who supported her during her old age; at the death of her first husband Qenherkhepshef the elder, she may have passed the documents to her subsequent husband Khamnun, as Pestman argues (Pestman 1982: 161), if not directly to their son Amennakht and his brother(s). However, the absence of any reference to the papyri in her transfer may indicate a degree of ambiguity or complexity in the obligations and the rights of access surrounding such material. Nor is it yet clear which factors permitted any decision to recycle papyri or parts of papyri, demonstrated by at least two of the letters, or how many individuals might be involved in the decision.

The details in the history of the papyri require further research of the whole group, starting from new inspection of the present condition of all items. Nevertheless, the find remains notable in combining what Pestman calls 'semi-literary' and 'real literary' compositions. As he remarked:

> It is particularly interesting to find so many texts in the last-mentioned category in this archive. The fact that the owners of the archive collected so many of these texts shows their great interest in literary matters ... These facts are surprising, for even though *Kn-ḥr-ḫpš.f* was a 'scribe of the Tomb' by profession, one would certainly not expect to find a man with such intellectual interests in a community of stone-cutters. And it is still more surprising to note that the second principal custodian of the archive, *Imn-nḥtw*, who was a simple workman, must have had these very same interests, for he cherished and even enlarged the collection. (Pestman 1982: 166)

In view of the results of their draughtsmanship in the Valley of the Kings, the artists of the Project must have required greater talent than this assessment allows. Nevertheless, Pestman exposes a vital lesson from the group, that an accountant – that is the 'job' of Qenherkhepshef – might assemble, copy and bequeath a diverse collection of narrative tales, eulogies, teachings, hymns, ritual manuals, health incantations and healing prescriptions in the thirteenth century BC. This lesson from the New Kingdom might be drawn out to other periods, including back to the late Middle Kingdom, when one or more people were involved in depositing a box with a similar range of writings in a tomb slightly further north in Thebes. In the accounts on the Ramesseum Papyri I had sought a title which I could relate to the forms of the figurines found with them, and to the rituals and incantations among the writings: 'the recurrence of priestly titles perhaps indicates some connection with the owner of these papyri' (Quirke 1990: 190). Yet alongside the words I was translating as 'lector-priest' and 'pure-priest', is one ḥȝty-ꜥ 'mayor', and no title is given for either of the men listed beside the entry 'my house/estate' (Barns 1955: pl. 25, lines 83–4). Today, I try to search for ancient writers and readers with fewer assumptions, perhaps in the company of Qenherkhepshef, accountant of the royal Project, and Amennakht, carpenter on the Project. Nor am I sure that our words 'scribe', 'priest' and 'doctor' help towards understanding the assignment of activities or division of labour in the ancient society. Rather than projecting our sense of professional identities onto the people of Egypt of the second millennium BC, we might consider outlines of their own interests, as different expressions of other lives. I hope that this act of reconsideration strikes some chord with Rosalie, for her own work on the archaeology of health and of people, as a tribute to her dedicated commitment to the living Egypt, past and present.

Table 15.4   Papyri from a box at the bottom of a tomb shaft in the area later covered by the Ramesseum store-rooms

Papyrus Ramesseum	Content	Frames/ length[a]	Height of papyrus roll[b]	Script	Location, inv. no.
A	Tales of Khuninpu, Sanehat	8	¼	HT	ÄMP 10499
B	Senusret I statue ritual ('Dramatic Papyrus')	5	1	CHG	BM 10610
C	Nubian fortress dispatches/incantations	5	1 > ½[c]	HT	BM 10752
D	word-list (Onomasticon)	10	½	HT	ÄMP 10495
E	funerary liturgy for rites at a mastaba	9	½	CHG	BM 10753
I	Lament of Sasobek	19	1	HT	BM 10754

2	miscellaneous didactic maxims	2 (c.1.0 m)	½	HT	BM 10755
3	prescriptions/ incantations for mother and child, eyes	13 (c.1.8 m)	1	HT	BM 10756
4	as 3 (part of same roll?)	6 (c.0.75 m + x)	1	HT	BM 10757
5	prescriptions for ointments to relax muscles	6 (c.1.0 m)	½	CHG	BM 10758
6	hymns to Sobek	7	½	CHG	BM 10759
7	incantations (funerary formulae?)	11	½	CHG	BM 10760
8	incantations against headache 'Hedjhotep offerings'	14	½	HT	BM 10761
9	incantation to protect house against harmful forces	3	18 cm	HT	BM 10762
10	Incantation to protect body against snakes	6	½	HT	BM 10763
11	incantations for good health (or love charms?)	2	½	HT	BM 10764
12	incantations against fever	2	1?	HT	BM 10765
13	incantations for health, list of 77 days of purification	1	½	HT	BM 10766
14	incantations for good health	1	½	HT	BM 10767
15	incantations for good health	1	½	HT	BM 10768
16	incantations for protection including against bad dreams	29	½	HT	BM 10769
17	incantations for the five days on the end of the year	5	½	HT	BM 10770
18	as C recto (dispatches) – part of same roll?	2	(1>)½	HT	BM 10771
19	incantations for good health	3	½?	HT	BM 10772
–	literary lament/didactic same roll as 1?	1 fragment?		HT	in BM 10754.D
20?	grain accounts – from one of the above?	1 (6 fragments)	?	HT	ÄMP 10131

Abbreviations
ÄMP – Ägyptisches Museum und Papyrussammlung, Berlin

BM – British Museum, London
CHG – cursive hieroglyphs
HT – hieratic

Notes
a   Includes number of frames in which fragments are mounted: frames vary in size.
b   1 = full height *c*.25–30 cm; ½ = half-height; ¼ = quarter-height.
c   A roll used full-height for its first use, later torn in half lengthways for its second use.
d   *Sources*: Gardiner 1955; Parkinson 2009: 14653; British Museum 2014.

Table 15.5   Papyri from one(?) find in 1928 at Deir el-Medina

Chester Beatty	Contents	Location
1	Late Egyptian Tale of Horus and Seth, love songs	Chester Beatty Library and Gallery, Dublin
2	Late Egyptian Tale of Truth and Falsehood	British Museum EA 10682
3	Dream Book, eulogy of Ramesses II at Battle of Qadesh	British Museum EA 10683
4	hymns, didactic excerpts	British Museum EA 10684
5	Middle Egyptian Hymn to Nile Flood, didactic excerpts	British Museum EA 10685
6	prescriptions and incantations for good health	British Museum EA 10686
7	incantations for good health	British Museum EA 10687
8	incantations for good health	British Museum EA 10688
9	offering ritual for Amun in name of king Amenhotep I, incantations for good health	British Museum EA 10689
10	aphrodisiacs	British Museum EA 10690
11	incantations for good health including Tale of Isis and Ra, hymn to Amun	British Museum EA 10691
12–15	incantations for good health	British Museum EA 10692-10695
16	incantation for purity	British Museum EA 10696
17	excerpts from Late Egyptian Satirical Letter	British Museum EA 10697
18	didactic excerpts, incantations for good health	British Museum EA 10698
19	Middle Egyptian Teaching of Khety	British Museum EA 10699
other		Ashmolean Museum, Oxford, and Institut Français d'Archéologie Orientale
	Teaching of Any, incantations for good health	Institut Français d'Archéologie Orientale DeM 1

will of a woman named Niutnakht	Institut Français d'Archéologie Orientale DeM 2 and Ashmolean Museum, Oxford
letters	Institut Français d'Archéologie Orientale DeM 3–16, 21–2
list of bronze tools	Institut Français d'Archéologie Orientale DeM 17

Sources: Černý 1945; Gardiner 1935; Pestman 1982; Posener 1978.

References

Barns, J. (1955), *Five Ramesseum Papyri* (Oxford: Oxford University Press).

Berger-el Naggar, C. (2004). 'Des textes des Pyramides sur papyrus dans les archives du temple funéraire de Pépy Ier.', in S. Bickel and B. Mathieu (eds.), *D'un monde à l'autre: Textes des Pyramides et Textes des Sarcophages* (Cairo: Institut Français d'Archéologie Orientale), 85–90.

Bourriau, J. (1991), 'Patterns of change in burial customs during the Middle Kingdom', in S. Quirke (ed.), *Middle Kingdom Studies* (Reigate: SIA Publishing), 3–20.

British Museum (2014), www.britishmuseum.org/research/publications/online_research_catalogues/rp/the_ramesseum_papyri/the_catalogue.aspx (consulted 30 October 2014).

Černý, J. (1945), 'The will of Naunakhte and the related documents', *Journal of Egyptian Archaeology* 31, 29–53.

Černý, J. (1973), *A Community of Workmen at Thebes in the Ramesside Period* (Cairo: Institut Français d'Archéologie Orientale).

Cuvigny, H. (2009), 'The finds of papyri: the archaeology of papyrology', in R. Bagnall (ed.), *The Oxford Handbook of Papyrology* (New York: Oxford University Press), 30–58.

Gardiner, A. (1935), *Hieratic Papyri in the British Museum: Third Series, Chester Beatty Gift* (London: British Museum).

Gardiner, A. (1955), *The Ramesseum Papyri* (Oxford: Oxford University Press).

Gnirs, A. (2009), 'Nilpferdstosszähne und Schlangenstäbe: zu den magischen Geräten des so genannten Ramesseumsfundes', in D. Kessler *et al.* (eds.), *Texte-Theben-Tonfragmente Festschrift für Günter Burkard* (Wiesbaden: Harrassowitz), 128–56.

Grajetzki, W. (2007), 'Multiple burials in ancient Egypt to the end of the Middle Kingdom', in S. Grallert and W. Grajetzki (eds.), *Life and Afterlife in Ancient Egypt during the Middle Kingdom and Second Intermediate Period* (London: Golden House), 16–34.

Gutekunst, W. (1986), 'Zauber', in W. Helck and W. Westendorf (eds.), *Lexikon der Ägyptologie*, VI (Wiesbaden: Harrassowitz), cols. 1320–55.

Kemp, B. and Merrillees, R. (1980), *Minoan Pottery in Second Millennium Egypt* (Wiesbaden: Harrassowitz).

Mace, A. and Winlock, H. (1916), *The Tomb of Senebtisi at Lisht* (New York: Metropolitan Museum of Art).

Messiha, K. and Messiha, H. (1964), 'A new concept about the implements found in the excavations at Gîza', *Annales du Service des antiquités de l'Égypte* 58, 209–25.

Miniaci, G. and Quirke, S. (2009), 'Reconceiving the tomb in the late Middle Kingdom: the burial of the Accountant of the Main Enclosure Neferhotep at Dra Abu al-Naga', *Bulletin de l'Institut français d'archéologie orientale* 109, 339–83.

Parkinson, R. (2009), *Reading Ancient Egyptian Poetry: Among Other Histories* (Chichester: Wiley-Blackwell).

Pestman, P. W. (1982), 'Who were the owners, in the "community of workmen", of the Chester Beatty Papyri?', in R. Demarée and J. J. Janssen (eds.), *Gleanings from Deir el-Medina* (Leiden: Nederlands Instituut voor het Nabije Oosten), 155–72.

Petrie, W. (1897), *Six Theban Temples. 1896* (London: Bernard Quaritch).

Posener, G. (1978), 'Introduction', in J. Černý and G. Posener (eds.), *Papyrus hiératiques de Deir el-Medineh*, I (Cairo: Institut Français d'Archéologie Orientale).

Quibell, J. (1898), *The Ramesseum* (London: Bernard Quaritch).

Quirke, S. (1990), *The Administration of Egypt in the Late Middle Kingdom: The Hieratic Documents* (New Malden: SIA Publishing).

Quirke, S. (2015), *Birth Tusks: The Armoury of Health in Context – Egypt 1800 BC* (London: Golden House).

Seidlmayer, S. (2006), 'People at Beni Hassan: contributions to a model of ancient Egyptian rural society', in Z. A. Hawass and J. E. Richards (eds.), *The Archaeology and Art of Ancient Egypt: Essays in Honor of David B. O'Connor*, II (Cairo: Conseil Suprême des Antiquités de l'Égypte), 351–68.

Sommer, U. (1991), *Zur Entstehung archäologischer Fundvergesellschaftungen: Versuch einer archäologischen Taphonomie* (Bonn: Habelt).

Vernus, P. (1986), 'Le prêtre-ritualiste Hr-mni, rédacteur de la stèle de Hr-m-xaw.f', in A. Guillaumont *et al.* (eds.), *Hommages à François Daumas*, II (Montpellier: Université de Montpellier), 588–92.

Yoyotte, J. (1957), Review of Gardiner 1955, *Revue d'Égyptologie* 11, 172–5.

Zivie, A. (1990), *Découverte à Saqqarah: le vizir oublié* (Paris: Seuil).

16

Schistosomiasis, ancient and modern: the application of scientific techniques to diagnose the disease

Patricia Rutherford

Currently more than 300 million people worldwide are infected by schisto-somes, which cause the disease state of schistosomiasis. Infection is most evident in communities of the developing world that lie between the latitude lines of 36 degrees north and 34 degrees south where fresh water temperatures range between 25°C and 35°C, the perfect temperature in which the larvae and intermediate hosts can live (Strickland 1991: 781–808). Village communities that dwell by rivers constantly swim, fish and wash there, and this lifestyle, combined with increased irrigation and poor sanitation, makes them vulnerable to the cercariae (free-swimming larval stage). The parasitic *Schistosoma* lives and feeds upon the cells, blood, mucus and tissue fluids of its primary host and although most *Schistosoma* infect only animals, humans can be infected.

The three main species responsible for the infection are *Schistosoma mansoni*, *S. haematobium* and *S. japonicum*. As shown in Figure 16.1, *S. mansoni* and *S. japoni-cum* live primarily within the veins of the hepatic portal system, which drains the intestines, whereas *S. haematobium* live primarily in the veins draining the bladder. Schistosomes can live in humans for over twenty years, continually breeding and producing thousands of spiny ova, half of which are released back into the water via faeces or urine, depending on the worm's location in the body, while the other half remain in the body, causing damage to lung, neural and renal tissues. This mechanical damage is combined with immunological and pathologic reactions such as inflammation, fibrosis, cirrhosis, abdominal distension and hemorrhaging (Cheever 1969).

Although first described in detail in the early 1900s by Bilharz (1852, for *S. haematobium*), Sambon (1907, for *S. mansoni*) and Logan (1905, for *S. japonicum*), studies of ancient literature, artistic representations and physical remains have suggested that schistosomiasis is an ancient disease. For example one of the clas-sic symptoms, blood in the urine, is described in the Ebers Papyrus as the *aaa*

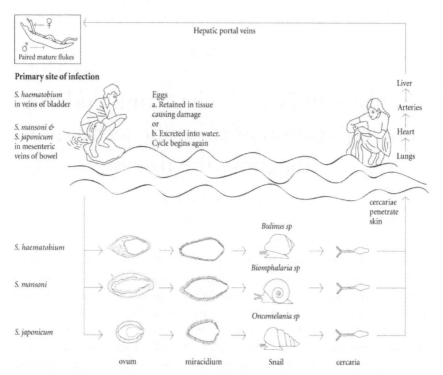

16.1 The lifecycle of S. mansoni, S. haematobium and S. japonicum. (Modified by the author and J. Sherry from the original by G. Barnish in Sturrock 2001: 9.)

disease (Farooq 1973: 1–16; Contis and David 1996). The ancient Egyptians also wrote that boys became men when blood was seen in their urine, and likened this to the young females' first menstruation (Hoeppli 1973: 2). Also, tissues dating as far back as 5,000 years have been positively diagnosed with the disease (Deelder *et al.* 1990).

Taking the aforementioned information into account, a joint project was born between the Manchester Museum Mummy Project, the Egyptian Reference Diagnostic Centre of the Egyptian Organization for Biological and Vaccine Production (VACSERA) and Medical Service Corporation International, Arlington, Virginia, USA (Contis and David 1996). The aim of the Schistosomiasis Research Project was to create an epidemiological profile of schistosomiasis in Egypt spanning 5,000 years. To fulfil this, ancient tissue samples from collections worldwide had to be acquired for testing (Lambert-Zazulak, Rutherford and David 2003; see also Lambert-Zazulak in Chapter 25). Once they were collected the development of robust, cost-effective, reproducible tests that could be applied to a large-scale study was needed (Rutherford 1997, 1999, 2000, 2002).

Diagnosis of schistosomiasis in modern patients can be achieved by radiology (which shows calcification of the bladder) and histology as well as molecular tests that detect antibodies towards schistosoma antigens, that is, the enzyme-linked immunosorbent assay (ELISA). Alternatively, ova can be observed microscopically in rectal snips, faeces or urine since the distinct ova shapes of each species can confirm which particular species has infected the host. Such microscopic analysis is the most common test used in the field today as it is quick and easy; however, such tests require body fluids, which are not available in mummified remains. Previous analyses of ancient remains for schistosomiasis also have limitations; for example, histology (Ruffer 1910; Millet *et al.* 1980), radiology (Isherwood, Jarvis and Fawcett 1979) and ELISA (Deelder *et al.* 1990; Miller *et al.* 1992; Miller *et al.* 1993: 55–60) can all be impractical when working with ancient tissues on a large scale as they may be very expensive (radiology and ELISA) or low in sensitivity (histology). Although histology would be the obvious choice for detecting ova in bladder and viscera samples, previous research has shown it to produce inconsistent results (Tapp 1979, 1984). Therefore, an alternative test was sought that would be cost-effective, reproducible and sensitive. Immunocytochemistry met all the aforementioned criteria, and was successfully applied to both modern and ancient tissues (Rutherford 1997, 1999, 2000, 2002). This immunosassay exploits the reaction between antibodies and antigens, as antibodies raised by infecting laboratory animals with the disease of interest can easily be isolated and conjugated to a tag that can be visualised directly or under a certain ultraviolet wavelength (Burry 2009: 1–4).

Previous research has applied immunocytochemistry to ancient tissues to reveal the presence of cellular components (Horton *et al.* 1983; Krypczyk and Tapp 1986; Fulcheri, Baracchini and Rabino Massa 1992; Nerlich *et al.* 1993) but not to demonstrate the disease. Studies have also embedded ancient samples in paraffin wax, a type of tissue preparation that has been successfully carried out for many years, predominately for histological purposes (Ruffer 1910; Tapp 1979: 95–102). However, the preparation in hot wax often has deleterious effects upon the tissue, causing diffusion, loss and even chemical alterations to the antigens of interest. As the ancient schistosoma antigens are already much degraded and are present only in very small quantities, such high temperatures have to be avoided. Therefore in this study both modern and ancient tissues were embedded in a cold medium called glycol methacrylate (GMA; Taab, UK) which polymerises at 4°C. The hardened resin allowed much thinner tissue sections to be cut (2 μm), which enhanced the sensitivity of immunocytochemistry tests and provided more support for the fragile ancient samples (Rutherford 1999).

Modern controls

A protocol had to be established using modern samples known to be infected with schistosoma before investigating finite ancient samples. Once procedures were established with the modern samples, such positive and negative modern samples then served as controls, which were directly compared with the ancient samples also being tested. In order to limit unnecessary sampling of ancient tissues an interim step was carried out to ascertain whether antisera would react with infected tissues that had been blocked in wax, and then poorly stored for over fifty years. Infected bladder tissue taken from an Egyptian cadaver over fifty years ago was the specimen utilised. If positive results were not achieved with this sample then the probability of antigens being present in the ancient samples would be low (Rutherford 1997, 1999, 2000, 2002).

Using an array of antisera directed towards an array of epitope sites found on *S. mansoni* (raised in rabbit) and *S. haematobium* (raised in hamster), antigens were used. Rabbit and hamster serum taken from unimmunised rabbits (Sigma Diagnostics, UK) was also used to ensure the reactivity of the antisera. As an indirect immunostaining protocol was used, the secondary antibody was conjugated to biotin (i.e. donkey biotinylated anti-rabbit, Amersham, UK, and goat biotinylated anti-hamster, Jacksons, USA). To visualise the reaction, the protein streptavidin conjugated with fluorescein (FITC; Amersham, UK), was used. Before any antiserum was applied to the sections, a blocking serum was applied (10 ml PBS pH 7.4, 0.05 g Bovine Serum Albumin, 150 μl donkey serum (*S. mansoni*) or goat serum (*S. haematobium*), 50 μl Triton X).

Preparation of ancient samples

Experimental designs for the ancient samples were approached cautiously with earlier research being taken into account; for example, in previous histological studies of ancient mummified tissues the most commonly used rehydrating solutions were those developed by Ruffer (1921: 11–17) and Sandison (1955). However, a comparative study done by Turner and Holtom (1981) had shown that these solutions do not always produce suitable tissue samples for sectioning, when compared with the use of a fabric conditioner trade-named Comfort® (Lever Bros). However, as the type of experiments undertaken in this study were predominately immunological, the colour, preservatives and perfumes found in the Comfort® fabric conditioner were unacceptable, as they may have interfered with the immunocytochemistry in some way. Therefore, an alternative conditioner, which contains no perfume, preservatives or colour, was selected (Surfacem, UK).

There was a marked difference between preparations of modern and ancient samples for immunocytochemistry. Unfortunately, only a few ancient samples were prepared with the same ease as the modern tissues. One Pharaonic example was a sample of liver tissue taken from a canopic jar discovered in an unopened tomb at Rifeh. The jar, which contained no debris or resins, belonged to the 12th Dynasty mummy of Nakht-Ankh. This tissue was easily sectioned, demonstrated good tissue integrity and also supported other researchers' results (Tapp 1979: 95–102).

The remaining ancient samples had varying degrees of mummification resins and gritty particles enmeshed within them, and such artefacts inhibited the sectioning process markedly. As the gritty particles were siliceous in nature a very dilute solution of hydrofluoric acid (2.5 per cent) was used to remove the silica (sand) particles from the ancient samples, thus enabling very thin (2 μm), flat, intact sections to be cut with ease. This was chosen following the example of palaeobotanists, who use hydrofluoric acid to decalcify ancient petrified seeds and plant material without damaging delicate specimens (F. Barnett, personal communication, 1997). Experiments with both modern and ancient tissues showed that at the correct dilution of 2.5 per cent, the acid does not disrupt the antigenic epitopes, as positive staining still occurred. A range of knives were also explored. If no silica was present, glass Ralf knives were used as tungsten knives were easily damaged. If silica was evident, a diamond knife was used, but even after hydrofluoric acid treatment the knife was often still damaged.

Results of immunostaining

Between 1995 and 2002 fifty samples were tested, and the results obtained from immunostaining and other reinforcing analyses indicated a positive result in 36 per cent of the cases (Rutherford 2002). One such example is that of a Roman Period mummy in the Manchester Museum (no. 1766) which had displayed calcified bladder tissue in previous X-ray studies (Tapp 1979: 95–102; Tapp 1984: 78–95). Discrete staining to both ova and worms was seen. These results were assessed by experts in this field at VACSERA, Egypt, who confirmed these to be *S. haematobium* ova and worms (Al Sherbiny, personal communication, 1999). The ELISA discussed below also supported these results indicating a positive result for circulating anodic antigens (CAAs) (80 ng/ml). Details of each sample, its provenance status and its results can be seen in Rutherford (2002).

Other diagnostic tests

Although immunocytochemistry was the first protocol used upon samples and became the mainstay of the research, other diagnostic tests were also investigated; for example reagents to perform the ELISA were kindly provided by

Professor Deelder. As the ELISA target is a CAA regurgitated from the worms' gut, it should be present in all vascular tissues of the body, in contrast to the ova and worms that are found only in specific sites (Deelder *et al.* 1990; Miller *et al.* 1992; Miller *et al.* 1993: 55–60). Therefore the ELISA was initially used to both reinforce immunostaining results and increase the sample number, as there are many body parts in collections around the world. The test, however, does have limitations: the CAAs are present only during the occurrence of an active infection as they are degraded each day by the liver (Deelder *et al.* 1990).

Other tests such as histology, enzyme-linked immunoelectro-transfer blot (EITB) (Al Sherbiny *et al.* 1999) and DNA analysis were also explored as additional techniques when immunostaining results were positive. Histology was used to demonstrate the general morphology of tissue samples and DNA content, whereas the EITB targeted antibodies rather than antigens in the tissue. However, the EITB test was quickly discarded from the study as it targeted antibodies rather than antigens in the samples and was also found to be less sensitive than the antigen tests (Rutherford 2002).

The results of the immunostaining also dictated whether DNA analysis was carried out. Although such analysis could identify the actual species that had caused the infection, the decision to destroy finite samples should always be approached with caution, not only from an ethical point of view but also because of the considerable difficulties associated with the analysis of ancient DNA (Pääbo 1989; Pääbo *et al.* 2004). Again, the most obvious limitation was the availability of suitable samples, as the ancient schistosome DNA can be extracted only from tissue that harbours the ova and worms. Therefore, only a few of the available mummy tissue samples were selected for testing in the schistosomiasis study for the schistosoma parasite at the DNA level.

DNA studies

This area of study was just as challenging as the immunocytochemistry research. The first question that had to be addressed was 'Is mummified tissue suitable for DNA analysis?' Desiccated mummies are often well preserved because of the lack of moisture, and as the action of damaging nucleases is dependent upon moisture, the DNA molecule may incur less nucleotide damage. Also, as the mummification process used natron, an alkaline compound, then this is beneficial to the survival of the acidic DNA molecule. Air-tight tombs in which some mummies have been discovered also inhibit certain chemical reactions and decomposition by aerobic micro-organisms. Additionally low temperatures, dry air in the tomb, desiccation and alkalinity of the natron provide good preservation conditions for the DNA molecule (Lindahl 1993; Burger *et al.* 1999; Willerslev and Cooper 2005). Some researchers have gone on record stating that 'aDNA investigations in pharaonic mummy tissue samples is indeed not senseless' (Zink and Nerlich 2003: 110).

At the time of the study (1997), several reports with promising results began to appear and diagnosis of disease in ancient remains were being described; for example, Sallares *et al.* (2000) reported that they had amplified part of the 18s ribosomal DNA specific for *Plasmodium falciparum* which causes the disease malaria. Guhl *et al.* (1999) stated that 330 base pairs of *Trypansoma cruzi* DNA were amplified in order to confirm the presence of Chagas' disease. Other diseases such as plague (Drancourt *et al.* 1998), leprosy (Montiel *et al.* 2003) and tuberculosis (Donoghue *et al.* 1998) were identified. Also, the DNA of bacteria *Vibrio* was found in the gut flora of the Tyrolean Iceman by Cano *et al.* (2000) and *E. coli* in the Lindow Man by Fricker *et al.* (1997). Such positive results inspired optimism about the DNA study, which after considerable research produced some positive results. In particular, 236 base pairs of the *S. haematobium* cytochrome oxidase C fragment were sequenced from the bladder tissue of an Egyptian mummy known as Besenmut, a priest in the temple of Min in Akhmim, now in Leicester (700 BC). This allowed the parasite to be located to an area and time. Other tests such as immunocytochemistry supported this result (Rutherford 2002).

Today ancient DNA work is widely reported, but at the time of the schistosomiasis project (1995) the research was still in its infancy. Accounts of the problems and solutions at that time influenced the protocols adopted by the writer, for example, as only 1–2 per cent of the DNA yield that is expected from modern samples is extracted from ancient tissues (Pääbo 1989; Pääbo 1990: 159–66; Pääbo *et al.* 2004). Many researchers have concentrated on targeting mitochondrial DNA (mtDNA), as there are several hundred copies of this genome per cell in contrast to two copies of each gene locus in the nuclear genome (Stone *et al.* 1996). It also has the bonus of being inherited exclusively through the maternal line and is therefore used in sibship studies.

Another advantage is its circular structure, which is supercoiled, in contrast to the linear nuclear DNA, which is easily degraded. This supercoiling seems to protect the mtDNA from excessive cleaving, thus producing fragment lengths of between 100 and 500 base pairs (Hagelberg 1994: 195–204; Pääbo *et al.* 2004). However, in general only small fragments of ancient DNA survive albeit from the nucleus or organelle, the average size being about 200–300 base pairs (Kaestle and Horsburgh 2002: 92–130). Therefore, despite mtDNA being present in high copy numbers the amount of damage is the same. One could hypothesise that the histones present in the nucleus serve to protect the DNA wrapped around them (approximately 200 base pairs) in the same way as supercoiling protects mitochondrial DNA, and that therefore the only real advantage to working with mtDNA is its abundance.

The small amounts of degraded DNA present have to be amplified for analysis, and this is achieved by using the polymerase chain reaction (PCR) devised
by Mullis and Faloona (1987). Although this was primarily devised for modern
DNA amplification, small intact copies of DNA can be amplified alongside the
badly degraded DNA molecules, thus eliminating many modification problems
(Rutherford 2002).

Modern DNA controls

Before ancient samples were analysed protocols had to be established upon
modern samples. *S. mansoni* and *S. haematobium* worm, cercarea and ova DNA
were obtained from the Christie Hospital, Manchester, to use as positive controls. Negative controls were also incorporated into the study, that is, distilled
water and reagents only. Positive controls were amplified and extracted in
a different area from the ancient samples, which were studied in a separate
laboratory. All steps were done under sterile conditions. Experiments were also
repeated to confirm the results if possible (Rutherford 2002).

When DNA is extracted from a modern sample, visual assessment of the
sample plays an important part in obtaining a clear, uncontaminated extract.
When one is working with ancient mummy tissues this is very difficult to achieve
as the mummification resin, dirt and salts present are released into the solutions
being used. Therefore, several centrifugation steps are sometimes necessary.
Even after this, the preparation would often be still slightly brown in colour
which obscured spectrometry readings. The use of silica beads was considered
in order to further clean up the samples, but as Hoss and Pääbo (1993) reported
additional loss of DNA with such beads, it was therefore decided not to pursue
this option (Rutherford 2002).

After extraction from modern samples the DNA is often visible to the naked
eye as small strands. However, it is often not visible in ancient extracts, owing
to the discoloration of extraction solutions. Therefore, caution was always taken
when separating the organic and inorganic phases with pipettes. There was only
one example where the ancient DNA was visible after extraction, that being a
sample from the liver of the 12th Dynasty mummy of Nakht-Ankh. This was
not surprising as this sample appeared similar to modern liver after having been
treated with conditioning solution.

Several ancient samples yielded DNA but, unfortunately, contamination
inhibited amplification and sequencing of the DNA except for the 236 base
pair segment previously mentioned, that belonged to *S. haematobium* cytochrome
oxidase C. The sequence was subjected to a BLAST (Basic Local Alignment
Search Tool) search that confirmed a 97 per cent match to *S. haematobium*.
However, the ethics of total destruction of samples should be addressed, as in

these situations there is often no material left for replication of results. To simply destroy a sample for a meagre 200–300 base pairs of DNA seems excessive and so alternatives should always be considered first. Therefore, only a select few of the mummy tissue samples available for testing in the schistosomiasis study were investigated for the schistosoma parasite at the DNA level.

Conclusion

Although the ideal samples for these investigations are tissues that harbour ova and worms from provenanced mummies, such criteria were only partially met. Several samples were collected to establish what experimental formats were the most appropriate, and only when standard procedures had been determined did sample collection shift in context, to only provenanced samples that could be documented to a certain place and time. The study did however place the presence of schistosomiasis in ancient Middle and Upper Egypt (see Rutherford 2002).

To study the distribution patterns of any infection such as schistosomiasis, the provenance of the sample being investigated is required: a criterion that many isolated body parts do not meet. Therefore, large-scale epidemiological studies must aim to collect provenanced samples. There is little purpose in destroying ancient tissue samples that may well provide results, but which are then unable to be applied to a particular place in time or area. Unfortunately, many museums house high numbers of body parts in comparison to whole mummies, and although such artefacts have served in establishing optimum protocols, such samples have limits in relation to epidemiology studies. The subsequent collection of medieval samples from Sudanese Nubia dating to around AD 500 and samples from the forty-eight Graeco-Roman mummies found in the Dakhleh Oasis have addressed this issue. This particular group is an excellent source of material as many of the samples have been taken from the liver, colon, intestines and even coprolites, which harbour not only schistosome worms and ova but other diseases that warrant investigation.

This research project was able to produce a list of what was practical as well as highlighting many limiting factors. The established protocols are now recorded so that investigators can draw upon them and adapt them to their own research, thereby, it is hoped, saving time and protecting the finite ancient remains from unnecessary destruction.

Acknowledgements

The author would like to acknowledge the contributions of the following: the Kay Hinckley Charitable Trust; Professor M. J. Ferguson; Professor A. R. David;

Dr P. Lambert Zazulak; the Egyptian Reference Diagnostic Centre of the Egyptian Organization for Biological and Vaccine Production (VACSERA); and Professor M. Doenhoff, University of Bangor, Wales. Special thanks must be expressed to all depositors of tissue for testing, and particularly to Professor D. Van Gervan and Professor A. Aufderheide for donating a large number of samples.

References

Al-Sherbiny, M. M., Osman, A. M., Hancock, K., Deelder, A. M. and Tsang, C.W. (1999), 'The application of immunodiagnostic assays: detection of antibodies and circulating antigens in human schistosomiasis and correlation with clinical findings', *American Journal of Tropical Medicine and Hygiene* 60, 960–6.

Bilharz, T. M. (1852), 'Ferere Beobachtungun uber das die Pfortader des Menschen bewohnende *Distomum haematobium* und sein Verhaltniss zu gewissen pathoogishen Bildungen aus brieflichen Mitheilungen an Professor v. Sielbold vom 29 März 1852', *Zeitschrift für wissenschaftliche Zoologie* 4, 72–6.

Burger, J., Hummel, S., Hermann, B. and Henke, W. (1999), 'DNA preservation: a microsatellite DNA study on ancient skeletal remains', *Electrophoresis* 20, 1722–8.

Burry, R. W. (2009), *Immunocytochemistry: A Practical Guide for Biomedical Research* (New York: Springer).

Cano, R. J., Pioner, H. N., Pieniazek, N. J., Acra, A. and Poiner, G. O. Jr (1993), 'Amplification and sequencing of DNA from a 120–135 million year old weevil', *Nature* 363, 536–8.

Cheever, A. W. (1969), 'Quantitative comparison of intensity of *Schistosoma mansoni* infections in man and experimental animals', *Transactions of the Royal Society of Tropical Medicine and Hygiene* 63, 781–95.

Contis, G. and David, A. R. (1996), 'The epidemiology of *Bilharzia* in ancient Egypt: 5000 years of schistosomiasis', *Parasitology Today* 12 (7), 253–5.

Deelder, A. M., Miller, R. L., Dejonge, N. and Krijger, F. W. (1990), 'Detection of shistosome antigens in mummies', *The Lancet* 335 (8691), 724–5.

Donoghue, H. D., Spigelman, M., Zias, J., Gemaey-Child, A. M. and Minnikn, D. E. (1998), '*Mycobacterium tuberculosis* complex DNA in calcified pleura from remains 1400 years old', *Letters in Applied Microbiology* 27, 265–9.

Drancourt, M., Aboudharam, G., Signol, M., Dutour, O. and Raoult, D. (1998), 'Detection of 400 year-old *Yersinia pestis* DNA in human dental pulp: an approach to the diagnosis of ancient septicemia', *Proceedings of the National Academy of Sciences of the USA* 95, 12637–40.

Farooq, N. (1973) 'Historical development', in N. Ansari (ed.), *Epidemiology and Control of Schistosomiasis (Bilharziasis)* (Basel: S. Karger), 1–16.

Fricker, E. J., Spigelman, M. and Freicker, C. R. (1997), 'The detection of *Escherichia coli* DNA in the ancient remains of Lindow Man using the polymerase chain reaction', *Letters in Applied Microbiology* 24 (5), 351–4.

Fulcheri, E., Baracchini, P. and Rabino Massa, E. (1992), 'Immunocytochemistry in histopaleopathology', in A. C. Aufderheide (ed.), *Abstract in Proceedings of the First*

World Congress of Mummy Studies, II (Tenerife: Archaeological and Ethnographical Museum of Tenerife), 559.

Guhl, F., Jaramillo, C., Vallejo, G. A., Yockteng, R. and Cárdenas-Arroyo, F. (1999), 'Isolation of *Trypanosoma cruzi* DNA in 4,000-year-old mummified human tissue from northern Chile', *American Journal of Physical Anthropology* 108, 401–7.

Hagelberg, E. (1994), 'Mitochondrial DNA from ancient bones', in B. Herrmann and S. Hummel (eds.), *Ancient DNA* (New York: Springer-Verlag), 195–204.

Higuchi, R., Bowman, B., Freiberger, M., Ryder, O. A. and Wilson, A. C. (1984), 'DNA sequences from the quagga, an extinct member of the horse family', *Nature* 312, 282–4.

Hoeppli, R. (1973), 'Morphological changes in human schistosomiasis and certain analogues in ancient Egyptian sculpture', *Acta Tropica* (Basel) 30, 1–11.

Horton, W. A., Dwyer, C., Goering, R. and Dean, D. C. (1983), 'Immunohistochemistry of types I & II collagen in uncalcified skeletal tissues', *Journal of Histochemistry & Cytochemistry* 31 (3), 417–25.

Hoss, M. and Pääbo, S. (1993), 'DNA extraction from Pleistocene bones by a silica based purification method', *Nucleic Acids Research* 21 (16), 3913–14.

Isherwood, I., Jarvis, H. and Fawcett, R. A. (1979), 'Radiology of the Manchester mummies', in: A. R. David (ed.), *The Manchester Museum Mummy Project: Multidisciplinary Research on Ancient Egyptian Mummified Remains* (Manchester: Manchester University Press), 25–64.

Kaestle, F. A. and Horsburgh, K. A. (2002), 'Ancient DNA in anthropology: methods, applications and ethics', *Yearbook of Physical Anthropology* 45, 92–130.

Krypczyk, A. and Tapp, E. (1986), 'Immunocytochemistry and electron microscopy of Egyptian mummies', in A. R. David (ed.), *Science in Egyptology: Proceedings of the 'Science in Egyptology' Symposia* (Manchester: Manchester University Press), 361–5.

Lambert-Zazulak, P. I., Rutherford, P. and David, A. R. (2003), 'The International Ancient Egyptian Mummy Tissue Bank at the Manchester Museum as a resource for the palaeoepidemiological study of schistosomiasis', *World Archaeology* 35 (2), 223–40.

Lindahl, T. (1993), 'Instability and decay of the primary structure of DNA', *Nature* 362, 709–15.

Logan, O. T. (1905), 'A case of dysentery in Hunan Province caused by the trematode *Schistosoma japonicum*', *Chinese Medical Journal* 19, 243–5.

Miller, R. L., Armelagos, G. J., Ikram, S., Dejonge, N., Krijer, F. W. and Deelder, A. M. (1992), 'Palaeoepidemiology of *Schistosoma* infection in mummies', *British Medical Journal* 304, 555–6.

Miller, R, L., Dejonge, N., Krijger, F. W. and Deelder, A. M. (1993), 'Predynastic schistosomiasis', in W. V. Davies and R. Walker (eds.), *Biological Anthropology and the Study of Ancient Egypt* (London: British Museum Press), 55–60.

Millet, N. B., Hart, G. D., Reyman, T. A., Zimmerman, M. R. and Lewin, P. K. (1980), 'ROM1: mummification for the common people', in A. Cockburn and E. Cockburn (eds.), *Mummies, Disease and Ancient Cultures* (Cambridge: Cambridge University Press), 71–84.

Montiel, R., Garcia, C., Canadas, M. P., Isidro, A., Guijo, J. M. and Malgosa, A.

(2003), 'DNA sequences of *Mycobacterium leprae* recovered from ancient bones', *FEMS Microbiology Letters* 226 (2), 413–14.

Mullis, K. B. and Faloona, F. A. (1987), 'Specific synthesis of DNA in *vitro* via a polymerase-catalysed chain reaction', *Methods in Enzymology* 155, 335–50.

Nerlich, A. G., Parsche, F., Kirsch, T., Wiest, I. and von der Mark, K. (1993), 'Immunohistochemical detection of intestinal collagens in bones and cartilage tissue remnants in an infant Peruvian mummy', *American Journal of Physical Anthropology* 91 (3), 269–85.

Pääbo, S. (1989), 'Ancient DNA: extraction, characterization, molecular cloning, and enzymatic amplification', *Proceedings of the National Academy of Sciences of the USA* 86, 1939–43.

Pääbo, S. (1990), 'Amplifying ancient DNA', in M. A. Innis, D. H. Gelfand, J. J. Sninsky, T. J. White (eds.), *PCR Protocols: A Guide to Methods and Applications* (San Diego: Academic Press,), 159–66.

Pääbo, S., Pioner, H., Serre, D., Jaenicke-Despres, V., Hebler, J., Rohland, N., Kuch, M., Krause, J., Vigilant, L. and Hofreiter, M. (2004), 'Genetic analysis from ancient DNA', *Annual Review of Genetics* 38, 645.

Ruffer, M. A. (1910), 'Note on the presence of "Bilharzia haematobia" in Egyptian mummies of the Twentieth Dynasty 91250–1000 BC)', *British Medical Journal* 1 (2557), 16.

Ruffer, M. A. (1921), *Studies in Palaeopathology of Egypt* (Chicago: University of Chicago), 11–17.

Rutherford, P. (1997) 'The Diagnosis of Schistosomiasis by Means of Immunocytochemistry upon Appropriately Prepared Modern and Ancient Mummified Tissues' (MSc thesis, University of Manchester).

Rutherford, P. (1999), 'Immunocytochemistry and the diagnosis of schistosomiaisis: ancient and modern', *Parasitology Today* 15 (9), 390–1.

Rutherford, P. (2000), 'The diagnosis of schistosomiasis in modern and ancient tissues by means of immunocytochemistry', *Chungara: Revista de antropologia Chilena* 32 (1), 127–31.

Rutherford, P. (2002), 'Schistosomiasis: The Dynamics of Diagnosing a Parasitic Disease in Ancient Egyptian Tissue' (PhD dissertation, University of Manchester).

Sallares, R., Gomzi, S., Richards, A. and Anderung, C. (2000), 'Evidence from ancient DNA for malaria in antiquity', paper presented at the Fifth International Ancient DNA Conference, Manchester.

Sambon, L. W. (1907), 'Remarks on *Schistosoma mansoni*', *Journal of Tropical Medicine and Hygiene* 10, 303–4.

Sandison, A. T. (1955), 'The histological examination of mummified material', *Stain Technology* 30 (6), 277–83.

Stone, A. C., Milner, G. R., Paabo, S. and Stoneking, M. (1996), 'Sex determination of ancient human skeletons using DNA', *American Journal of Physical Anthropology* 99, 231–8.

Strickland, G. T. (1991) (ed.), *Hunter's Tropical Medicine*, 7th edn (London: W. B. Saunders Company).

Sturrock, R. F. (2001), 'The schistosomes and their intermediate hosts', in A. A. F. Mahmoud (ed.), *Schistosomiasis* (London: Imperial College Press), 7–84.

Tapp, E. (1979), 'Diseases in the Manchester Mummies', in A. R. David (ed.) *The Manchester Museum Mummy Project: Multidisciplinary Research on Ancient Egyptian Mummified Remains* (Manchester: Manchester University Press), 95–102.

Tapp, E. (1984), 'Disease in the Manchester mummies: the pathologist's role', in A. R. David and E. Tapp (eds.), *Evidence Embalmed: Modern Medicine and the Mummies of Ancient Egypt* (Manchester: Manchester University Press), 78–95.

Turner, P. J. and Holtom, D. B. (1981), 'The use of a fabric softener in the reconstitution of mummified tissue prior to paraffin wax sectioning for light microscopical examination', *Stain Technology* 56 (1), 35–8.

Willerslev, E. and Cooper, A. (2005), 'Ancient DNA', *Proceedings of the Royal Society of Biological Sciences* 272 (1558), 3–16.

Zink, A. and Nerlich, A. G. (2003), 'Molecular analysis of the Pharaohs: feasibility of molecular studies in ancient Egyptian material', *American Journal of Physical Anthropology* 121, 109–10.

17

An unusual funerary figurine of the early 18th Dynasty

John H. Taylor

The small wooden figurine which is the subject of this chapter is a carved and painted representation of an anthropoid coffin of a type which can be dated to the earlier part of the 18th Dynasty. Containers in the form of miniature coffins are examples of a well-known class of object which have been found in funerary contexts at several sites in Egypt and Sudan, where they were used as receptacles for human remains, for the figurines which are conventionally termed shabtis and occasionally for other objects, but the present example is unusual in having been carved in a single piece, without a cavity. Its date and possible function will be considered below. It is a pleasure to dedicate this article to Rosalie David, whose pioneering multi-disciplinary research has inspired a generation of younger scholars to apply innovative scientific methods to the study of mummies and grave goods to enhance our understanding of life and death in the ancient Nile valley.

Acquisition

The figurine entered the collections of the British Museum, London, in 1915, when it was purchased from the Cairo antiquities dealer Panayotis Kyticas. It was assigned the number EA 53995, but no provenance was recorded in the acquisitions register of the then Department of Egyptian and Assyrian Antiquities. Described there simply as a 'painted wooden ushabti figure', it was acquired from Kyticas among a group of eighty-seven miscellaneous objects (EA 1651–2, 53966–54050) which included shabtis of various periods, bronze figurines and utensils and Coptic antiquities, none of which appear to have any strong contextual affinity with the item here under discussion. The figurine has so far received only a single brief notice in print (Taylor 2001b: 177, n. 15). Although it

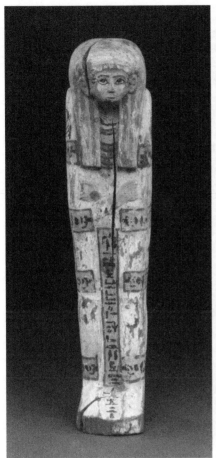
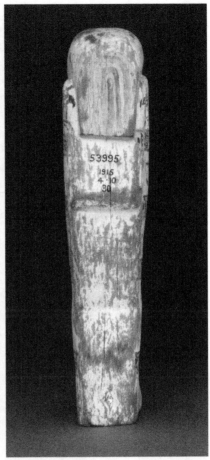

17.1 Figurine of Senty-resti, front view. British Museum EA 53995. (Courtesy of the Trustees of the British Museum.)

17.2 Figurine of Senty-resti, rear view. British Museum EA 53995. (Courtesy of the Trustees of the British Museum.)

has hitherto been classed among shabtis in the collections of the British Museum, it is not a conventional shabti and its true function requires further elucidation.

Description

The figurine (see Figures 17.1–6 and Plate 7) is carved from a single piece of wood, identified microscopically as *ficus sycomorus* by Caroline Cartwright of the Department of Conservation and Scientific Research at the British Museum. It measures 21.1 cm in length, with a maximum width of 5.0 cm and a maximum depth of 4.9 cm. The head, carved in the round, occupies a relatively low position in relation to the shoulders. The face is oval, with large protruding ears, the skin is coloured yellow, and the eyes and eyebrows are painted in black and white. A tripartite wig or headdress, painted with blue and yellow stripes, extends over the breast and down the back to a point midway between the shoulders and the buttocks. The rows of a broad collar are represented between the wig lappets as bands of blue and yellow, outlined in black. These rows are not continued on the outer edges of the figure, but large collar terminals in the shape of falcon-heads are represented in black outline at the shoulders. Below the collar the two hands are depicted carved in lightly raised relief, crossing on the breast with the right hand uppermost, the skin painted yellow.

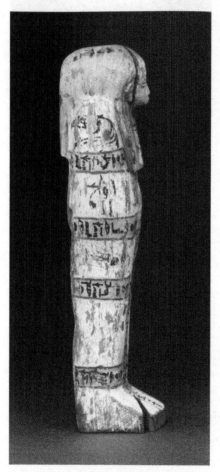 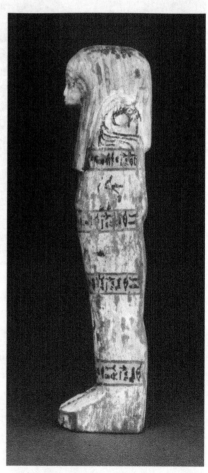

17.3 Figurine of Senty-resti, right side. British Museum EA 53995. (Courtesy of the Trustees of the British Museum.)

17.4 Figurine of Senty-resti, left side. British Museum EA 53995. (Courtesy of the Trustees of the British Museum.)

The remainder of the surface of the figure has a white-painted background. Below the hands is a central band of yellow, with red frame-lines containing a hieroglyphic inscription in black; the band ends at the level of the ankles, but below this the inscription has been continued on the plain white ground as far as the toes. On each side of the figurine are four lateral bands, again containing texts drawn in black on yellow backgrounds with red frames. These bands extend down the sides of the body, the inscriptions being orientated so as to be legible when the figure is in a recumbent position. No attempt has been made to represent the line which would mark the point of contact between the lid and case of a full-size coffin. On each side, the space between the first and second lateral bands is occupied by a large *wedjat* eye, and that between the second and third bands by a male human figure (one of the Sons of Horus?), represented standing and facing towards the head. There are no traces of any similar figures in the remaining compartments, although the painted surfaces here are fairly well preserved. A figure of Isis with upraised arms, standing on a *neb* basket, is painted on the top of the head directly overlaying the stripes of the headdress. The figure is flanked by an inscription in two short vertical lines of hieroglyphs. On the base of the feet is a similar figure of Nephthys, with a short inscription to her right. On the rear of the wooden figure the buttocks and the depressions at the back of the knees have been carefully modelled, but there are no painted images or inscriptions in this area. The entire surface of the figurine has been painted but no traces of varnish can be detected.

Inscriptions

Central text:

> *ḏd mdw in Nwt di̓.s ꜥwy.sy ḥr¹ snty-rs.ti m3ꜥ-ḫrw in[?] s3.s [?] tti̓[?]*
> Words spoken by Nut: She places her two arms over Senty-resti, true-of-voice. It is her son [?]Teti [?]²

---

1   Damaged sign, perhaps *ḥr* (Gardiner sign list D 2), followed by vertical stroke.
2   The signs following *m3ꜥ-ḫrw* appear to begin *in* and end with the name of the dedicator. Although the second sign in this name is slightly larger than the first, both are probably the flat loaf (Gardiner sign list X 1), indicating that the name is Teti. Preceding this name is a damaged and rather unclear group, possibly to be rendered *s3.s*, but this is uncertain. Such dedication formulae occur at the end of the texts on a number of 'stick' shabtis of the late 17th to early 18th Dynasty (Whelan 2007: pls. 5, 6, 8). Although Whelan translates the '*in*' in these formulae as 'by', Harco Willems has pointed out that they are examples of participial statements (Willems 2009: 515 and n. 10). Hence the present text ought to be rendered as 'It is her son Teti [sc. 'who makes her name live']'.

Proper right side:

> 1. *ỉm3ḫyt ḫr dw3–mwt.f snty-rs.t[i]*
> Revered before Duamutef, Senty-rest[i]

> 2. *ỉm3ḫyt ḫr wsir snty-rs.t[i]*
> Revered before Osiris, Senty-rest[i]

> 3. *ỉm3ḫyt ḫr inpw snty-rs.ti*
> Revered before Anubis, Senty-rest[i]

> 4. *ỉm3ḫyt ḫr qbḥ-snw.f snty-rs.ti*
> Revered before Qebhsenuef, Senty-resti

Proper left side:

> 1. *ỉm3ḫyt ḫr [i]mst[y] snty-rs.ti*
> Revered before Imsety, Senty-resti

> 2. *ỉm3ḫyt ḫr wsir snty-rs.ti*
> Revered before Osiris, Senty-resti

> 3. *ỉm3ḫyt ḫr inpw snty-rs.ti*
> Revered before Anubis, Senty-resti

> 4. *ỉm3ḫyt ḫr ḥpy snty-rs.[ti]*
> Revered before Hapy, Senty-res[ti]

Top of head:

> 1. *ỉm3ḫyt ḫr 3st ...*
> 2. *snty-...*

> Revered before Isis ... , Senty-[resti]'

Base of foot:

> *ỉm3ḫyt ḫr nbt-ḥwt snty-rs.ti*
> Revered before Nephthys, Senty-resti

Iconography and date

The figure is an accurate copy of a type of anthropoid coffin which is attested only in the Theban necropolis during the earlier years of the 18th Dynasty. This type represented the deceased person in the form of the *sˁḥ* – the individual cocooned in linen wrappings or a shroud, with the exposed head framed by a tripartite headdress. The *sˁḥ* form represents the dead person having undergone ritual transformation into an eternal being with divine attributes, and since the

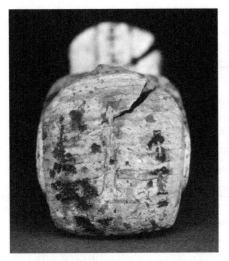 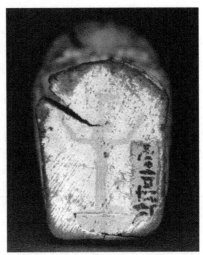

17.5 Figurine of Senty-resti, top of head. British Museum EA 53995. (Courtesy of the Trustees of the British Museum.)

17.6 Figurine of Senty-resti, base of foot. British Museum EA 53995. (Courtesy of the Trustees of the British Museum.)

First Intermediate Period it had become customary to fashion the mummy itself into this image (Seidlmayer 2001: 230). The early anthropoid coffins, of the 12th to 13th Dynasties, imitated the same model, and it was also used for funerary images of the deceased both as integral elements of stelae and individually as shabti-figures (Schneider 1977: I, 65–7, 160–1). The arms might be covered by the wrappings or depicted as folded on the breast, sometimes holding objects in the hands. Other attributes of the *sꜥḥ*, found on mummies and anthropoid coffins, were a broad collar and bands arranged vertically and laterally on the body.

This iconography is attested on anthropoid coffins of the Middle Kingdom, and was succeeded (at least at Thebes) by the feathered *rishi* pattern in the 17th and early 18th Dynasties, but contemporary with the later *rishi* coffins there emerged a new type in which typical features of the older Middle Kingdom model were reintroduced and combined with elements of design adapted from the exterior surface decoration of rectangular coffins (texts inscribed on the bands, divine figures). The most distinctive feature of these early 18th Dynasty coffins is their coloration, with polychrome decoration on a white background, a blue and white striped headdress and yellow bands on the body (Lapp and Niwinski 2001: 283). The background colour has given rise to the name by which these coffins are now generally known: the 'white'-type. In a study by Miroslaw Barwik the period of use of the 'white'-type has been defined as from the reign of Tuthmosis I (or perhaps slightly earlier) to the joint reign of Hatshepsut and Tuthmosis III (Barwik 1999: 6–12, 19–20), a rather short period of perhaps not more than forty years.[3] The 'white'-type of coffin has been regarded as the precursor of the much longer-lived 'black'-type which was in use from the reign of Tuthmosis III to that of Ramesses II, if not later (Taylor 2001b: 167–8).

Although fewer than forty coffins of the 'white'-type are known, a classification of them has proved possible (Barwik 1999). The closest parallels to the British Museum figurine among the full-size coffins are those of Barwik's categories C and D, which are characterised by the inclusion of images (funeral scenes or standing deities) in compartments along the sides of the case, and figures of Isis and Nephthys at the head and foot ends (Barwik 1999: 16–19). Barwik regards these coffins as examples of the 'fully developed "white"-type', noting that the programmatic arrangement of divine figures (missing from other 'white' coffins) was also a typical feature of the succeeding 'black' type. Certain more specific features of the British Museum model, when compared with full-size coffins, seem also to locate it towards the latter end of the 'white' coffin's phase of production. One of these features is the representation of the crossed hands on the breast, which is attested on two specimens of Barwik's group D (Cairo CG 61016 and Turin, Museo Egizio, Provvisorio 718). This is a rare attribute for the 'white'-type, and one which appeared more frequently on anthropoid coffins only as the 'black'-type became more widespread, from the reign of Tuthmosis III onwards. A second peculiarity of the British Museum model is the 'irregular' disposition of Isis and Nephthys at the head and foot respectively. This is a reversal of the stations of these goddesses, who were usually positioned with Nephthys at the head and Isis at the foot (as in the vignette of Book of the Dead, Spell 151). These are the positions which they occupy on most coffins and sarcophagi of the New Kingdom and later periods, and yet the unorthodox arrangement just mentioned is attested on at least two full-size coffins of the 'white'-type: New York, Metropolitan Museum of Art 12.181.298 and Paris, Musée du Louvre E14543. The New York coffin is admittedly not among the latest examples of the type, having been found in a closed burial context bearing a seal of Tuthmosis I, but the Louvre specimen can be dated from ceramic and scarab evidence to the joint reign of Hatshepsut and Tuthmosis III (Barwik 1999: 19). Hence, while not totally conclusive, the depiction of the hands on the British Museum model and the 'advanced' decorative programme of its surfaces appear to fit comfortably into the period of joint rule of Hatshepsut and Tuthmosis III.

3   Barwik's (1999: 12) suggestion of 'about a hundred years' seems too long.

The owner

The interpretation of the name of the owner of the British Museum model proposed here requires some explanation. It begins with a group reading *snty*, written as if a dual form; this is followed by a group of signs which varies in different
locations on the object, and which concludes with the suffix *.tí*. The central part
of the name comprises two signs, one of which is the eye (Gardiner sign list D
4), preceded in six places by a low horizontal sign resembling the 'portable seat'
(Gardiner sign list Q 2). Thus this central element appears to consist of the name
of the god Osiris, suggesting that the name as a whole was *snty-wsir.ti*, and this
indeed was the reading given by S. R. K. Glanville in a brief description of the
figurine written, probably in the 1920s, on a museum catalogue card, now in
the archives of the British Museum's department of Ancient Egypt and Sudan.
However, this rendering would yield a name of an otherwise unattested pattern
and moreover one whose interpretation is problematic since its elements do not
provide a clear meaning.

However, in four places on the object (left side, text 1, right side, texts 3 and
4, base of foot), the horizontal 'portable seat' sign in the name is replaced by the
'lashed pieces of wood' sign (Gardiner sign T 13). The association of this sign
with the eye-hieroglyph yields the perfectly intelligible reading *rs*, 'to be awake'
(sc. 'alive') and the name can be rendered as *snty-rs.tí*. A plausible explanation
for the scribe's vacillation between sign T 13 and the 'portable seat' hieroglyph
Q 2 can be offered. The semi-hieratic sign Gardiner U 40 was often used in place
of T 13 and is also attested in the 17th and early 18th Dynasties, juxtaposed with
the 'eye' as a substitute for the 'seat' sign Q 1 in writings of the name of Osiris
(for example, on some 'stick' shabtis of the late 17th to early 18th Dynasties and
on a *rishi* coffin: Whelan 2007: pls. 5, 7, 9; Miniaci 2011: 265, pl. 7.b.); the signs
look particularly similar in hieratic script. The scribe, perhaps working from
a draft in hieratic, appears to have misinterpreted the central element of the
personal name as the name of Osiris, and in several places wrote the name of
the god accordingly, using the alternative spelling with the 'portable seat' sign.

The reading 'Senty-resti' conforms to a name-pattern well attested in the
Second Intermediate Period and early 18th Dynasty, in which a subject is
placed before the verb *rs* in the stative: (m.) X-*rs(.w)* and (f.) X-*rs.ti*, that is,
'X is awake.' In some examples the first element, X, is a noun, such as *sn*
or *mwt*, with first-person possessive suffix either written or implied (cf. the
name Mutresti: Ranke 1935–52: I, 148, 10; Lapp 2004: 42–3). By analogy one
might take *snty* as a writing of *snt.í* and interpret the name as 'My sister is
awake.' A masculine counterpart to this, *sn.í-rs(.w)*, is attested (Ranke 1935–52:
I, 309, 12) and names modelled on the same pattern are attested in the Middle
Kingdom: *sn.í-ʿnḫ(.w)*, 'My brother lives', and *snt.í-ʿnḫ.t(í)*, 'My sister lives'

(Ranke 1935–52, I: 310, 12; 312, 3). However, there are also examples of the X-*rs(.w)*/X-*rs.ti* pattern in which the first element is itself a personal name, as in (among others) Iay-res, Iah-res, Iuwy-res, Ibia-res, Ibi-res, Ipu-resti, Ameny-shery-res, Teti-res, Ruiu-resti and Bebi-resti (Ranke 1935–52, I: 6, 3; 13, 7; 16, 17; 19, 5; 20, 11; 23, 13; 31, 16; 221, 6; 385, 5; II: 276, 31; Davies and Gardiner 1915: 63). Though the name Senty-resti has not been previously attested, Senti and Senty are known as independent feminine names (Ranke 1935–52, I: 312, 1, 5), and the existence of a compound form with *rs.ti* is perfectly in accordance with the naming traditions of the early 18th Dynasty.

Function and context

Small or miniature coffins, imitating those made for human bodies, were used to fulfil a number of different functions. They could serve to house the remains of young children or foetuses (Carter 1933: 88–9, pl. XXVI) or act as containers for the mummified viscera, in place of or in addition to canopic jars (Dodson 1994: 61 and n. 79; James 2007: 108–9). They also occur as representations of the *sꜥḥ*/mummy on the deck of model funerary barques (Glanville 1972: 12, 15, 19, pl. IIIa, b; Lacovara and Trope 2001: 46), as containers for shabtis (see below) and – less frequently – as receptacles for votive figures and other objects of magical power or special personal significance (Lilyquist 2003: 21, fig. 7b; James 2007: 134–5).

Senty-resti's model is simultaneously a *sꜥḥ*-image and, more specifically, a representation of a coffin, since features such as the divine figures on the sides, head and foot are proper only to coffins in the sphere of human images in Egyptian funerary iconography. Lacking a cavity, the model cannot have functioned in a practical sense as a receptacle, and hence its role should be sought in the context of funerary magic or ritual. The date of the figure eliminates the possibility that it might have formed part of the accoutrements of a model funerary boat, since such models fell out of use in the late 12th Dynasty and are not attested in burials of the early New Kingdom. Its dating to the early 18th Dynasty, its scale and the inclusion of the name of a dedicator in the inscription all indicate that its function was probably related to the use of shabtis.

In the early 18th Dynasty, the shabti, as a *sꜥḥ*-image, served primarily to enable its owner to participate vicariously in activities which would be beneficial to her or him. These included the familiar agricultural tasks mentioned in Book of the Dead Spell 6, which provided food in the afterlife, and also the participation in rituals at important cult-places, such as at Abydos, the traditional burial place of Osiris, where a share of the god's offerings might be obtained at his annual festival. Thus the shabti's primary role was to serve its owner 'as a bearer of his extended identity', giving him access to the divine (Assmann 2005: 111). Senty-resti's figurine is not a shabti *per se*, but it can be related to the function of such images since in this period shabtis were commonly placed in individual miniature coffins, emphasising the close association between the figurine and the person whom it represented (Schneider 1977: I, 267; Aston 1994: 22; Whelan 2011). A shabti placed within a model coffin was treated exactly as the body of the deceased was treated, and equipped with the same magical capabilities. The protection and divine empowerment provided by the images of deities and the speech of Nut painted on the surface would be efficacious for the person represented by the figurine, just as the corresponding features of a full-size coffin would be for the mummified individual inside.

The use of miniature coffins to contain shabtis can be traced back to the origins of the figures. The non-mummiform wax figures ('proto-shabtis') of the First Intermediate Period and 11th Dynasty and the earliest 'true' shabtis of the 12th to 13th Dynasties were enclosed in small rectangular coffins (Taylor 2001a: 117, fig. 77; Arnold 1988: 34–9, 147–9, pls. 13–15). In the 17th and early 18th Dynasties both the crude 'stick' shabtis and the more carefully crafted examples in use at that time were regularly placed in miniature coffins, both rectangular and anthropoid (Newberry 1930–57: pls. I–II). These coffins vary in appearance from very simple, roughly carved specimens without decoration, to others which reproduce in greater or lesser detail the design features of full-size coffins of their period: miniature *rishi*, 'white'-type and 'black'-type coffins are all attested (Newberry 1930–57: 343, 347–8, pls. XI, XVII, XLV; d'Auria, Lacovara and Roehrig 1988: 136, no. 73; Whelan 2011). The size varies but most are between 20 cm and 35 cm in length (within which range British Museum EA 53995 also falls). There are even a few instances of coffin 'assemblages' for shabtis, comprising rectangular outer and anthropoid inner coffins (Pumpenmeier 1998; Taylor 2001a: 121, fig. 82).

The custom of placing shabtis in miniature coffins declined after the middle of the 18th Dynasty, a development which was probably linked with the changing status of the figures. The shabti's identification with its owner appears to have weakened and its role as surrogate agricultural labourer became more pronounced, a 'depersonalisation' which was manifested first in the appearance of tools for shabtis from the reign of Tuthmosis IV onwards (Spanel 2001: 568) and reflected in later references to the figures as *ḥmw*, slaves or servants (Schneider 1977: I, 261, 319). Although a few shabti coffins are attested as late as the Ramesside Period (e.g. Newberry 1930–57: 348–51, pl. XVII; Spanel 2001: 568, fig.), from the reign of Amenhotep III onwards they were increasingly replaced by shrine-shaped boxes containing larger numbers of figures (Aston 1994: 22).

In the early 18th Dynasty certain elements of iconography and text seem to have been applied indiscriminately to shabtis and their anthropoid coffins.

Some of the coffins possess features which properly belonged to shabtis, such as the text of Spell 6 of the Book of the Dead, while shabtis may display elements of s*ḥ* iconography which are otherwise found only on coffins (an example is the shabti of Renseneb, British Museum EA 57342). This phenomenon points to the existence of a particularly close identification between shabtis and shabti coffins at this date. Senty-resti's model is remarkable in that, while its solid form recalls that of the shabti, its external decoration is drawn entirely from the repertoire of the contemporary anthropoid coffin. Although rare, the model is not quite unique in this. A few other wooden figurines of this period, though crudely fashioned, also have the colour scheme and intersecting bands of the 'white'-type coffin, with the *ḥtp-dỉ-nsw* formula in the centre (Brunner-Traut and Brunner 1981: 267, Taf. 63; Whelan 2007: 26 (fig. 17, item 3), 27, 63–4; Whelan 2011: 18). A more detailed example, inscribed for a person named Djehutymose and formerly in the collection of Gustave Jequier, is a closer match for British Museum EA 53995; it had a central axial band of inscription containing the *ḥtp-dỉ-nsw* formula, transverse bands with *ỉmȝḥy ḥr* formulae and four figures of deities in the compartments between the lateral bands (Nash 1911: 35, pl. VIII, no. 48).

The existence of Senty-resti's model and its parallels raises the question: are they to be understood as variants of the conventional shabti, reflecting fluidity in the use of iconography and text in this period, or are they representations of a shabti or transfigured person (s*ḥ*/mummy) *within* a coffin? As a representation of a closed coffin, Senty-resti's figurine conforms to the principle which activated other 'models' from ancient Egypt, such as the miniature offering sets of the Old Kingdom, the dummy jars of the New Kingdom and the dummy canopic jars of the Third Intermediate Period. These items represent only the external form and appearance of a container, but conceptually they fuse both container and contents into a single crafted object. The existence of the contents is implicit and in a magical sense they are actually present, having been brought into existence by the fashioning and ritual activation of the enclosing form. As Susan Allen has observed of the model vessels that were commonly used in funerary contexts: 'it is their outward form that is symbolically important and their contents are implied by their shape' (Allen 2006: 20). The implied contents of Senty-resti's model coffin is an image of her as a s*ḥ*, a transfigured being.

It may be supposed that painting the exterior of a carved figure to make it a simulacrum of a coffin endowed it with a double power: the protective and transformative power of a full-size coffin, reduced to a miniature scale; and the efficacy of the s*ḥ*-image whose presence within is implied. With this in mind, Whelan's suggestion that the 'stick' shabtis of this period might have been made from 'waste' wood left over from coffin manufacture (Whelan 2007: 46–7) may be significant. If it is correct, it might be that such fragments were thought to contain magical potency which could be conveyed from a real coffin to its smaller copy.

The context of shabtis in the early 18th Dynasty

Information about the deposition of shabtis in the early 18th Dynasty is sparse, but it is apparent that in certain parts of the Theban necropolis at that period 'stick' shabtis were deposited in the above-ground parts of tombs. Whelan has assembled the evidence for this practice, noting the best-documented finds (Whelan 2007: 1–22; cf. Willems 2009: 513–19): a tomb found by Giuseppe Passalacqua in the 1820s, excavations by the Marquis of Northampton in 1898–99, Carter and Carnarvon's excavations at and around the tomb of Tetiky (Theban tomb 15) in 1908 and excavations by the Metropolitan Museum of Art, New York, at 'Tomb 37' (MMA 5) in 1915–16. All of these finds lay within a relatively small area encompassed by the pyramid tomb of Nubkheperre Intef at Dra Abu el-Naga and the eastern extremity of the Asasif, a region which was intensively used for burials in the 17th and early 18th Dynasties and where both *rishi* and 'white'-type coffins have been found. Contemporary records of these excavations indicate that the 'stick' shabtis and also others of more elaborate type, frequently enclosed in miniature coffins, were found in tomb courtyards, sometimes deposited in niches in the wall or in mud-brick shrines, or grouped around the mouth of a burial shaft. A distinctive feature was that the shabtis from a single location, such as those from the courtyard of the tomb of Tetiky, bore the names of many different individuals and were often accompanied by the name of a dedicator. In one exceptional instance the Northampton excavations brought to light a shabti which had been placed in a small coffin accompanied by four miniature jars, as if replicating the assemblage of a tomb (Northampton and Newberry 1908: 26–7; Whelan 2007: 10).

This manner of depositing shabtis, together with the frequent mentions of dedicators in the inscriptions, suggests that their function may have been analogous to that of other 'extra-sepulchral' shabtis, examples of which have been found buried at sites of special sanctity, such as Abydos, Giza and the Serapeum at Saqqara. These were places at which deities and/or deceased kings and sacred animals were the object of cult activity, and the deposition of shabtis at such locations was evidently intended to enable the owner to participate in the rituals and to receive a share of the offerings presented (Schneider 1977: I, 268–9; Pumpenmeier 1998: 75–8). Some of the figures, such as those of the high official Qenamun, bore dedicatory texts stating that they were the gift of the king as a special favour to a faithful servant (Pumpenmeier 1998: 47–8). The Theban shabtis discussed above may have fulfilled a similar function, enabling the persons they represented to share in the benefits of the funerary cult of the occupant near whose tomb they were buried. In this context the benefits were provided through the mediation not of the king, but of members of the deceased's own family or community. The figurines therefore acted as foci for beneficial interaction between the living and the dead. This integration of the deceased into the wider social group seems to have been a distinctive aspect of local burial practice at Thebes in the late Second Intermediate Period and early 18th Dynasty and is reflected in other aspects of mortuary practice there in the same period, such as the grouping of burial places around sites of communal cult activity (Seiler 2005: 197–8; Whelan 2007: 46).

It is into this context of mortuary practice that the figure of Senty-resti fits most comfortably. The date of its acquisition, 1915, associates it with a period when archaeological activity was taking place at Dra Abu el-Naga and the nearby areas: precisely the excavations which were yielding many early 18th Dynasty shabtis and coffins. The figure may even have been a 'stray' from Northampton's excavations or, perhaps more plausibly, those of Carter and Carnarvon, although proof is lacking.

Who were the dedicatees?

In discussions of the function of the 'stick' shabtis, Speleers and Erman considered that they were intended to give poorer people access to the privileged afterlife which the tomb owner enjoyed (cited in Whelan 2007: 45). Whelan questions the suggestion that this practice was restricted to the poorer classes, pointing out that some of the figures were dedicated by persons of high status, but this does not invalidate the general idea that the recipients of such dedications may have been persons who could not aspire to the full paraphernalia of formal burial, and that a key function of the objects was to enable these individuals to partake of the benefits of the funerary cult through another medium. Harco Willems has developed the idea further, suggesting that the 'stick' shabtis in miniature coffins may have been brought to tombs and dedicated to the deceased in the context of mortuary festivities which included music and feasting, a practice which may possibly have lain at the roots of statements by Herodotus and Plutarch that a figure of a corpse was sometimes exhibited at Egyptian feasts (Willems 2009: 516–19).

Where the dedicatees of the shabtis were actually buried is in most cases unknown, but there is a strong possibility that some were interred at or near the spot where their figures were deposited. The shabtis of the parents of Tetiky were placed around the shaft in the courtyard of his tomb, where there was also a chapel apparently for his father, suggesting that he was buried in the vicinity (Whelan 2007: 14). It may be, but cannot be proved, that the persons named on the other shabtis from this context were also buried there. Carter stated that the shabtis deposited around the shaft were 'dedicated to persons buried in the vaults below' (Carnarvon and Carter 1912: 13), although the report gives no description of what was found there, if indeed the shaft was excavated. Since Tetiky seems to have been the person who enjoyed the highest status among his immediate family it may be that his relatives had simpler funerary arrangements. Perhaps some were buried without full-size decorated coffins or their bodies were not fashioned into sꜥḥ-images; such simple burial treatment seems to have been accorded to members of the family of Senenmut before his rise to high office under Hatshepsut (Dorman 1988: 167–71; Dorman 2003: 32–4). The 'stick' shabtis and model coffins may then have taken the place of formal burial as a conduit to the benefits of the afterlife. It may be noted that in no case at this period is a full-size coffin known for an owner of a 'stick' shabti or model coffin (though, admittedly, few full-size coffins have survived from this period). Certainly, no other funerary equipment belonging to Senty-resti has come to light and, if the above suggestions are correct, it may be that her model coffin represented the totality of her formal burial accoutrements.

References

Allen, S. (2006), 'Miniature and model vessels in ancient Egypt', in M. Barta (ed.), *The Old Kingdom Art and Archaeology: Proceedings of the Conference held in Prague, May 31 – June 4, 2004* (Prague: Charles University), 19–24.

Arnold, D. (1988), *The South Cemeteries of Lisht*, I: *The Pyramid of Senwosret I* (New York: Metropolitan Museum of Art).

Assmann, J. (2005), *Death and Salvation in Ancient Egypt*, trans. David Lorton (Ithaca and London: Cornell University Press).

Aston, D. A. (1994), 'The shabti-box: a typological study', *Oudheidkundige Mededelingen uit het Rijksmuseum van Oudheden te Leiden* 74, 21–54.

Barwik, M. (1999), 'Typology and dating of the "White"-type anthropoid coffins of the early XVIIIth Dynasty', *Etudes et Travaux* 18, 7–33.

Brunner-Traut, E. and Brunner, H. (1981), *Die ägyptische Sammlung der Universität Tübingen* (Mainz: Philipp von Zabern).

Carnarvon, Earl of and Carter, H. (1912), *Five Years' Explorations at Thebes. A Record of Work Done 1907–1911* (London, New York, Toronto and Melbourne: Oxford University Press).

Carter, H. (1933), *The Tomb of Tut.Ankh.Amen*, III (London: Cassell).

D'Auria, S., Lacovara, P. and Roehrig, C. H. (1988), *Mummies & Magic: The Funerary Arts of Ancient Egypt* (Boston: Museum of Fine Arts).

Davies, N. de G. and Gardiner, A. H. (1915), *The Tomb of Amenemhet (No. 82)* (London: Egypt Exploration Fund).

Dodson, A. (1994), *The Canopic Equipment of the Kings of Egypt* (London and New York: Kegan Paul International).

Dorman, P. F. (1988), *The Monuments of Senenmut: Problems in Historical Methodology* (London and New York: Kegan Paul International).

Dorman, P. F. (2003), 'Family burial and commemoration in the Theban necropolis', in N. Strudwick and J. H. Taylor (eds.), *The Theban Necropolis: Past, Present and Future* (London: British Museum Press), 30–41, pls. 5–6.

Glanville, S. R. K. (1972), *Catalogue of Egyptian Antiquities in the British Museum*, II: *Wooden Model Boats* (London: British Museum).

James, T. G. H. (2007), *Tutankhamun: The Eternal Splendor of the Boy Pharaoh*, revised edn (Vercelli: White Star).

Lacovara, P. and Trope, B. T. (eds.) (2001), *The Realm of Osiris: Mummies, Coffins, and Ancient Egyptian Funerary Art in the Michael C. Carlos Museum* (Atlanta: Michael C. Carlos Museum, Emory University).

Lapp, G. (2004), *Catalogue of the Books of the Dead in the British Museum*, III: *The Papyrus of Nebseni (BM EA 9900)* (London: British Museum Press).

Lapp, G. and Niwinski, A. (2001), 'Coffins, sarcophagi and cartonnages', in D. B. Redford (ed.), *The Oxford Encyclopedia of Ancient Egypt* (Oxford and New York: Oxford University Press), I, 279–87.

Lilyquist, C. (2003), *The Tomb of Three Foreign Wives of Tuthmosis III* (New York: Metropolitan Museum of Art).

Miniaci, G. (2011), *Rishi Coffins and the Funerary Culture of Second Intermediate Period Egypt* (London: Golden House Publications).

Nash, W. L. (1911), 'Notes on some Egyptian antiquities IX', *Proceedings of the Society of Biblical Archaeology* 33, 34–9, pls. VIII–X.

Newberry, P. E. (1930–57), *Catalogue général des antiquités égyptiennes du Musée du Caire, Nos. 46530–48575. Funerary Statuettes and Model Sarcophagi* (Cairo: Imprimerie de l'Institut Français d'Archéologie Orientale).

Northampton, Marquis of, Spiegelberg, W. and Newberry, P. E. (1908), *Report on some Excavations in the Theban Necropolis during the Winter of 1898–9* (London: Archibald Constable and Co.).

Pumpenmeier, F. (1998), *Eine Gunstgabe von Seiten des Königs: ein extrasepulkrales Shabtidepot Qen-Amuns in Abydos* (Heidelberg: Heidelberger Orientverlag).

Ranke, H. (1935–52), *Die ägyptischen Personennamen*, I-II (Glückstadt and Hamburg: J. J. Augustin).

Schneider, H. D. (1977), *Shabtis: An Introduction to the History of Ancient Egyptian Funerary Statuettes with a Catalogue of the Collection of Shabtis in the National Museum of Antiquities at Leiden*, 3 vols (Leiden: Rijksmuseum van Oudheden).

Seidlmayer, S. J. (2001), 'Die Ikonographie des Todes', in H. Willems (ed.), *Social Aspects of Funerary Culture in the Egyptian Old and Middle Kingdoms* (Leuven, Paris and Sterling, VA: Peeters), 205–52.

Seiler, A. (2005), *Tradition & Wandel: die Keramik als Spiegel der Kulturentwicklung Thebens in der Zweiten Zwischenzeit* (Mainz: Philipp von Zabern).

Spanel, D. B. (2001), 'Funerary figurines', in D. B. Redford (ed.), *The Oxford Encyclopedia of Ancient Egypt* (Oxford and New York: Oxford University Press), I, 567–70.

Taylor, J. H. (2001a), *Death and the Afterlife in Ancient Egypt* (London: British Museum Press).

Taylor, J. H. (2001b), 'Patterns of colouring on ancient Egyptian coffins from the New Kingdom to the Twenty-Sixth Dynasty: an overview', in W. V. Davies (ed.), *Colour and Painting in Ancient Egypt* (London: British Museum Press), 164–81.

Whelan, P. (2007), *Mere Scraps of Rough Wood? 17th–18th Dynasty Stick Shabtis in the Petrie Museum and Other Collections* (London: Golden House Publications).

Whelan, P. (2011), 'Small yet perfectly formed – some observations on Theban stick shabti coffins of the 17th and early 18th Dynasty', *Egitto e Vicino Oriente* 34, 9–22.

Willems, H. (2009), '*Carpe diem*: remarks on the cultural background of Herodotus II.78', in W. Claes, H. de Meulenaere and S. Hendrickx (eds.), *Elkab and Beyond. Studies in Honour of Luc Limme* (Leuven, Paris and Walpole: Peeters), 511–20.

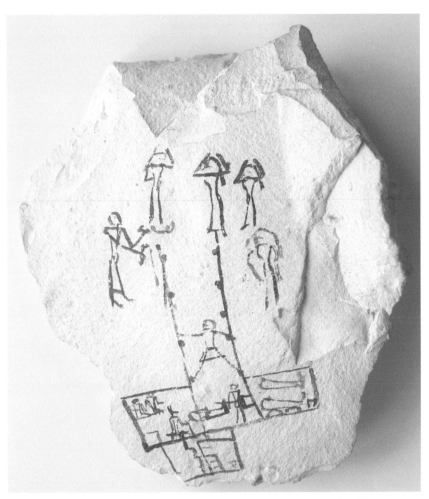

1 The Manchester 'funeral' ostracon. Manchester Museum 5886. (Courtesy of Manchester Museum, University of Manchester. Photograph by the author.)

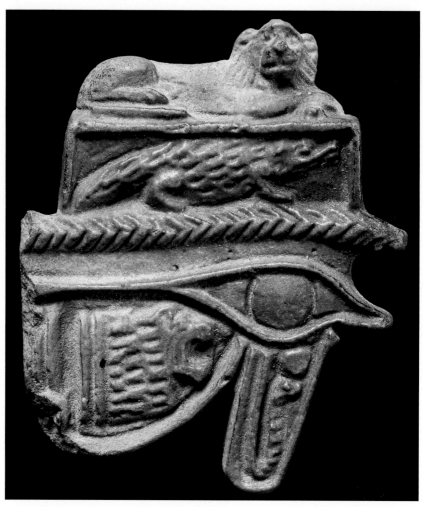

2 Wedjat eye, British Museum EA 26586. (Courtesy of the Trustees of the
British Museum.)

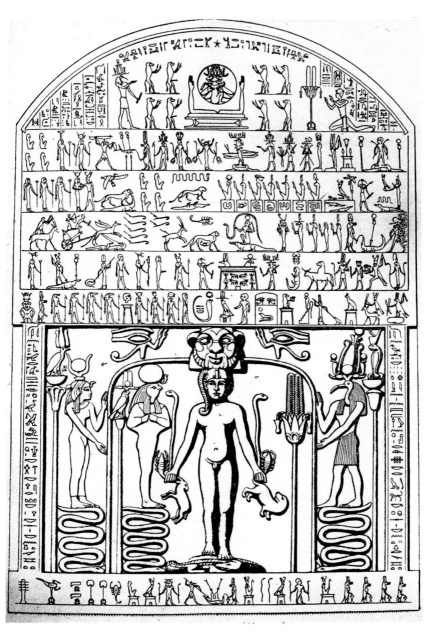

3 Metternich Stela. (After Golenischeff 1877: Taf. 1.)

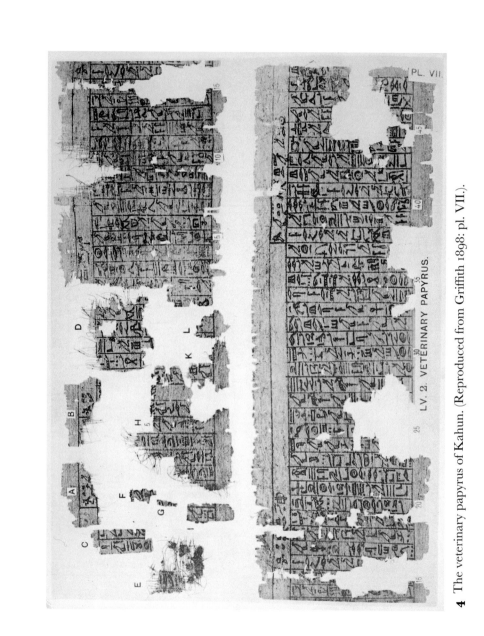

4 The veterinary papyrus of Kahun. (Reproduced from Griffith 1898: pl. VII.).

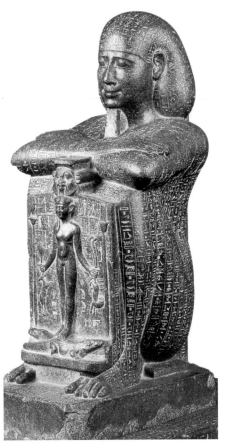

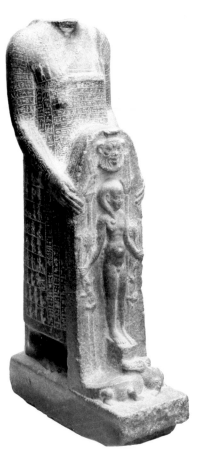

5 Healing statue of Djedhor, JE 46341, Egyptian Museum, Cairo. (Courtesy of Manchester Museum, University of Manchester.)

6 Healing statue of Hor, Turin 3030. (Courtesy of the Museo Egizio. Photograph by Simon Connor.)

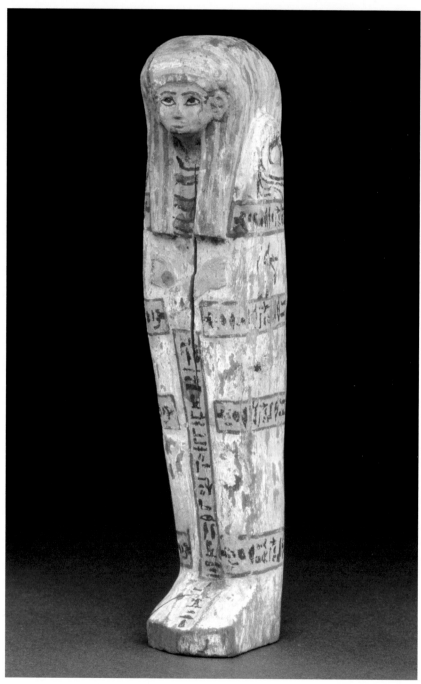

7 Figurine of Senty-resti, British Museum EA 53995. (Courtesy of the Trustees
of the British Museum.)

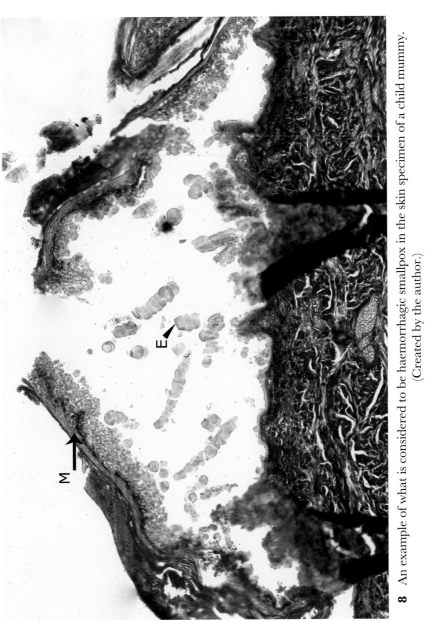

8 An example of what is considered to be haemorrhagic smallpox in the skin specimen of a child mummy. (Created by the author.)

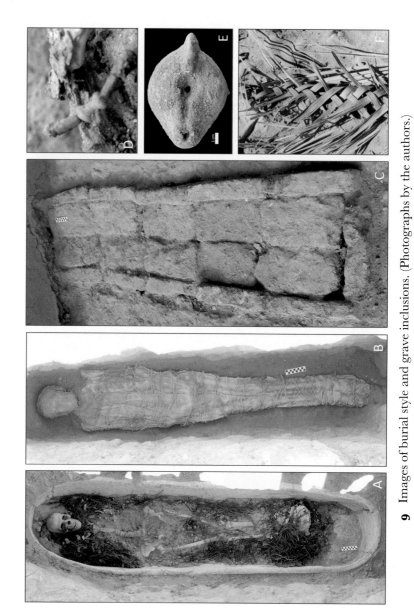

9 Images of burial style and grave inclusions. (Photographs by the authors.)

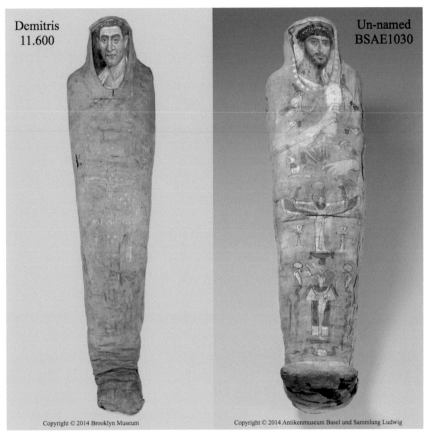

10 Two examples of Red Shroud mummies: Demetris, 11.600 (courtesy of Brooklyn Museum), and BSAE 1030 (courtesy of Antikenmuseum Basel und Sammlung Ludwig).

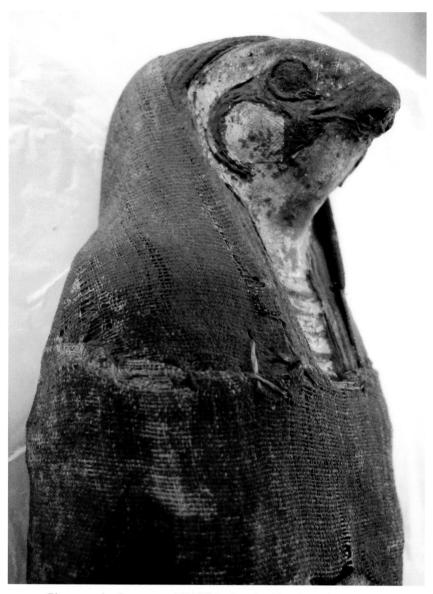

11 Photograph of mummy AEABB81 showing the shrouded post-cranial aspect and the elaborate gilded head and breastplate. (Courtesy of Manchester Museum, University of Manchester.)

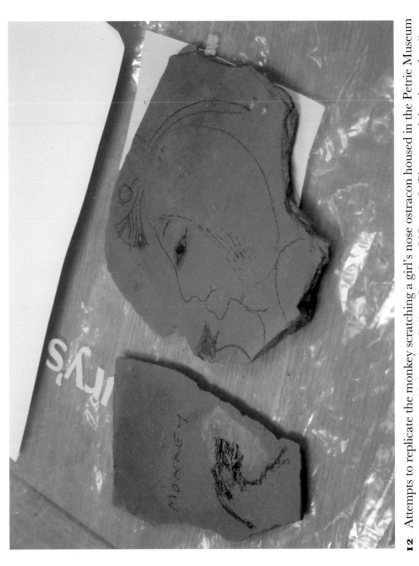

12 Attempts to replicate the monkey scratching a girl's nose ostracon housed in the Petrie Museum of Egyptian Archaeology, University College London, UC 15946. (Photograph by the author.))

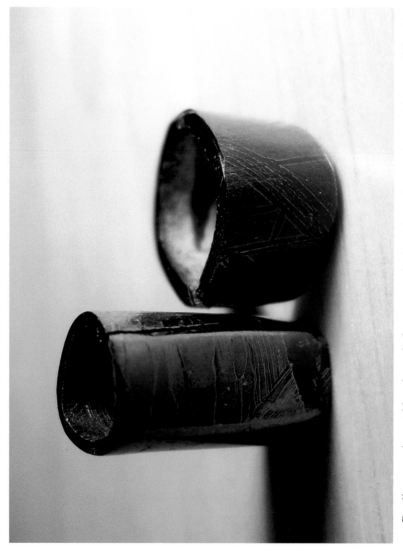

13 Replica experimental beads made from meteorite iron, heated to produce a thin colourful oxide: Seymchan pallasite iron (left), Muonionalusta octahedrite iron (right). (Photograph by the author.)

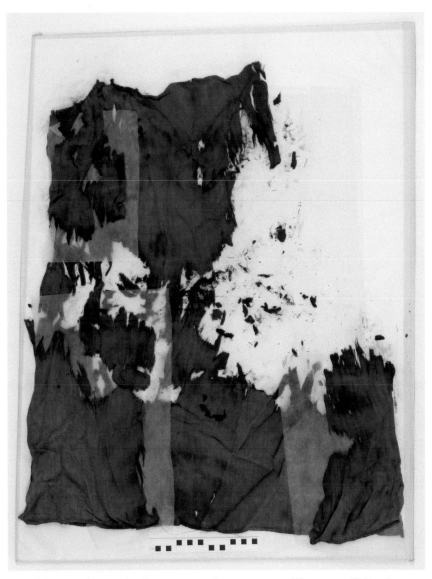

14 The 1770 bag-tunic after conservation treatment. (Courtesy of Manchester Museum, University of Manchester. Photograph by the author.)

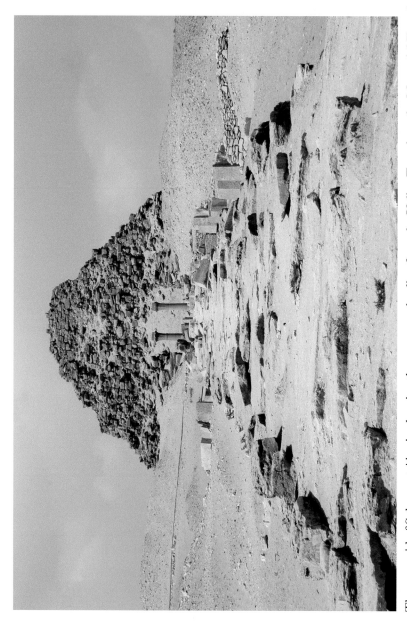

15 The pyramid of Sahura at Abusir, showing the causeway leading from the Valley Temple to the Memorial Temple. (Photograph by the author.)

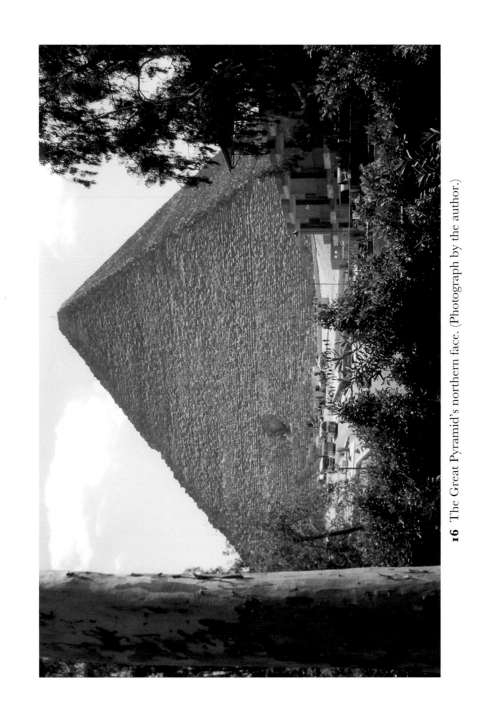

16 The Great Pyramid's northern face. (Photograph by the author.)

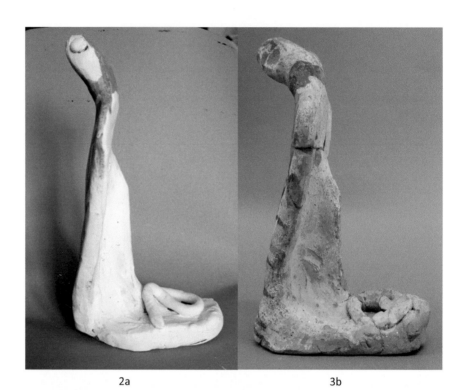

2a   3b

17 (a) Replica cobra produced by Alicja Sobczak. (Photograph by the author.)
(b) Amarna cobra, Berlin, Ägyptisches Museum und Papyrussammlung
21961. (Courtesy of Ägyptisches Museum und Papyrussammlung.
Photograph by the author.)

PART III

Understanding Egyptian mummies

18

The biology of ancient Egyptians and Nubians

Don Brothwell

Since Napoleonic times, there has been a constant interest in not only the art and architecture of Egypt and Nubia, but also the mummies and skeletons discovered there. Early studies, such as Nott and Gliddon (1857), lacked scientific rigour, but by the end of the nineteenth century, there was concern to improve scientific accuracy in reporting and increase sample sizes. Examples of this improved standard of research are provided by Elliot Smith and Wood Jones (1910) and Oetteking (1908) on Egyptian and Nubian material. As a young graduate, I became increasingly aware of Elliot Smith, not only his skeletal and cultural studies (Smith 1923), but also the excellent work on mummies (Smith 1912; Smith and Dawson 1924). In fact, he was one of a group of scientists at the turn of the twentieth century helping to reshape studies on earlier human populations (see Cockitt, Chapter 30, in this volume). The irascible mathematician Karl Pearson had used Naqada and Nubian data in estimating stature (Pearson 1898), although height estimation is still problematic today.

Elliot Smith was an old-fashioned anatomist who believed in observation by eye rather than multivariate analysis. In his book *The Ancient Egyptians and the Origin of Civilization* (1923), for instance, he picks out skulls and mandibles which he considers to indicate foreign elements in the population. There is a resounding silence from him on the work of Karl Pearson, who encouraged osteometric research on the Egyptians. In fact, both professors were yards away from one another at University College London. So much for senior academic behaviour. Elliot Smith was certainly more interested in the mixing of these earlier populations, and this has been a recurring question in various studies subsequently. Strouhal (1968), for instance, considered the question of population mixing and viewed the X group people of Wadi Qitna to be a mixed group, but mainly black Africans. Without far more population studies, the people extending along the Nile might be thought of as purely North African and Mediterranean in appearance. In fact, the degree of homogeneity and the origins of the genes of these peoples are likely to be far more complex and debatable. South of the early Egyptian and Nubian societies, in the region of the White Nile, south of Khartoum, are some of the tallest black populations in Africa, such as the Dinka and Shilluk. Male stature in these groups can commonly exceed 180 cm. Mixing with shorter Mediterranean people resulted in a range of body forms along the Nile.

There is also evidence of gene frequency clines, or gradations, from north to south, as for instance in the Rhesus blood group gene C (Mourant 1954). Also, more recently, Hassan and colleagues (2008) studied Y-chromosome haplogroup variation in a number of Sudanese populations and found significant correlations between genetic variation and the regional and linguistic differences. So we can see in modern genetic data evidence of group differentiation, and one of the jobs of bio-Egyptology is surely to link this evidence to old bones and teeth. Clearly the demography of these ancient populations is important, and yet, after the many cemetery surveys in Egypt and Nubia, we have remarkably few studies of this kind. In terms of overall population size, it seems likely that during Predynastic and earlier Dynastic times total numbers remained low. But later dynasties could have seen increases and greater fluctuations, as Hollingsworth (1969) has suggested (Figure 18.1).

Fluctuations can also be seen in city numbers; the population of Alexandria, for instance, is thought to have declined from 600,000 or so to 100,000 between 600 and 800 AD. Life expectancy at birth is unlikely to have been more than twenty years, and the Christian cemetery at Meinarti in Sudan had an estimate of 19.2 years (Swedlund and Armelagos 1976). Today in Egypt it is fifty-four years, but in regions of Sudan it varies between twenty-two and fifty-eight years. This kind of variation could well have occurred in the past, and mortality patterns could have changed rapidly, as at Meinarti between 1050 and 1150 AD (Swedlund and Armelagos 1976). Such differences could well be reflected in some of the pathology, and we need to keep this in mind when considering prevalence changes in such pathology as orbital cribra and enamel hypoplasia.

Who exactly were the ancestors of the people we are considering here? By the end of the Pleistocene, new peoples and their domestication ideas were spreading westwards and south in Africa. Some skeletal material, including an Olduvai skull (Mollison 1929), was wrongly labelled 'White', but is Caucasian. This kind of research has rather fogged our understanding of the evolutionary differentiation and spread of black Africans, but clearly they were well established in the Sudan by Mesolithic times. Data from ancient DNA and isotope studies will be vital to address research questions for those working in Egypt and Nubia in the future. Questions about ancient mating patterns will have to be asked as well (Strouhal 1968). Today in Nubia, over 50 per cent of marriages

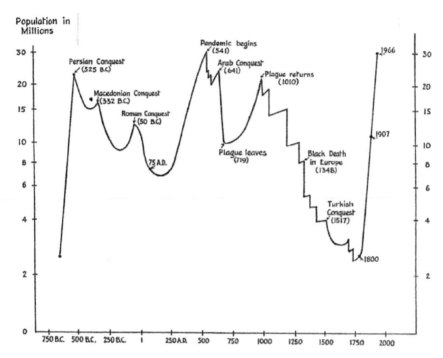

18.1 Population fluctuations in early Egypt, from the 26th Dynasty to recent times. (Created by the author after Hollingsworth 1969.)

are of first cousins, and the rest are usually of relatives (Geiser 1989). In the past, this kind of endogamous behaviour could have accelerated the emergence of regional distinctiveness. In his Nubian studies, Nielsen (1973) makes another demographic point for consideration. He suggests that the degree of physical variation he was noting between males and females might in some cases be indicating that immigrant males were taking 'native', that is indigenous, wives.

In the nineteenth century, Darwin's cousin Francis Galton emphasised the importance of measurement in the study of biological variation. Since then, there has certainly been a flurry of measuring as regards Nubian and Egyptian bones. Batrawi's (1935) stature estimates on C-group and New Kingdom individuals gives a male mean of 167 cm. Robins and Shute (1986) give Naqada males a mean height of 170 cm, but surprisingly view the limb proportions to be 'super-negroid'. So stature does not suggest strong black African influence, but limb proportions can. We need to investigate this further.

Because the morphology of the head is more variable than that of other parts of the body, the skull has been studied extensively. Fifty years ago, the Nubian Jebel Moya group were studied in detail (Mukherjee, Rao and Trevor 1955). It can be seen that by the multivariate analysis of a series of measurements, Jebel

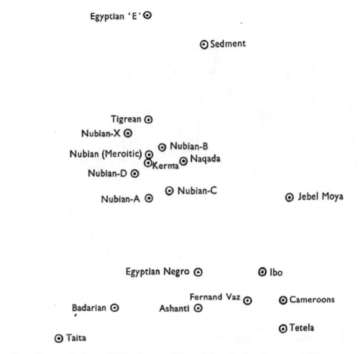

Egyptian 'E' ⊙

⊙ Sedment

Tigrean ⊙
Nubian-X ⊙
                ⊙ Nubian-B
Nubian (Meroitic) ⊙   ⊙ Naqada
              ⊙ Kerma
Nubian-D ⊙

              ⊙ Nubian-C
Nubian-A ⊙   ⊙ Jebel Moya

Egyptian Negro ⊙   ⊙ Ibo

              Fernand Vaz ⊙   ⊙ Cameroons
Badarian ⊙   Ashanti ⊙

                              ⊙ Tetela
⊙ Taita

18.2 General plan of D² relationships of the distinctive Jebel Moya population
in comparison with Nubian and other groups. (Created by the author
after Mukherjee, Rao and Trevor 1955.)

Moya is somewhat distinctive, being positioned between black African and
more northern Egyptian groups (Figure 18.2).

David Carlson's (1976) study of various early Nubian samples also reveals
differences, but in this case he argues that these could be due to local micro-
evolution, and not group movements, mixing or replacements. It is certainly
important to remember that isolation, endogamy, founder effect and selection
pressures can result in subtle changes. Dental measurements can at times also
be revealing, and Joel Irish (2006) has argued for greater homogeneity from
this evidence. In a novel study by Frederik Rösing (1986), family clusters were
isolated in two Aswan cemeteries. This statistical method, combined with DNA
results, could be very revealing in the future.

In recent years, another form of population analysis has developed, based
on the variable occurrence of non-metric or epigenetic traits. Early Nubian
excavation reports did note some of these traits, but later it became clearer
that some traits, especially when considered multifactorially, could help to dis-
criminate between populations. Caroline and Sam Berry with Peter Ucko (1967)
considered twelve Egyptian populations in this way and, although there were

some regional differences, concluded that overall there was no evidence for significant mixing and change. Using a different order of analysis, the Dutch biologist Agatha Knip (1970) considered two early Christian cemeteries facing one another on each side of the Nile. Employing non-metric traits, she found the differences to be highly significant, which raises the question of how far the Nile can not only allow the movement and mixing of peoples, but at times result in isolation, perhaps influenced by other factors, religious, marital or administrative. Non-metric traits on teeth have also been used, and Johnson and Lovell (1995) suggested on this type of evidence that two Nubian groups separated by a thousand years were nevertheless probably both derived from the same ancestral population.

Let me turn now to the questions of health. Since the days of the early Nubian reports, there has been gradual improvement in diagnosis and analysis. The first few researchers probably had good knowledge of dry bone pathology and pseudo-pathology. In his 1935 report, Batrawi mistakes rodent gnawing for some form of disease. He also misses the fact that the skull of a young Meroitic female (grave 174/94) displays changes which may well indicate a malignant tumour. His case of 'amputation' of the toes could well be leprosy and needed X-raying. Oral pathology began to be studied in a little more detail early on, and Ruffer published on it by 1908. Leigh was tabulating data by 1934, and his oral pathology tables demonstrated that abscesses were caused in his sample mainly by severe tooth wear and pulp exposure, rather than by caries. Consequent tooth loss especially affected the molars. By the 1960s comparative studies, especially of caries, were being published with again the molars being most susceptible. Social and environmental factors clearly needed to be considered, as seen in the contrasts shown in Figure 18.3a between the 1st–2nd Dynasty royal tombs of Abydos, with their notably low prevalences, and the increase and divergence in the late Dynastic series (Brothwell 1963).

A consideration of oral pathology has of course always been relatively easy compared with the diagnostic problems of many palaeopathological specimens. I'm not sure if Elliot Smith and his young colleague Wood Jones thought it all to be easy, but I think that some cases really did puzzle Batrawi. Even today, diagnosis may be difficult. In the case of bone changes from mycotic infection, I wonder how often it has been identified as a tumour. There is one Nubian foot (Brothwell 1996) which is a classic case of Madura foot. Rare inherited anomalies can of course occur, as indicated by the bones of two Nubians who showed multiple fracturing in all limbs, surely a strong indication of osteogenesis imperfecta (Brothwell 1973).

Since Ruffer and Willmore described a pelvic tumour in 1914, at least eighteen types of tumour have been described from Egypt and Nubia, although the diagnoses are mainly tentative. In one or two cases, the diagnosis has been

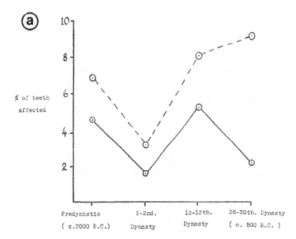

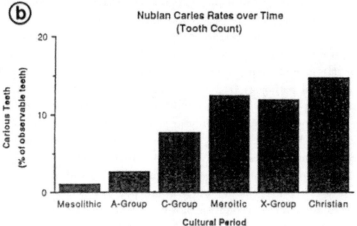

18.3 (a) Changes in the prevalence of pulp exposure (—) and chronic abscesses (--) in some early Egyptian populations. (Reproduced from Brothwell 1963.) (b) Changes in caries rates in relation to agricultural intensification through a sequence of cultural periods in Nubia. (Created by the author after Beckett and Lovell 1994.)

changed, as in the 5th Dynasty femur bone mass originally named as an osteosarcoma, but now accepted as an osteochondroma (see Brothwell 2008: 264, fig. 12.5). Prevalence of tumours in the past is unlikely to have reached the high values seen today, because life expectancy was so much lower, but there was the occasional exception.

Irrigation and agriculture may have impacted on disease in various ways. For instance, caries prevalence (Figure 18.3b) in Nubia was affected (Beckett and Lovell 1994). Patterns of joint disease could also have radically changed.

Did irrigation further encourage the survival of the mosquito and increase its occurrence? We now have evidence of malaria confirmed by molecular analysis (Rabino Massa, Cerutti and Savoia 2000), but we still need to know more about the degree of causal linkage with porotic changes in the skull and orbital cribra. The differentiation of the anaemias by pathology and molecular analysis is still a major problem.

In the area of serious infectious diseases, DNA studies have, for the first time, identified *Corynbacterium* (? *diptheriae*) in a Theban mummy (Zink *et al.* 2001). Tuberculosis, especially in the spine, has been described over many years. The bone pathology can now be supported by molecular evidence (Zink *et al.* 2007), and one interesting question we can now ask is whether ancient DNA studies might show more microevolutionary variation in this disease than previously surmised. And what populations is tuberculosis hitting, urban or rural, stressed or otherwise? In notable contrast is the relative lack of evidence of the other mycobacterial disease, leprosy. Why is it that a cold northern country like Britain has far more evidence of it than Egypt and Nubia together? Could this be linked to the way the disease was moved, perhaps by Roman expansion, into Europe? As for syphilis and its clinical relatives, they remain a complete mystery.

Evidence of schistosomiasis was found by Ruffer ninety years ago, and now we have not only evidence from eggs in mummy viscera and bladder wall calcification but also antigen evidence of the parasite extending back to Predynastic times (Rutherford 2008; Chapter 16, in this volume). Without doubt, this has been another major cause of poor health throughout the development of these early Nilotic societies. The significant changes in climate and environment along the Nile raise other epidemiological questions. In parts of East Africa, sleeping sickness (trypanosomiasis) is linked to the distribution of the Tsetse fly. It was a serious condition in Uganda, but the fly also extends into the cattle country of southern Sudan. In the past, with a more favourable environment, could its impact have extended further north, even beyond Khartoum?

It is worth mentioning here that we tend to assume that museum material which has been studied and reported on is unlikely to yield further important new information. But restudies can be very worthwhile and can even raise questions about diseases not yet recognised in the past. For instance, I was interested to find a skull in the London Natural History Museum from late Predynastic El Amrah (Af.11.2.125). It displays clear bone changes in the nasal area (Figure 18.4), with irregular new bone in the nasal cavity, and a remodelling laterally of the nasal aperture on the left side. The new bone extended back above the bones of the palate, and at one point the palate has been perforated. This could be an infected trauma, but the bone in this region of the face is thin, and there is no evidence of breakage. Another interesting diagnostic possibility is that this is the first evidence of aspergillosis. Sandison and colleagues (1967)

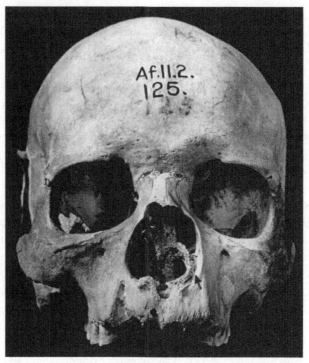

18.4 Facial view of a late Predynastic skull from El Amrah (Af.11.2.125) displaying nasal changes possibly indicating infection by Aspergillus. (Courtesy of the Natural History Museum.)

describe the condition in living northern Sudanese cases, and clearly the environment in this area is ideal for the development of nasal and orbital lesions from infection by Aspergillus.

Finally, a brief word on trauma and surgery. Evidence of broken bones is easy to detect, and they have been described since the first Nubian reports. But now total trauma evidence is considerable and there is growing interest in their analysis (see Forshaw, Chapter 11 in this volume). To give but one recent study, Margaret Judd (2006) has shown contrasting injury profiles in urban and rural people living near Kerma (*c*.2500–1500 BC). The rural group had significantly more non-violence-related injuries, suggesting more occupational accidents.

Regarding direct evidence of surgery on these ancient bodies, there is remarkably little. There are very few cases of skull surgery (trephination), which contrasts significantly with the many cases from Europe. In one Nubian case trephining is associated directly with a compressed fracture and in another with infection of the middle ear and temporal bone, whereas most European cases could be purely of ritual significance.

Conclusions

From the nineteenth-century beginnings of studies on human remains from Egypt and Nubia, the subject has been greatly transformed. What began as a fascination with mummies and pyramids has broadened out into a truly scientific evaluation of past populations. Early visual appraisal of skulls gave rise to more careful osteometric comparisons and a consideration of the health status of these ancient peoples. Non-metric traits on bones and teeth were eventually added to the methodology by which communities could be compared. Early crude attempts to blood group ancient remains have now given way to more refined ancient DNA and other molecular analyses. Other studies, including selected isotope analyses, indicate clearly the extent of modern scientific enquiries, and we can be optimistic about the future of human bio-Egyptology.

Acknowledgments

I am most grateful for permission to reproduce Figures 18.1, 18.2 and 18.3. I am also grateful to the Trustees of the Natural History Museum for Figure 18.4.

References

Batrawi, A. M. (1935), 'Report on the human remains', *Mission archéologique de Nubie 1929–1934* (Cairo: Government Press).

Beckett, S. and Lovell, N. C. (1994), 'Dental disease evidence for agricultural intensification in the Nubian C-Group', *International Journal of Osteoarchaeology* 4, 223–40.

Berry, C. A., Berry, R. J. and Ucko, P. J. (1967), 'Genetical change in ancient Egypt', *Man* 2, 551–68.

Brothwell, D. R. (1963), 'The macroscopic dental pathology of some earlier human populations', in D. R. Brothwell (ed.), *Dental Anthropology* (Oxford: Pergamon), 271–88.

Brothwell, D. R. (1973), 'The evidence for osteogenesis imperfecta in early Egypt', in S. Basu, A. K. Ghosh, S. K. Biswas and R. Ghosh (eds.), *Physical Anthropology and its Extending Horizons* (Calcutta: Longman), 45–55.

Brothwell, D. R. (1996), 'Is this ancient Nubian foot a possible early example of mycotic infection?', *Journal of Paleopathology* 8, 187–9.

Brothwell. D. R. (2008), 'Tumours and tumour-like processes', in R. Pinhasi and S. Mays (eds.), *Advances in Human Palaeopathology* (Chichester: Wiley), 253–81.

Carlson, D. (1976), 'Temporal variation in prehistoric Nubian crania', *American Journal of Physical Anthropology* 45, 467–84.

Geiser, P. (1989), *The Egyptian Nubian: A Study in Social Symbolism* (Cairo: American University in Cairo Press).

Hassan, H. Y., Underhill, P. A., Cavalli-Sforza, L. C. and Ibrhahim, M. E. (2008),

'Y-chromosome variation among Sudanese: restricted gene flow, concordance with language, geography, and history, *American Journal of Physical Anthropology* 137, 316–23.

Hollingsworth, T. H. (1969), *Historical Demography* (London: Hodder and Stoughton).

Irish, J. D. (2006), 'Who were the ancient Egyptians? Dental affinities among Neolithic through post-dynastic peoples', *American Journal of Physical Anthropology* 129, 529–43.

Jonson, A. L. and Lovell, N. C. (1995), 'Dental morphological evidence for biological continuity between the A-Group and C-Group periods in Lower Nubia', *International Journal of Osteoarchaeology* 5, 368–76.

Judd, M. A. (2006), 'Continuity of interpersonal violence between Nubian communities', *American Journal of Physical Anthropology* 131, 324–33.

Knip, A. S. (1970), 'Metrical and non-metrical measurements on the skeletal remains of Christian populations from two sites in Sudanese Nubia', *Koninkl Nederland Akademie van Wetenschappen* 73, 433–68.

Leigh, R. W. (1934), 'Notes on the somatology and pathology of ancient Egypt', *Publications in American Archaeology and Ethnology* 84, 1–54.

Mollison, T. (1929), 'Untersuchungen über den Oldowayfund: der Fossilzustand und der Schädel', *Verhandlungen der Gesellschaft für physische Anthropologie* 3, 60–7.

Mourant, A. E. (1954), *The Distribution of the Human Blood Groups* (Oxford: Blackwell).

Mukherjee, R., Rao, C. R. and Trevor, J. C. (1955), *The Ancient Inhabitants of Jebel Moya (Sudan)* (Cambridge: Cambridge University Press).

Nielsen, O. V. (1973), 'Population movements and changes in ancient Nubia with special reference to the relationship between C-group, New Kingdom and Kerma', *Journal of Human Evolution* 2, 31–46.

Nott, J. C. and Gliddon, G. R. (1857), *Indigenous Races of the Earth* (Trübner: Philadelphia).

Oetteking, B. (1908), 'Kraniologische Studien an Altägyptern', *Archive für Anthropologie* 8, 1–10.

Pearson, K. (1898), 'Mathematical contributions to the theory of evolution', *Philosophical Transactions of the Royal Society of London* 192, 169–244.

Rabino Massa, E., Cerutti, N. and Savoia, M. D. (2000), 'Malaria in Ancient Egypt: paleo-immunological investigation on Predynastic mummified remains', *Revista de antropologia chilena* 32, 7–9.

Robins, G. and Shute, C. D. (1986), 'Predynastic Egyptian stature and physical proportions', *Human Evolution* 1, 313–24.

Rösing, F. W. (1986), 'Kith or kin? On the feasibility of kinship reconstruction in skeletons', in A. R. David (ed.), *Science in Egyptology* (Manchester: Manchester University Press), 223–37.

Ruffer, M. A. (1908), 'Abnormalities and pathology of ancient Egyptian teeth', *American Journal of Physical Anthropology* 3, 335–82.

Ruffer, M. A. and Willmore, J. G. (1914), 'Note on a tumour of the pelvis dating from Roman times', *Journal of Pathology and Bacteriology* 18, 480–4.

Rutherford, P. (2008), 'The use of immunocytochemistry to diagnose disease in mummies', in R. David (ed.), *Egyptian Mummies and Modern Science* (Cambridge and New York: Cambridge University Press), 99–115.

Sandison, A. T., Gentles, J. C., Davidson, G. M. and Branko, M. (1967), 'Aspergilloma of paranasal sinuses and orbit in northern Sudanese', *Journal of the International Society for Human and Animal Mycology* 6, 57–69.

Smith, G. E. (1912), *The Royal Mummies* (Paris: Imprimerie de l'Institut Français d'Archéologie Orientale).

Smith, G. E. (1923), *The Ancient Egyptians and the Origin of Civilization* (London: Harper).

Smith, G. E. and Dawson, W. R. (1924), *Egyptian Mummies* (London: Allen and Unwin).

Smith, G. E. and Jones, F. W. (eds.) (1910), '*The Archaeological Survey of Nubia, Report for 1907–1908*, II: *Report on the Human Remains* (Cairo: National Printing Department).

Strouhal, E. (1968), 'Une contribution à la question du caractère de la population préhistorique de la Haute-Égypte', *Anthropologie* 6, 19–22.

Swedlund, A. C. and Armelagos, G. J. (1976), *Demographic Anthropology* (Dubuque: Brown).

Zink, A. R., Molnar, E., Motamedi, N., Palfy, G., Marcsik, A. and Nerlich, A. G. (2007), 'Molecular history of tuberculosis from ancient mummies and skeletons', *International Journal of Osteoarchaeology* 17, 380–91.

Zink, A., Reischl, U., Wolf, H., Nerlich, A. G. and Miller, R. (2001), 'Corynebacterium in ancient Egypt', *Medical History* 45, 267–72.

19

Further thoughts on Tutankhamun's death and embalming

Robert Connolly and Glenn Godenho

In 1966 the late Professor R. G. Harrison made a surprise appointment to the long-vacant lectureship in physical anthropology in the University of Liverpool's Department of Anatomy. The person appointed was young Robert Connolly from the Pathology Department. Professor Harrison had – at the suggestion of Professor Fairman in the Egyptology Department – investigated the burial remains in Tomb 55 (KV 55) in the Valley of the Kings, and declared them to be Smenkhkare (Harrison 1966). There had previously been several other suggestions, but at the time Smenkhkare fitted the bill satisfactorily and (on not very secure grounds) conclusively. The identity of Smenkhkare is still a matter of wide debate (e.g. Dodson 2009: 30ff). An association between Connolly, Harrison and Fairman, plus several former research students from the Department of Anatomy, continued over the next few years. This association culminated in 1968 with Professor Harrison, a small group from Liverpool and a very large television team entering KV 62 and conducting a detailed study of the mummy of Tutankhamun (Connolly 2010). Some tissue samples were returned to Liverpool, and it was Connolly's task to determine the blood-group of Tutankhamun and of the KV 55 remains (Harrison, Connolly and Abdalla 1969). The fact that both were A_2 and MN seemed at the time to be convincing evidence that Tutankhamun and the occupant of KV 55 were brothers (Harrison, Connolly and Abdalla 1969). Fairman dispatched his new research student, Rosalie David, across to Anatomy to find out what they were doing. She was not quite prepared for a disquisition on Sephadex gel-filtration columns and the affinity for specific glycosphingolipids and the erythrocyte membrane. However, she reported back to Fairman who soon after the meeting said to Harrison, 'Science is Science and Egyptology is Egyptology, there is nothing that science can do for us' (despite his complementary remarks in *Antiquity* (Fairman 1972)). Rosalie and many others would disagree now! This chapter is the result of collaborative teaching at the University of Liverpool between science and humanities, where the authors have discussed the case of Tutankhamun's mummy with undergraduates for the past few years. Of course, any discussion of Egyptian mummies necessarily involves reference to Professor Rosalie David's contributions to the field, and it is the authors' pleasure to have worked with her in teaching and research matters over the years. We hope that this chapter appeals to the Professor not only in terms of subject, but also as a demonstration of the value of teaching in research development – a cause that she has championed with great success, as can be seen in her development of Egyptology teaching at the University of Manchester.

The 2005 computed tomography (CT) scans of Tutankhamun produced under the direction of Dr Zahi Hawass (Hawass *et al.* 2009) have instigated a series of studies hypothesising on how possible peri-mortem damage to the body affected the mode of mummification, the extent to which that damage might reveal cause of death, and the likelihood that some of the visible damage relates to post-mortem (ancient and modern) activity (see Ikram 2013 for a review of the salient research). A recent paper by W. Benson Harer (2011) on the condition of the mummy of Tutankhamun is a most welcome addition to our understanding of the possible circumstances surrounding his death and subsequent embalming. However, Harer's use of the CT images bears some interesting comparisons with the conventional flat-plate photographic film X-ray images taken by the late Professor R. G. Harrison in 1968. On 4 December 1968 Professor Harrison and his photographer and radiographer, Mr Lynton Reeve, both from the Department of Anatomy at the University of Liverpool, entered KV 62 accompanied by Dr Z. Iskander, Mr A. Tahl and Mr S. Osman from the Department of Antiquities in Cairo, and Professor A. Abdalla from the Department of Anatomy at Cairo University (among others, including a BBC television recording crew). Several X-ray pictures were taken in extremely cramped conditions, amid the TV team and scientists plus the usual crowds of tourists. They were of course rewarded with the first almost public viewing of the actual mummy of Tutankhamun since 11 November 1925 when Douglas Derry attempted his famous autopsy (see Derry 1927 for a report and Leek 1972 for a more comprehensive account). The 35 cm × 43 cm photographic X-ray plates were, with no little trepidation, developed by Mr Reeve in a blacked-out bathroom in the Winter Palace Hotel in Luxor with the chemicals laboriously but carefully brought from Liverpool. The images were excellent and the films are still in pristine condition, being continuously maintained and archived by the Victoria Gallery and Museum, University of Liverpool. Professor Harrison and Professor Abdalla published the preliminary findings in 1972 (Harrison and Abdalla 1972). The findings concerning the probable cause of death of King Tutankhamun and the reasons for his 'bizarre embalming' do not differ from the views of this article's first author as a result of discussions with Professor Harrison prior to his death in 1982 and subsequent study of digitally enhanced copies of the original X-ray films (Connolly 2010).

Comparisons of the CT scans and the flat plates merit discussion. Harer states that the royal embalmers made a first attempt to remove the brain via the standard, but not universal, route of breaking through the very fragile cribriform plate of the ethmoid bone which separates the cranial cavity from the nasal cavity (Harer 2011: 229). Certainly the 2005 CT scans show some minor damage in this region, but it is insufficient to suggest that the brain was removed through the nasal cavity; brain removal through the nasal cavity would require that the whole cribriform plate structure is completely destroyed. Interestingly, extensive study of the digitally enhanced copies of the original 1968 plates in 2003 (Boyer *et al.* 2003) shows no damage at all in the region (Figure 19.1).

The difference, it is now suggested, is simply some damage to the ethmoid bone during handling of the head either at, or since the 1968 examination. The bone is very fragile, particularly in specimens of this antiquity, and simply moving the head could cause the damage noted by Hawass *et al.* (2009: 163) rather than being the work of the royal embalmers. If, as is suggested, Tutankhamun had been dead for some time before reaching the embalming workshop, the brain could have begun to liquefy and could easily be drained out of the foramen magnum in the base of the skull. Derry (1927) reports the skull being only loosely attached to the cervical vertebrae in 1925 and indeed

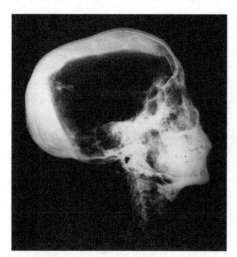 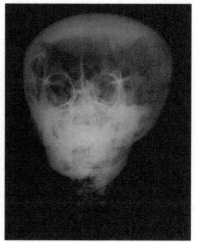

19.1 Tutankhamun, lateral skull X-ray. (Courtesy of the University of Liverpool, image produced by Lynton Reeve.)

19.2 Tutankhamun, frontal skull X-ray. (Courtesy of the University of Liverpool, image produced by Lynton Reeve.)

several fragments from the first cervical vertebra are loose in the cranial cavity, appearing in different orientations in different X-ray images (see Figures 19.1 and 19.2). These fragments could only have been released by Derry, not the royal embalmers, for otherwise they would be embedded in the layers of resin which both Harer and Harrison report (Harrison and Abdalla 1972: 11; Harer 2011: 229; Boyer *et al.* 2003: 1143–6; Hawass *et al.* 2009: 164).

The two layers of resin in the vertex and occiput, although unusual, are possibly not unique. However the amount of resin used is relatively small. The mummy of Yuya – Tutankhamun's grandfather or great-grandfather (Connolly, Harrison and Ahmed 1976), generally now reckoned to be the latter (Dodson 2009: 15–16 and 95–8) – shows vastly more resin in the cranial cavity but only a trace in the vertex (Figure 19.3). Surely by *c.*1400 BC, the principles of royal embalming were established (Ikram and Dodson 1998: 118).

Harer's description of the thorax merits detailed comparison with the 1968 plates (Figure 19.4) and some comment. Both the CT scans and the flat plates show clearly that some ribs are cut and some broken, and we are in absolute agreement over which ribs are intentionally severed and which are broken, and that the cutting or sawing must have been the work of the royal embalmers (Harer 2011: 228–9).[1] Furthermore, if it were necessary or desirable to remove the anterior thoracic wall at embalming, it would have been easier to cut or saw through the ribs than to break them away from the soft tissue. This strongly supports the supposition that many of the ribs – especially, but not exclusively on the left side of the body – were broken before reaching the royal embalmers, presumably as a result of a very serious and probably lethal traumatic event (intoned also by Harer 2011: 229 and 233). It cannot be assumed with certainty however from the evidence we have, that the heart and sternum were entirely absent from the body when it reached the embalming workshop. Surely, following the traumatic event, Tutankhamun's followers would have wrapped the king in the damaged remnants of his clothes and almost certainly additional drapery and would not have disposed of any of his royal body. Unless the trauma was so violent as to distribute body parts far from their source or was perhaps an animal attack, both of which seem unlikely from the evidence, then it would be more reasonable to suppose they were delivered to the royal embalmers. What however could have been the condition of the sternum and heart?

The units of the sternum of an eighteen-year-old youth may not have been completely fused and may still be joined together only in a fragile manner by cartilage and fibrous tissue, and thus severe trauma could very easily separate

---

[1] But see also the alternative suggestion previously made by Forbes, Ikram and Kamrin (2007: 51–2) and reinforced by Ikram (2013: 295) that the ribs may have been damaged at some point after the modern rediscovery.

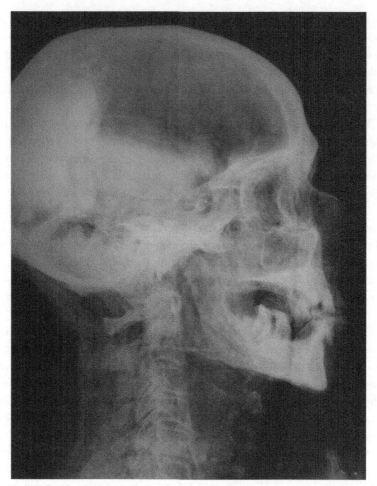

19.3 Yuya, lateral skull X-ray. (Courtesy of the University of Liverpool, image produced by Lynton Reeve.)

the individual units (Figure 19.4), possibly breaking individual units as well as dissociating them. Reconstruction at this stage would be very difficult and probably unnecessary, hence the practical value of the gold and blue glass beaded collar being used to cover the extensive damage to the thorax. This beaded collar is now absent; however, the 1968 X-ray image clearly shows a total of twenty-three beads distributed between the upper thorax and the upper arms. Figure 19.4 shows the beads very clearly, and on the right side the penetrating thread-holes of some are notably visible. Similar X-ray opaque white spots appear in Harer's figure 1 in exactly the same location on the 1968 plates and are certainly beads embedded in the mummy, but not identified as such or commented upon. In addition, a single bead is visible on the right arm (Figure 19.5).

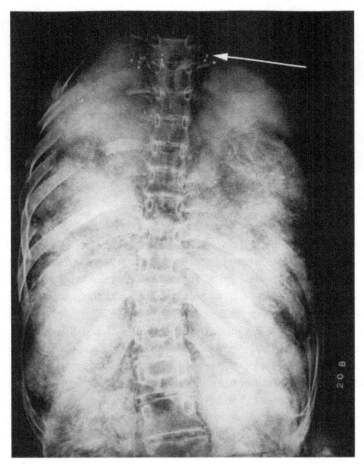

19.4 Tutankhamun, thorax X-ray. (Courtesy of the University of Liverpool, image produced by Lynton Reeve.)

It is difficult to say with certainty that this demonstrates that Tutankhamun's arms were originally crossed over the chest (rather than beside the body where they are now located), because, as Ikram (2013: 293–4) demonstrates, Burton's photographs and Derry's description show that Tutankhamun's arms were not discovered crossed over his chest, but were instead folded over his abdomen. Presumably these beads are the remnants of the unofficial disinterment of Tutankhamun's body at some time between Carter's 1926 and Harrison's 1968 examinations, as suggested by Forbes, Ikram and Kamrin (2007: 56).

The problem of the heart is carefully discussed by Harer (2011: 232) but whether it was disposed of by the royal embalmers must remain an open question. The human heart is remarkably small in comparison with the body size

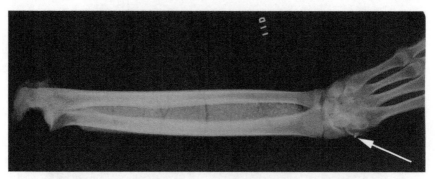

19.5 Tutankhamun, right arm X-ray. (Courtesy of the University of Liverpool, image produced by Lynton Reeve.)

(Gray 1913: 562). The fully grown adult male heart measures about 12 cm from base to apex, 8–9 cm transversely at its broadest part and 6 cm anteroposteriorly and weighs between 280 and 340 g. Tutankhamun was of small stature, perhaps 150–60 cm, and of slight build as he appears in mummified form and so his heart (assuming cardiac development was the same in antiquity as it is now) would have been at the low range of size and weight – small. Such a structure, if extensively damaged in a serious traumatic incident would, like the sternum, be unreconstructable and hence possibly discarded in fragments by the royal embalmer. Why no substitute heart or heart scarab was included by the embalmers is a matter of debate, and Ikram (2013: 296–8) discusses the possibilities fully.

The interesting state of the diaphragm described by Harer (2011: 230–1) is not visible on the flat-plate X-ray images. The comparison of the pelvic region is however of considerable interest. The 1968 flat plate (Figure 19.6) clearly shows the pelvic cavity to be very tightly packed with presumably resin-soaked linen. Harer reports no packing in the pelvis (2011: 231). Is this an aberration of the resolution of CT scanning from the choice of attenuation factors and window-width, or is the packing no longer present? This can be answered only by direct examination of the mummy. Also, Figure 19.6 shows distinctly that most of the left side of the bony pelvis is absent. Harrison noted this (Harrison and Abdalla 1972: 12) and its significance is noted by Connolly (2010). It is broken, not cut or sawed. The pubic bones are missing, and a large proportion of the ilium and adjoining bones from the left side are also absent. It is probably important that this damage is on the same side as the most extensive destruction to the thorax and was thus presumably incurred in the same incident. The unusual position of the embalming incision (Harer 2011: 230; Ikram 2013: 294) could thus be explained by the supposition that the royal embalmers could have extracted the pelvic viscera and inserted the packing through an existing traumatic wound. In the context of trauma, it is noteworthy that the fractured femur reported by

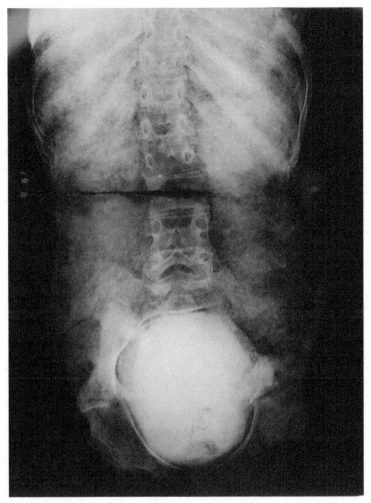

19.6 Tutankhamun, pelvis X-ray. (Courtesy of the University of Liverpool, image produced by Lynton Reeve.)

Harrison and Abdalla (1972: 12) and extensively discussed by Hawass *et al.* (2009: 163) is also on the left side of the body.

Unless textual evidence becomes available, the actual cause of death and the state of the body at embalming will probably never be known with certainty, but fatal thoracic trauma is high on the list of priorities as determined from the evidence available. It should be noted, however, that only a very small proportion of causes of death will actually be visible on X-ray analysis, and so even thoracic trauma may be far from the actual facts. However, this offers opportunities for further collaboration between science and Egyptology.

References

Boyer, R. S., Rodin, E. A., Grey, T. C. and Connolly, R. C. (2003), 'The skull and cervical spine radiographs of Tutankhamun: a critical appraisal', *American Journal of Neuroradiology* 24, 1142–7.

Connolly, R. C. (2010), 'The X-ray plates of Tutankhamun: A reassessment of their meaning and significance', in J. Cockitt and R. David (eds.), *Pharmacy and Medicine in Ancient Egypt: Proceedings of the Conferences Held in Cairo (2007) and Manchester (2008)* (Oxford: Archaeopress), 46–50.

Connolly, R. C., Harrison, R. G. and Ahmed, S. (1976), 'Serological evidence for the parentage of Tutankhamun and Smenkhkare', *Journal of Egyptian Archaeology* 62, 184–6.

Derry, D. (1927), 'Report upon the examination of King Tutankhamen's mummy', in H. Carter, *The Tomb of Tut.ankh.Amen*, II: *The Burial Chamber* (London: Cassell), 143–61.

Dodson, A. (2009), *Amarna Sunset: Nefertiti, Tutankhamun, Ay, Horemheb, and the Egyptian Counter-Reformation* (Cairo: The American University in Cairo Press).

Fairman, H. W. (1972), 'Tutankhamun and the end of the 18th Dynasty', *Antiquity* 46, 15–8.

Forbes, D., Ikram, S., and Kamrin, J. (2007), 'Tutankhamun's missing ribs', *KMT* 18 (1), 50–6.

Gray, H. (1913), *Anatomy: Descriptive and Applied* (Philadelphia and New York: Lee and Febiger).

Harer, W. B. (2011), 'New evidence for King Tutankhamen's death: his bizarre embalming', *Journal of Egyptian Archaeology* 97, 228–33.

Harrison, R. G. (1966), 'An anatomical examination of the pharaonic remains purported to be Akhenaten', *Journal of Egyptian Archaeology* 52, 95–119.

Harrison, R. G., and Abdalla, A. B. (1972), 'The remains of Tutankhamun', *Antiquity* 46, 8–14.

Harrison, R. G., Connolly, R. C. and Abdalla, A. B. (1969), 'Kinship of Smenkhkare and Tutankhamun affirmed by serological micromethod', *Nature* 224, 325–6.

Hawass, Z., Shafik, M., Rühli, F. J., Selim, A., El-Sheikh, E., Abdel Fatah, S., Amer, H., Gaballa, F., Gamal Eldin, A., Egarter-Vigl, E. and Gostner, P. (2009), 'Computed tomographic evaluation of Pharaoh Tutankhamun, ca. 1300 BC', *Annales du Service des antiquités de l'Égypte* 81, 159–74.

Ikram, S. (2013), 'Some thoughts on the mummification of King Tutankhamun', *Études et travaux* 26 (1), 292–301.

Ikram, S. and Dodson, A. (1998), *The Mummy in Ancient Egypt: Equipping the Dead for Eternity* (London: Thames and Hudson).

Leek, F. F. (1972), *The Human Remains from the Tomb of Tut'ankhamūn* (Oxford: Griffith Institute).

20

Proving Herodotus and Diodorus? Headspace analysis of 'eau de mummy' using gas chromatography mass spectrometry

David Counsell

Herodotus was a pre-eminent historian of the ancient world, as evidenced by his surviving, important interpretations of ancient history, yet the authenticity of his work has often been questioned over the centuries since his death. Born around 484 BC in Halicarnassus (modern-day Bodrum in Turkey), Herodotus wrote his great work *The Histories* in the early fifth century BC, reputedly after years of travelling, patient research and recording. Unfortunately, his 'strong sense of the marvellous' and 'interest in the unusual or the fantastic' led to accusations, even in antiquity, that he was little more than a teller of tall stories rather than a serious historian (De Sélincourt and Marincola 1994: xv). This tarnished reputation has led to him being dubbed the 'father of history' by many, but described by others as the 'father of lies' because of his apparently extraordinary accounts (De Sélincourt and Marincola 1994: xv; Shaw and Nicholson 1995: 126). Without doubt the reliability of *The Histories* has long been questioned; it has even been suggested that Herodotus may have compiled his history 'second hand', never having visited many of the places he claimed (De Sélincourt and Marincola 1994: xxvii).

Ancient descriptions of the mummification process

Featuring prominently among the many 'marvellous' and 'fantastic' accounts from Herodotus's *Histories* are his descriptions of the mummification of ancient Egyptians, which must have seemed unbelievable to many, but the details of which we now know largely to be true. In these accounts Herodotus describes three techniques of embalming used, which depended upon the wealth of the individual and his family (De Sélincourt and Marincola 1994: 115–16). Of these the first description by Herodotus; 'the most perfect process' (II, 86) runs as follows:

> As much as possible of the brain is extracted through the nostrils with an iron hook, and what the hook cannot reach is rinsed out with drugs; next the flank is laid open with a flint knife and the whole contents of the abdomen removed; the cavity is then thoroughly cleansed and washed out, first with palm wine and again with an infusion of pounded spices. After that it is filled with pure bruised myrrh, cassia, and every other aromatic substance with the exception of frankincense, and sewn up again, after which the body is placed in natron, covered entirely over, for seventy days never longer. When this period, which must not be exceeded, is over, the body is washed and then wrapped from head to foot in linen cut into strips and smeared on the under side with gum, which is commonly used by the Egyptians instead of glue. (De Sélincourt and Marincola 1994: 115)

The failure of early attempts to emulate this description of mummification did little to improve Herodotus's reputation, although this may in part have been due to early translations of *The Histories* describing the use of a natron solution. Modern investigations have proved that dry natron rather than a natron solution must have been used (Garner 1979: 19–23). This has prompted conclusions that 'Herodotus is a more trustworthy source than used to be thought' (Andrews 1984: 11).

This principal technique of mummification, though described during the fifth century BC, probably differs little in principle from the technique used during the New Kingdom, though evidence abounds of experimentation in the pursuit of excellence. Different packing materials were tried, different gums and resins were employed, wigs were used, and in the case of Amenhotep III and some of the later mummies from the 21st Dynasty, subcutaneous packing was inserted in an attempt to provide a more lifelike appearance (Smith 1912).

Herodotus goes on to describe two further, simpler and less expensive methods of embalming that were available for the non-elite who may not have been able to afford the full procedure. The second of these mentions the use of cedar oil as a purge of the intestines. Both of these methods record the use of natron for preservation but do not include details of the use of other herbs and spices in the process, though this is considered likely to have occurred (De Sélincourt and Marincola 1994: 115–16).

In addition to the descriptions of the mummification process by Herodotus, we get further information from a later source in the work of Diodorus Siculus, a Syrian living about 40 BC (Shaw and Nicholson 1995: 86). In his account Diodorus describes how the priest who defiled the body, by incising and eviscerating the corpse, was ritually stoned from the embalmers' tent by his colleagues after his unpleasant task was completed. He also recorded that the embalmer's incision was usually made in the left flank (Andrews 1984: 17; Shaw and Nicholson 1995: 86). Importantly, Diodorus also reports the use of aromatic herbs and spices in the mummification process but specifies only cinnamon and myrrh, which were used to rub the body after treatment with natron (Manniche 1993: 90).

Hypothesis

The classical accounts of mummification by Herodotus and Diodorus are consistent in their description of the use of herbs and spices in the embalming process. Anyone who has spent time with mummies will be familiar with the not unpleasant but complex, musty smell that many of them retain to this day. This chapter attempts to identify residual volatile components in the 'eau de mummy' fragrance to confirm the use of herbs and spices as described in antiquity, thereby providing further support to the authenticity of Herodotus's and Diodorus's historical descriptions. Some agents are mentioned by name as being used; these are cassia, cinnamon and importantly myrrh, which was the only specific agent identified by both ancient commentators; Herodotus singled out frankincense as not being used. It may therefore be possible to identify specific chemical moieties in the mummy aroma that would confirm the presence of these and other residual materials from the mummification process.

The chemistry of volatile substances in herbs and spices

The principal volatile compounds responsible for scent and flavour in plants are the product of two biosynthetic pathways that together are capable of producing a vast range of natural compounds.

The shikimate pathway provides a route to the formation of aromatic heterocyclic compounds, particularly amino acids, and is not found in animals (Dewick 2009: 137). A central intermediary in this pathway is shikimic acid, and products of this pathway in plants and microbes include the essential amino acids phenylalanine, tyrosine and tryptophan, a number of vitamins including B vitamins, folate and the coumarin anticoagulants. This pathway is also responsible for a group of compounds called phenylpropenes, which are contained in the volatile oils from a number of plants including fennel, cinnamon, aniseed and cassia. These include cinnamyl compounds and eugenol (Dewick 2009: 156–9).

The mevalonate biochemical pathway is responsible for the synthesis of terpenoids and steroids. Acetate metabolism using three molecules of Acetyl coenzyme A produces mevalonic acid. The five-carbon isopentyl diphosphate or pyrophosphate (IPP) units subsequently derived from six-carbon mevalonic acid provide the building blocks for the terpenoid chain structures that are required for the production of myriad natural compounds, including diterpenoids (twenty carbon atoms) and steroids (thirty carbon atoms). In addition terpenoid chains produced by this pathway are added to carbon skeletons produced by the other biochemical pathways to supply important supplemental elements. Two IPP molecules are used to produce a monoterpene with a ten-carbon (C_{10}) structure which is a common component of volatile oils used in flavouring and perfumery. Cyclisation reactions extend the range of monoterpene structures considerably, leading to the production of monocyclic structures such as limonene and bicyclic ring structures such as borneol and camphor. The mevalonate pathway does produce a small number of monoterpene-based aromatic compounds such as the phenol-based cymene, thymol and carvacrol, the latter two being found in thyme (*Thymus vulgaris*) (Dewick 1995: 507–34; Dewick 2009: 187–310).

Not surprisingly, many of the plants used as herbs or in perfume manufacture are rich in these natural compounds. The presence of residual terpenes or phenylpropenes in 'eau de mummy' would therefore confirm the use of herbs and spices in the embalming process.

Methods

A novel technique was employed to collect the volatiles exuding from a mummy sample by allowing them to accumulate in the 'headspace' of a sealed container and then sampling these volatiles for analysis using gas-chromatography–mass spectrometry (GCMS).

The sample

A particularly pungent sample of mummy tissue was selected for this work from the International Ancient Egyptian Mummy Tissue Bank at Manchester University, originally removed from a mummy in the collection of the New Walk Museum, Leicester, UK. The sample used was from the male mummy of Bes-en-Mut (MMTB no. 528/1981.1885). He was a priest in the temple of Min at Akhmim (Egyptian: Khent-Min) in Upper Egypt in about 700 BC, around 250 years before Herodotus's descriptions of mummification.

Headspace analysis using solid phase microextraction

It has long been known that volatile substances are adsorbed onto absorbent materials and that the adsorbed compounds can be released by reheating the material, a process known as desorption. Solid phase microextraction (SPME) was first developed at the University of Waterloo in Ontario, Canada, and it employs this principle in a simple re-usable system. The system has a wide range of applications including food technology (Sides, Robards and Helliwell 2000:

322–9), pharmaceuticals (Penton 1997: 10–12) and toxicology (Yashiki *et al.* 1995: 17–24). It has also been used extensively for aroma analysis of food, for example cheese (Chin, Bernhard and Rosenberg 1995: 1118–29), and plant materials such as quaver fruit (Paniandy, Cane-Ming and Pieribattesti 2000: 153–8). I believe this to be its first application in archaeology.

Headspace SPME analysis was used to identify volatile agents from mummified tissue using a SUPELCO™ (Bellefonte, PA 16823-0048, USA) fibre and manual fibre holder combined with GCMS. This is a needle-based system that can be inserted through a seal into the headspace of a sealed container holding the material of interest. The SUPELCO™ system used comprises a 1 cm long, 100 μm diameter, fused silica fibre bonded to a stainless steel plunger. The fibre is coated with a stationary phase, namely polydimethylsiloxane (PDMS), that absorbs the analytes from the sample. The coated fibre is contained within a self-sealing needle system, whereby the plunger can be used to advance and withdraw the fibre into and out of a protected environment. Once inserted into the headspace vial the absorbent fibre is advanced from the needle into the headspace gases, where analytes are adsorbed into the PDMS coating. Gentle heat can be applied to facilitate vaporisation of volatile compounds in the sample. After a given time, overnight in this study, the adsorbent fibre is drawn back into the needle, where it is re-sealed. The needle can then be withdrawn from the sample vial with the sampling fibre protected from contamination in the ambient environment. For analysis, the needle is introduced through a seal into the sample port of the GCMS analyser, where the fibre is re-exposed and heated to desorb the analytes contained in the PDMS coating. The manual fibre holder can be adjusted to facilitate correct placement of the fibre within the gas chromatography sample port. Both the holding device and the fibre are re-usable, the fibre being recommended for replacement after every fifty uses.

Prior to use, the needle system was first purged or desorbed of any volatile materials adsorbed into the PDMS coating from the storage environment. This was achieved by exposing the fibre in the gas chromatography sample port and heating it through a short cycle to 300°C. The fibre was then retracted into the needle, which, after cooling, was removed from the gas chromatography port and immediately inserted into the headspace vial, where the fibre was exposed to the aroma surrounding the mummified sample. The open sample container and lid had previously been heated to 300°C and allowed to cool before insertion of the sample to remove any volatile contaminants.

The needle was left in situ overnight (eighteen hours) at an ambient temperature of 30°C. After the extraction period, the fibre was retracted into the needle and the needle removed from the headspace vial. Sample stability at this point is good, and there is no immediate need to run the sample, but in this case the GCMS analysis was carried out on the following day.

The analysis was run by first heating the needle casing, in the GCMS sample port, over a short cycle to 300°C with the source gas running to purge any contaminant volatile compounds that might be present on the needle exterior. After cooling back to 40°C, the fibre was exposed and the full GCMS analysis performed. A temperature gradient was used, starting at 45°C for one minute and climbing by 8°C per minute to a maximum temperature of 300°C, which was held for seventeen minutes. This is shorter than the one-hour cycle used for other analyses as the SPME system readily desorbs the analytes into the system, allowing separation by the gas chromatography over a shorter period.

The system used was a Fisons GC8000 gas chromatograph linked to a Fisons MD800 quadrupole mass spectrometer using electron ionisation (EI) and an electron multiplier detection system. The gas chromatography column used was a GC-1™(GC² Chromatography, Unit A, Millbrook Business Centre, Floats Road, Manchester, UK). This is a fused silica column 25 m in length and 0.25 mm in internal diameter internally coated with a 0.25 µm thick film of 100 per cent PDMS as the stationary phase. Computer analysis of the results was facilitated using MassLynx software (Waters, Micromass, Wythenshawe, Manchester, UK). This allows refinement by subtraction of ions from adjacent areas of the chromatogram to produce clean mass spectra that can then be automatically compared with known spectra in libraries such as those compiled by the National Institute of Standards and Technology (NIST) (1998) and John Wiley & Sons, Scientific Publishers (McLafferty 2013). These libraries were developed for use principally with electron ionisation.

Results

Analysis of the headspace results reveals the presence of a number of terpenoids and phenylpropene compounds. A selection of these is identified on the gas chromatogram in Figure 20.1. Figure 20.2 shows confirmatory mass spectra for these compounds.

Some of these substances are closely derived from common biochemical pathways, for example borneol and camphor (Dewick 2009: 196). Additional finds of naphthalene derivatives and a range of butyl and isobutyl compounds are most likely to be products from the breakdown and degeneration (diagenesis) of other compounds over time (Figure 20.3). In this process slow chemical reactions take place over long time periods, including oxidation and cross reactivity between compounds in the mummy itself or introduced as contaminates from fungal or bacterial infestations. This process produces new chemical moieties not necessarily present in the original mummy or the materials applied during the mummification process, making the interpretation of GCMS results more complex. Larger, more complex compounds were also found in the sample, for

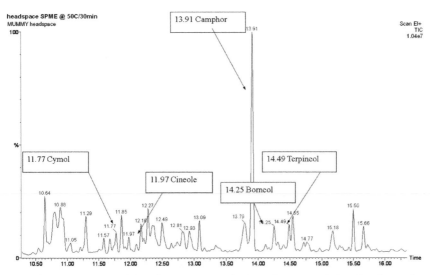

20.1 Section of the total ion chromatogram for 'eau de mummy' showing the peaks for selected compounds of interest. (Created by the author.)

example sesquiterpenoids with seven-member rings such as aromadendrene and longiborneol shown in Figure 20.4.

In total the following compounds were identified in the sample in order of their position on the chromatogram: phenol (10.80), cymol (11.77), limonene (11.85), geranyl isobutyrate (11.86), cineole (11.97), cinnamyl isobutyrate (12.82), camphor (13.91), borneol (14.24), terpineol (14.49), naphthalene (14.54), phenyl butyrate (14.77), methylnaphthalene (16.34), copaene (17.01), aromadendrene (17.98), α-muuroline (18.57), calamenene (18.87), longiborneol (20.08) and cadalin (20.62). Many of these substances are likely to be of plant origin, in particular the terpenoids, such as borneol, camphor and terpineol and the cinnamyl component of cinnamyl isobutyrate.

The analysis above was originally undertaken for my doctoral research in 2006 (Counsell 2006). For the purpose of this chapter a further analysis of the original results has been undertaken to look more specifically at the named herbs from the classical descriptions.

According to Dewick (2009: 158), cinnamaldehyde, molecular weight 132, is the major constituent of both cassia and cinnamon oils making up 70–90 per cent of their composition. A search of the gas chromatogram was undertaken using fragment masses of 131, 103 and 77 in addition to the molecular weight of 132 as indicated by the NIST Library. No cinnamaldehyde was found in the sample.

Verghese *et al.* (1987: 99–102) have demonstrated that there are chemical moieties such as boswellic acids that are unique to *Boswellia spp.* and are

Mass spectrum for 11.77 – para cymene, aka. cymol (NIST).

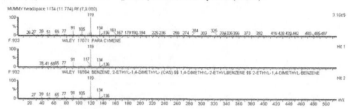

Mass spectrum for 11.97 – cineole.

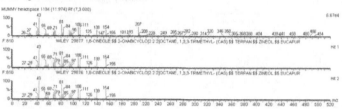

Mass spectrum for 13.91 – camphor.

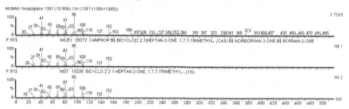

Mass spectrum for 14.25 – borneol.

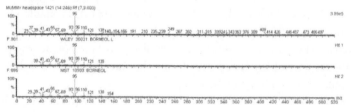

Mass spectrum for 14.49 – terpineol.

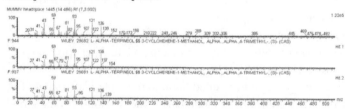

20.2 Confirmatory mass spectra for selected chromatography peaks in 20.1.
(Created by the author.)

Mass spectrum for 11.86 - Geranyl isobutyrate

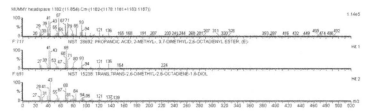

Mass spectrum for 10.80 - phenol

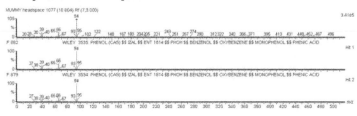

Mass spectrum for 14.54 - naphthalene

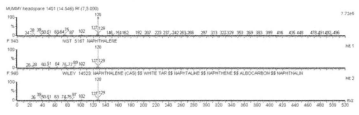

Mass spectrum for 16.34 - methyl naphthalene

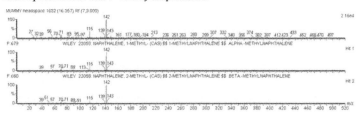

Mass spectrum for 12.82 – cinnamyl isobutyrate.

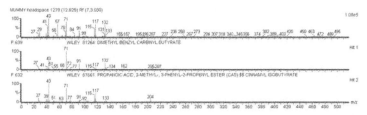

20.3 Mass spectra of breakdown and diagenesis products. (Created by the author.)

Mass spectrum for 17.01 - copaene

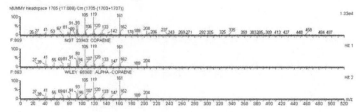

Mass spectrum for 18.57 - alpha muuroline

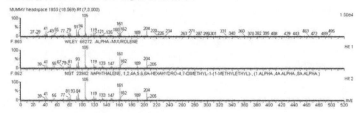

Mass spectrum for 18.87 – calamenene.

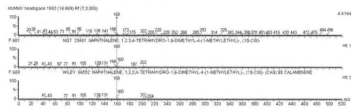

Mass spectrum for 17.98 - aromadendrene

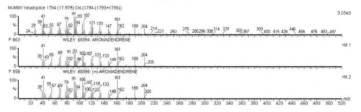

Mass spectrum for 20.08 – longiborneol

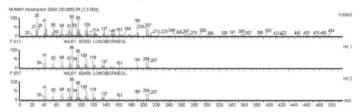

20.4 Mass spectra of selected complex volatiles. (Created by the author.)

contained only in frankincense resin but not in the extracted oil. No compounds of molecular weight 456 were detectable in the sample, nor were mass spectra available for boswellic acids in the available NIST database.

Apart from limonene, none of the compounds found to date in this sample are found in myrrh (Duke n.d., s.v. 'African myrrh'). A specific search for three further compounds found in but not unique to myrrh, namely α-bisabolene, cadinene and cinnamaldehyde, was undertaken but none were found in the sample.

Discussion

This simple technique has identified key constituents of the typical mummy smell or 'eau de mummy'. Some of these compounds, for example camphor, phenol and naphthalene, are stable products often found at the end of a degradation sequence from other less stable compounds including diterpenes and steroids as well as terpenes. Of the isolated compounds camphor was the most abundant, which probably explains the 'mothball-like' aroma experienced in the presence of many mummies. The variety of these compounds and the residual presence of such a wide range of plant-based chemical moieties confirm the use of a range of plant materials applied during the mummification process.

A number of herbs and spices are known to have been used by the Egyptians. These are summarised in Table 20.1, along with some of the known chemicals that make up their composition. The list is by no means exhaustive in either the herbs and spices known to the Egyptians or the chemical components of these herbs and spices. It serves, however, to illustrate the widespread nature of these compounds and the difficulty, therefore, of specifying that a particular plant or plants was present in the mummification materials. What it does confirm is that Herodotus and Diodorus are both correct in describing a mixture of herbs and spices being used in the mummification process.

When considering more specifically those plants that were named by the classical authors, it is possible to make the following comments. Cinnamon (*Cinnamonium zeylanicum.*) and cassia (*Cinnamonium cassia*) were probably both known to the ancient Egyptians but as they are very similar plants it is unclear whether the Egyptians were aware of the botanical distinction (Manniche 1993: 88–91). Both contain a range of the compounds identified in the sample but the principal component of the essential oil derived from both plants is cinnamaldehyde (Dewick 2009: 156). Unfortunately, cinnamaldehyde, or its alcohol and ester derivatives, could not be found. However, cinnamyl isobutyrate, which was found in the sample, has not been reported to date in any plant species (Duke n.d., s.v. 'Cinnamyl isobutyrate'), so one can speculate that its presence is likely to be due to diagenesis of cinnamaldehyde, possibly by microbial activity,

Table 20.1   Chemical constituents of common herbs and spices known to the ancient Egyptians that were found in 'eau de mummy'

Common name	Latin name	Known constituents found in mummy sample	Page reference in Manniche 1993
Rosemary	*Rosmarinus officinalis*	calamenene, cineole, borneol and camphor	144
Marjoram	*Origanum majorana*	calamenene with thymol, α-muurolene, 3-carene and aromadendrene reported in some species	129–30
Thyme	*Thymus spp.*	thymol and camphor	150
Basil	*Ocimum basilicum*	camphor, α-muuroline, borneol	128
Myrtle	*Myrtus communis*	calamenene, copaene, camphor and α-muurolene.	124–5
Juniper	*Juniperus spp.*	calamenene, aromadendrene, longiborneol and borneol with α-muurolene reported in some species	110–12
Cardamon	*Ellettaria cardamomum*	borneol and cineole	100
Cumin	*Cumin cyminum*	copaene and cineole	96–8
Coriander	*Coriandrum sativum*	camphor and borneol	94

Sources: 'Dr Duke's Phytochemical and Ethnobotanical Database' (Duke n.d.); Dewick 2009: 200–2.

over the centuries. This would support but not confirm the use of cinnamon and/or cassia in the embalming process.

Biblical frankincense, *Boswellia carteri*, and myrrh, *Commiphora spp.*, were both known to the ancient Egyptians (Manniche 1999: 26). It is interesting that Herodotus singles out frankincense as excluded from the mixture. Frankincense is known to contain α-muuroline, aromadendrene, α-copaene and borneol but this does not necessarily prove the presence of frankincense without the isolation of boswellic acids to confirm it. Regarding myrrh, only one of the compounds reported from the headspace test appears in the known constituents of the plant according to Dr Duke (Duke n.d., s.v. 'African myrrh'). The absence of other compounds present in myrrh would suggest that it is unlikely that myrrh was used on the Leicester mummy but further mummy studies would be required to refute its use absolutely.

Among the plants listed above it is possible to make a clear identification of one plant. According to Akiyoshi, Erdtman and Kubota (1960) longiborneol is identical to the compound juniperol, and juniperol is reported to be found only in the wood of *Juniperus communis*, the common juniper (Duke n.d., s.v. 'Juniperol'), which would appear to confirm the use of juniper oil in the embalming process. According to Manniche (1999: 119) Dioscorides refers to juniper oil prepared from the resin that 'was in most demand for anointing the dead'. Manniche goes on to suggest that it was juniper and not cedar oil that was referred to in the 'mummification literature', by which one assumes she means the classical descriptions of Herodotus, suggesting therefore that he was incorrect in his description of the purgative use of cedar oil, having mistaken it for juniper oil – unless of course this too is a faulty translation.

Despite this, the overall findings of this work confirm the use of a range of herbs and spices and give further support to the accuracy of the ancient accounts of mummification and in particular those of Herodotus. Perhaps as a result of this work his 'trustworthiness' (Andrews 1984: 11) will be further enhanced.

Acknowledgements

Thanks are due to Dr Vic Garner for his support and encouragement and to Drs Keith and Tony Hall of Hall Analytical Laboratories, Manchester, UK, for their invaluable assistance with the GCMS analysis.

References

Akiyoshi, S., Erdtman, H. and Kubota. T. (1960), 'Chemistry of the natural order cupressales-XXVI: the identity of junipene, kuromatsuene and longifolene and of juniperol, kuromatsuol, macrocarpol and longiborneol', *Tetrahedron* 9 (3), 237–9.

Andrews, C. (1984), *Egyptian Mummies* (London: British Museum Press).

Chin, H., Bernhard, R. and Rosenberg, M. (1995), 'SPME for cheese volatile compound analysis', *Journal of Food Science* 61, 1118–29.

Counsell, D. J. (2006). 'Intoxicants in ancient Egypt: The Application of Modern Forensic Analytical Techniques to Ancient Artefacts and Mummified Remains in the Evaluation of Drug Use by an Ancient Society. An Historical and Scientific Investigation' (PhD dissertation, University of Manchester).

De Sélincourt, A. (trans.) and Marincola, J. M. (ed.) (1994), *Herodotus: The Histories* (London: Penguin).

Dewick, P. M. (1995), 'The biosynthesis of C5–C20 terpenoid compounds', *Natural Product Reports* 12, 507–34.

Dewick, P. M. (2009), *Medicinal Natural Products: A Biosynthetic Approach*, 3rd edn (Chichester: John Wiley and Sons).

Duke, J. (n.d.) 'Dr Duke's Phytochemical and Ethnobotanical Databases', www.ars-grin.gov/duke (last accessed 28 October 2014).

Garner, R. (1979), 'Experimental mummification', in A. R. David (ed.), *The Manchester Museum Mummy Project: Multidisciplinary Research on Ancient Egyptian Mummified Remains* (Manchester: Manchester University Press), 19–24.

Manniche, L. (1993), *An Ancient Egyptian Herbal* (London: British Museum Press).

Manniche, L. (1999), *Sacred Luxuries: Fragrance, Aromatherapy and Cosmetics in Ancient Egypt* (London: Opus Publishing).

McLafferty, F. W. (2013), *Wiley Registry of Mass Spectral Data* (Hoboken, NJ: John Wiley and Sons).

National Institute of Standards and Technology (1998), *The NIST Mass Spectral Search Program*, Version 1.6 (Gaithersburg: US Secretary of Commerce).

Paniandy, J., Cane-Ming, J. and Pieribattesti, J. (2000), 'Composition of the essential oil and headspace SPME of the quava fruit', *Journal of Essential Oil Research* 12, 153–8.

Penton, Z. (1997), 'Determination of residual volatiles in pharmaceuticals with auto-mated SPME', *Chemistry New Zealand* 61, 10–12.

Shaw, I. and Nicholson, P. (1995), *The British Museum Dictionary of Ancient Egypt* (London: British Museum Press).

Sides, S., Robards, K. and Helliwell, S. (2000), 'Developments in extraction tech-niques and their application to analysis of volatiles in food', *Trends in Analytical Chemistry* 19, 322–9.

Smith, G. E. (1912), *The Royal Mummies* (Paris: Institut Français d'Archéologie Orientale).

Verghese, J., Joy, M., Retamar, J., Melinskas, G., Catalan C. and Gross, E. (1987), 'A fresh look at the constituents of Indian olibanum oil', *Flavour and Fragrance Journal* 2 (3), 99–102.

Yashiki, N., Magasawa, T., Kojima, T., Miyazaki, T. and Iwasaki, Y. (1995), 'Rapid analysis of nicotine and cotinine in urine using head space solid phase micro-extraction and selected ion monitoring', *Japanese Journal of Forensic Toxicology* 13, 17–24.

21

Science in Egyptology: the scientific study of Egyptian mummies, initial phase, 1973–79

Alan Curry

Ancient Egypt and its highly developed civilisation often captivate us. However, the scientific study of ancient Egyptian artefacts and mummies was uncommon before 1970. Enter Dr Rosalie David, who was appointed as Assistant Keeper of Archaeogy at the Manchester Museum in 1972. The Manchester Museum has been closely associated with the University of Manchester since the university's inception in 1824 (Rothwell 2012: 6). Shortly after her appointment, it was therefore natural that Rosalie should approach academics, mainly but not exclusively within university departments, to undertake a scientific study of the ancient Egyptian mummies and associated artefacts held within the Manchester Museum. This team of investigators utilised various 'cutting edge' methods available at the time.

The 'core team' in 1975 consisted of the following:

Dr Rosalie David, Assistant Keeper of Archaeology, Manchester Museum (Figure 21.1)
Dr Eddie Tapp, Consultant Histopathologist, Withington Hospital, Manchester (Figure 21.2)
Professor Ian Isherwood, head of the Department of Diagnostic Radiology, University of Manchester
Dr R. A. Fawcitt, Senior Lecturer, Department of Diagnostic Radiology, University of Manchester
Mr Frank Filce Leek, retired dental surgeon, Tring, Hertfordshire (Figure 21.2)
Mr Richard Neave, Assistant Director, Department of Medical Illustration, Manchester Royal Infirmary
Dr David Dixon, Lecturer in Egyptology, University College London
Mr Roy Garner, conservator, Manchester Museum
Mr G. Benson, Pharmacy Department, University of Manchester
Detective Chief Inspector (DCI) A. Fletcher, Greater Manchester Police

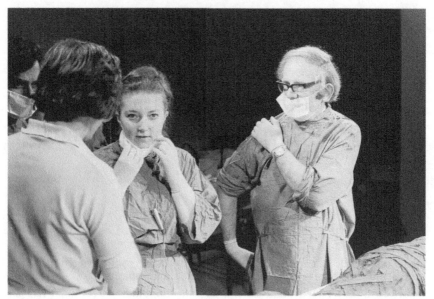

21.1 Rosalie David at the unwrapping of mummy 1770 at the new Manchester University Medical School in June 1975. (Photograph by Alan Curry.)

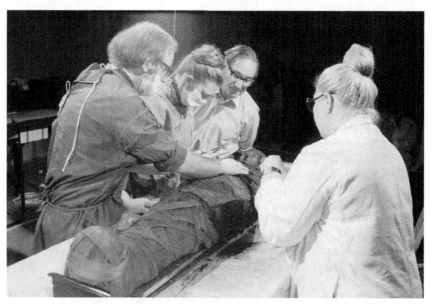

21.2 Eddie Tapp, Rosalie David and Frank Filce Leek just after the first bandages had been cut on mummy 1770. (Photograph by Alan Curry.)

Dr Sarah Hemingway, Pharmacy Department, University of Manchester
Miss Hilary Jarvis, radiographer, Manchester Royal Infirmary
Dr F. Leach, Drug Information Centre, St Mary's Hospital, Manchester
Dr G. Newton, Chemistry Department, University of Manchester
Mr K. C. Hodge, Chemistry Department, University of Manchester
Dr J. P. Wild, Department of Archaeology, University of Manchester
Mrs Cheryl Anfield, histology and electron microscopy laboratory techni-
cian, Withington Hospital, Manchester
Dr Ali Ahmed, pathologist, Department of Pathology, University of
Manchester Medical School
Professor William Kershaw, tropical parasitologist, Salford University
(Figure 21.3)
Dr Alan Curry, Senior Scientific Officer, Electron Microscopy Unit,
Department of Histopathology and Public Health Laboratory, Withington
Hospital, Manchester

In addition to the core members, many other individuals, particularly
laboratory staff (for example, Mr Ken Hollins, Senior Chief Technician in
Histology at Withington Hospital) and other professionals, were involved in
this project.

The project expanded further to include individuals not involved in the main
investigations. This was mainly due to team members meeting and exchanging
views, knowledge and experiences. An example of this was illustrated when
Frank Filce Leek (a delightful man who sadly died in 1985) made contact with
Dr Geoffrey Hosey of Bolton Institute of Technology in order to examine the
plant constituents of animal coprolites found at Amarna in Egypt and to try
to identify the animal species that produced these coprolites (Kemp 1984: 58).
Geoff Hosey (now Professor Hosey, Bolton University), who as a PhD student at
the University of Manchester was a contemporary of the author of this chapter,
Alan Curry, had as part of his PhD studies used the distinctive pattern of cells
and stomata in plant epidermal remains found in faeces to identify the plant diet
of roe deer, and so he possessed the necessary skills to undertake this additional
project (Hosey 1981: 276).

A summary of some of the significant scientific results

Radiocarbon dating (carbon-14 dating)

The unwrapping of mummy 1770 was central to the project, and this particular
mummy was selected because of its limited documentation and overall poor
state of preservation. The radiocarbon dating results indicated that the bones
of mummy 1770 were significantly older (c.1000 BC) than the bandages (c.AD
380), leading to the conclusion that the body had been re-wrapped at some time
during its history (Hodge and Newton 1979: 137). This result seemed to confirm

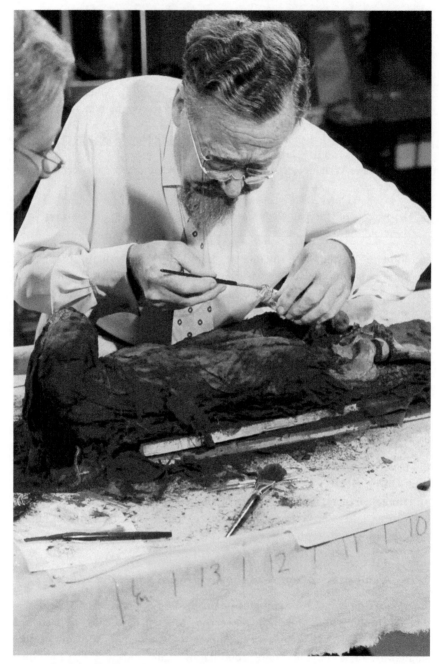

21.3 Professor William Kershaw removing insect remains from mummy 1770 for
identification. (Photograph by Alan Curry.)

some of the unusual findings (the presence of both gold nipple covers and an artificial phallus) discovered during the unwrapping of mummy 1770 (Tapp 1979b: 83), although recent results have shown that both body and wrappings are likely to be contemporary (Cockitt, Martin and David 2014: 95–102).

New and established non-invasive radiological techniques

The use of some of the radiological techniques (e.g. X-ray technology) in the study of mummies was well established (X-rays had been used at the end of the nineteenth century), but the application of new and emerging radiological techniques (such as tomography, computed tomography and orbiting equipment) was state-of-the-art. It was remarkable that this new and expensive equipment was made available to this study, and this is to the credit of both Rosalie and Ian Isherwood (and his enthusiastic colleagues, Hilary Jarvis and R. A. Fawcitt). There was one problem, however: the equipment used was large, complex and heavy, meaning that the mummies had to be taken to the Department of Diagnostic Radiology. The Zoology Department helped with this by providing transport from the Manchester Museum to the Medical School, which was located in the Stopford Building on the University of Manchester campus.

The radiological examination of the Manchester mummy collection allowed visualisation of the interior of the mummies, which sometimes permitted the determination of age, sex, disease development and the success of the embalming process (Isherwood, Jarvis and Fawcitt 1979: 25). However, it was the application of 'new' techniques such as computed tomography (CT, also called computerised axial tomography or CAT scans) that was a significant part of the radiological examination of the mummies. This expensive technique is, even today, available only in larger radiology departments, but has been significantly refined and developed since the mid-1970s.

The work of Ian Isherwood and his team was pioneering at the time. The recent exhibition 'Ancient Lives, New Discoveries' at the British Museum, London (2014–15), shows how the evolution and development of CT techniques have progressed, particularly in terms of computer capabilities, since the mid- to late 1970s (Taylor and Antoine 2014: 18). Without requiring the unwrapping of a mummy, one can visualise the outer coverings, including the coffin and bandages, and progressively view internal details (including remaining tissues and organs) in a seamless and continuous fashion. Artificial coloration enhances this visual experience. If this modern CT technology had been available in the mid-1970s, then the unwrapping of mummy 1770 might have been unnecessary (apart from tissue sampling for dating and microscopy), although its poor internal preservation would have limited the value of the internal revelations offered by this imaging technology. Such is the rapid and dynamic progress of science and technology.

Experimental mummification

The mummification process was known to involve the use of natron, a mixture of sodium carbonate and sodium bicarbonate with 'impurities' consisting of sodium chloride and sodium sulphate, which is found in natural deposits. However, as no full accounts of the mummification process have survived from ancient times, it was not clear whether natron was used as a solution or in its natural dry state. Various investigations using laboratory rats and mice by Roy Garner (Garner 1979: 19) showed that dry natron salts, rather than a solution, were needed for adequate mummification to occur without bodily fragmentation. This was a significant and important result. Roy also found that insect attack was a problem during the mummification of the experimental animals (see below).

Fingerprinting

DCI Fletcher and his team used this opportunity to fingerprint a mummy to improve their own techniques when dealing with long-deceased individuals. The fingerprints provided by the mummy Asru had to be taken using a special technique involving a flexible, quick-setting putty-like material (silicone) which was used in the dental profession, together with acrylic paint (Fletcher 1979: 79). Certainly, DCI Fletcher had a sense of humour when he claimed that if Asru had been a burglar in ancient Egypt, he could have provided fingerprint evidence. DCI Fletcher was able to determine from fingerprints and footprints that Asru had not done hard manual work during her life and that she was not a dancer. This work seems to confirm that Asru had been a high-status individual, although nowhere in the hieroglyphic inscription on her coffin are her job titles mentioned (Price 2013).

Analysis of mummy wrappings and textiles

The linen wrappings of various mummies investigated were found to be of extremely high quality (Wild 1979: 133). The wrappings were also found to be impregnated with other substances (e.g. beeswax) and to have been applied to the mummified body in a fairly dry state (Benson, Hemingway and Leach 1979: 119). Overall, these findings indicated that textile technology was highly developed in ancient Egypt.

Dental studies

Caries (tooth decay) was commonly present in Ptolemaic mummies (332–30 BC) but not in mummies from the Early Dynastic Period (c.3000–2686 BC) and Middle Kingdom Period (2055–1650 BC). These differences were possibly related to the type of food consumed during those periods. Evidence was also found of some of the teeth having been extracted, but no hints of the techniques used or instruments for removal were found. Perhaps predictably, wear to the cusps of teeth was seen in all mummies and was related to food contamination by abrasive particles such as quartz in wind-blown sand (also seen in the lungs: see below).

Of particular interest, one of the mummies, Khnum-Nakht, was found to have a rare tooth abnormality (double gemination or fusion of the upper central incisors), a finding which makes the relatively small Manchester mummy collection very important in the field of ancient Egyptian dental history (Leek 1979: 65). This genetic abnormality suggests that Nekht-Ankh, thought to have been the 'brother' of Khnum-Nahkt, may not have been related at all. More recent studies of the genetic relationship, or otherwise, of these 'Two Brothers' have produced mixed results: one study using mitochondrial DNA indicated a maternal relationship, whereas a second investigation, using the polymerase chain reaction (PCR) to sequence extracted DNA, found no evidence of a genetic relationship (David 2007: 133). The use of DNA from ancient sources (molecular ancient DNA technology) remains a field fraught with technical problems although DNA can often be successfully extracted from skeletal remains (Kaestle and Horsburgh 2002: 92). DNA degrades (fragments) over time, the yield is generally low, and extreme care has to be taken to avoid modern contamination (so confirming the authenticity of the sequence data produced). Techniques are being developed to compensate for this degradation and make ancient genomes more useful for many forms of analysis. These molecular studies on Khnum-Nakht and Nakht-Ankh highlight the need for better samples containing more intact DNA. Teeth would be the most obvious choice as they appear to 'protect' DNA to some extent from degradation as a result of hydroxyapatite adsorbtion (Kemp and Smith 2005: 53). As the remains of Khnum-Nakht and Nakht-Ankh are now largely skeletal, their teeth are likely to be the best source of relatively intact DNA. Modern surface contamination and microbial DNA contamination on the teeth can be eliminated by use of hypochlorite (bleach), thus providing better-preserved internal DNA samples (Kemp and Smith 2005: 53). If this is sanctioned, positive results could perhaps provide a definitive answer of their genetic relationship; offering a possible avenue for future research. As with later phases of the Mummy Project, such work would be for others to comment on.

Reconstruction of skulls and faces

Following the unwrapping of mummy 1770, Richard Neave reassembled the skull and expertly recreated the facial features on a cast of this reconstructed skull. This required accurate knowledge of tissue and muscle thicknesses over the skull (Prag and Neave 1997: 20). A wax model head complete with nose, eyes, hair and make-up was undoubtedly one of the highlights of this project

and, in a way, reincarnated mummy 1770 (Neave 1979: 149). The faces of
Khnum-Nakht and Nakht-Ankh were also impressively reconstructed as part of
the project (Neave 1979: 149).

Insects associated with the mummified tissues

Various insect remains associated with the mummified tissues were also investigated. Once recovered these remains were largely identified by Colin Johnson
and Alan Brindle of the Department of Entomology, Manchester Museum.
Not surprisingly, many insects familiar to us today such as cockroaches, blow-
flies, houseflies, pests of stored food and woodworm were also problematic for
Egyptian embalmers (Hinton 1945; Curry 1979: 113).

Histological evidence of disease

An important process in histologically examining tissue samples was immersion
of the dried samples in 10 per cent formol saline (buffered formaldehyde) for
twenty-four to forty-eight hours. This fixative, which was used for both histological and electron microscopy investigations, not only preserved what remained
of the cellular constituents within dried tissues, but also rehydrated them and
inhibited microbial growth. Such was the effectiveness of this procedure that
some rehydrated lung tissue from a canopic jar appeared to be almost freshly
removed from a living body (Tapp 1979a: 95).

Birefringent (crystalline) particles were found in histological sections of
fibrotic lung tissue from a canopic jar associated with the mummy of Nekht-
Ankh. These particles were analysed using analytical electron microscopy
(AEM; see below) and were found to contain the elements silicon, iron and
titanium, indicating inhalation of sand particles. These findings indicated that
Nakht-Ankh suffered from 'desert lung' (more technically called 'sand pneumo-
coniosis') and that this disease was of considerable antiquity (Tapp, Curry and
Anfield 1975: 276; Curry, Anfield and Tapp 1979: 103).

Evidence of parasitic infections

Not unexpectedly, evidence of parasite infection was found during some of
the investigations. The radiological examination of the mummies provided
some convincing evidence of parasite infections (Isherwood, Jarvis and Fawcitt
1979: 25). Calcified remains of the guinea worm (*Dracunculus medinensis*) were
found in mummy 1770, and evidence of schistosomiasis (*Schistosoma haematobium*) was found in the bladder wall of mummies 1766 (an adult female)
and 1775 (an adult male, named Artemidorus). Histological examination of
some of the rehydrated tissue samples from canopic jars also showed evidence of parasitic infections, such as *Strongyloides* and the guinea worm (Tapp
1979a: 95).

However, tissue samples prepared for transmission electron microscopy showed structures which, at the time, were also interpreted as evidence of parasitic infection (Curry, Anfield and Tapp 1979: 103). These results now appear rather speculative as they were based on poorly preserved cellular details. A modern-day analogy would be the difficulties surrounding the interpretation of extracted and fragmented DNA sequences from ancient Egyptian remains (see above). Other, different, but more appropriate methods of detection, such as immunological methods, have been developed and successfully used to detect some types of parasite infection (David 2008: 8).

Electron microscopy
The application of electron microscopy to this palaeopathological study of ancient Egyptian material could also be considered technologically advanced for the era. The senior histopathology consultant at Withington Hospital, Dr Eddie Tapp, became involved in the Egyptology project, and he expected the hospital's newly established electron microscopy unit (set up in 1972) to be involved as well. However, the electron microscopy unit could undertake only transmission electron microscopy. Fortunately, the close proximity of the Associated Electrical Industries (AEI) factory at Urmston, Manchester, meant that the Withington electron microscopy unit had access to other electron microscopy techniques in development there, such as analytical electron microscopy and scanning electron microscopy. AEI had been one of the early pioneers of electron microscopy (as Metropolitan Vickers) and was still developing new instruments with enhanced capabilities (Mulvey 1964: 1; Agar 1996: 415). At this time, AEI was developing variants of a new transmission electron microscope, named Corinth. In particular, an analytical derivative named CORA (Corinth Analytical) was in development which enabled elemental (chemical) analysis of the constituents of a specimen section to be determined. In addition, a scanning development of Corinth, termed CESA (Corinth Electron Scanning Attachment), was in development. This technique allowed the external features of specimens to be examined at high resolution and with a great depth of focus. Access to these new instruments was facilitated by the AEI demonstration staff, Dawn Chescoe and Madeline Samuels, but also by some of the developmental staff, such as Peter Kenway. Sadly AEI stopped its development work and production of electron microscopes in the late 1970s.

As expected, cell and cellular organelle preservation within the mummified tissues was generally found under the electron microscope to be very poor. In addition, bacterial spores and fungal hyphae were relatively commonly encountered, indicating some degree of putrefaction. However, there were some surprises, particularly the discovery of well-preserved centrioles in a piece of liver tissue (Curry, Anfield and Tapp 1979: 103). Centrioles are cell organelles that organise the mitotic spindle used to separate chromosomes during cell division. That these centrioles were preserved may have been due to the breakdown of haemoglobin in the blood-rich liver, thus allowing release of reactive hydroxyl radicals that would cause cross-linking of molecules, in a process analogous to the reaction of chemical fixatives used in histological tissue preparation procedures. Such chemical reactions involving iron have been postulated to explain the preservation of certain biological molecules and proteins in a few dinosaur fossils (Schweitzer 2014: 104).

To sum up the usefulness of the electron microscopy techniques used, transmission electron microscopy was found to be of limited value because of poor cellular preservation. Analytical electron microscopy was useful in elemental analysis of specimens, as was scanning electron microscopy in examining insect remains (see Figure 21.4).

Films, books and an exhibition

A number of factual films were made highlighting the results from the Mummy Project, two educational films and also a BBC *Chronicle* programme. The educational films produced by the Audio-Visual Department of the University of Manchester won awards from the British Association for the Advancement of Science (David 2008: 6):

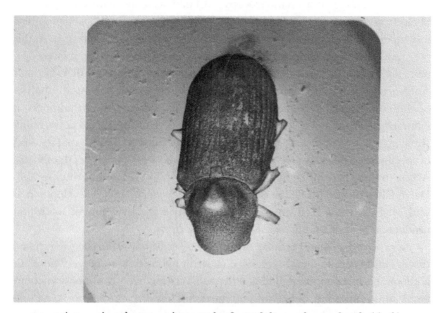

21.4 A scanning electron micrograph of an adult woodworm beetle (*Anobium punctatum*) found in a wooden coffin. (Photograph by Alan Curry.)

Revelations of a Mummy (alternative title *Life and Death in Ancient Egypt*), a BBC
Chronicle programme, first broadcast in early 1977
Unwrapping of 1770
Manchester Techniques and Scientific Investigations

In addition, it is perhaps little known that a film company, the Orion Picture
Company, also made contact, as a Philips electron microscope was to be
used as an investigative tool in a fictional horror film. *The Awakening*, involving the discovery of a tomb and mummy (belonging to 'Queen Kara', who
is reincarnated), was possibly inspired by the Mummy Project films outlined
above. The Histology Department at Withington Hospital supplied a sample
specimen grid. In the film, 'a virus' is discovered contaminating the mummy
and its wrappings. The use of an electron microscope to discover viruses is
appropriate, but, unfortunately, viruses replicate only in living cells. The film,
which starred Charlton Heston, Susannah York, Jill Townsend and Stephanie
Zimbalist, was released in 1980, is entertaining but completely fictitious. The
project is not credited.

The results were also published as a popular book, academic book and as the
proceedings of an international conference:

Mysteries of the Mummies: The Story of the Manchester University Investigation, edited
by A. R. David (London: Book Club Associates, 1978)
*The Manchester Museum Mummy Project: Multidisciplinary Research on Ancient
Egyptian Mummified Remains*, edited by A. R. David (Manchester: Manchester
University Press, 1979).
Science in Egyptology: Proceedings of the 'Science in Egyptology' Symposia, edited by
A. R. David (Manchester: Manchester University Press, 1986)

An exhibition of the results of this initial phase of the study was displayed at the
Manchester Museum.

Assessment of the project overall

Overall the project was a great success and generated considerable interest.
Egyptology had been about history, religious beliefs, art and surviving artefacts,
but now this fascinating civilisation could be carefully scrutinised by scientific
methods, many of which were developed or employed in conjunction with this
project (and developed further since this initial phase). Utilisation of these scientific investigations has given us new insights into the lives, diseases, parasites,
insect pests, dental problems, diet and customs of the ancient Egyptians. As a
result of the various investigations undertaken during the Mummy Project, it
was clear that life in ancient Egypt was less than idyllic.

Conclusion

This scientific study of Egyptian mummies was initiated and wonderfully organised by Rosalie David and shows her knowledge, competence and organisational skills. It is unlikely that National Health Service facilities could be used in the same way today, and dedicated laboratories would have to be established. The team Rosalie assembled in the 1970s, and their associates, are to be congratulated for what they achieved with the techniques and resources that were available at the time.

References

Agar, A. W. (1996), 'The story of European commercial electron microscopes', in T. Mulvey (ed.), *The Growth of Electron Microscopy: Advances in Imaging and Electron Physics* (London: Academic Press), 415–584.

Benson, G. G., Hemingway, S. R. and Leach, F. N. (1979), 'The analysis of the wrappings of mummy 1770', in A. R. David (ed.), *The Manchester Museum Mummy Project: Multidisciplinary Research on Ancient Egyptian Mummified Remains* (Manchester: Manchester University Press), 119–31.

Cockitt, J. A., Martin, S. O. and David, A. R. (2014), 'A new assessment of the radiocarbon age of the mummy no. 1770', in *Yearbook of Mummy Studies* 2 (Munich: Verlag Dr Friedrich Pfeil), 95–102.

Curry, A. (1979), 'The insects associated with the Manchester mummies', in A. R. David (ed.), *The Manchester Museum Mummy Project: Multidisciplinary Research on Ancient Egyptian Mummified Remains* (Manchester: Manchester University Press), 113–17.

Curry, A., Anfield, C. and Tapp, E. (1979), 'Electron microscopy of the Manchester mummies', in A. R. David (ed.), *The Manchester Museum Mummy Project: Multidisciplinary Research on Ancient Egyptian Mummified Remains* (Manchester: Manchester University Press), 103–11.

David, A. R. (2007), *The Two Brothers: Death and the Afterlife in Middle Kingdom Egypt* (Bolton: Rutherford Press).

David, R. (2008), 'The background of the Manchester Mummy Project', in R. David (ed.), *Egyptian Mummies and Modern Science* (Cambridge and New York: Cambridge University Press), 3–9.

Filce Leek, F. (1979), 'The dental history of the Manchester mummies', in A. R. David (ed.), *The Manchester Museum Mummy Project: Multidisciplinary Research on Ancient Egyptian Mummified Remains* (Manchester: Manchester University Press), 65–77.

Fletcher, A. (1979), 'The fingerprint examination', in A. R. David (ed.), *The Manchester Museum Mummy Project: Multidisciplinary Research on Ancient Egyptian Mummified Remains* (Manchester: Manchester University Press), 79–82.

Garner, R. (1979), 'Experimental mummification', in A. R. David (ed.), *The Manchester Museum Mummy Project: Multidisciplinary Research on Ancient Egyptian Mummified Remains* (Manchester: Manchester University Press), 19–24.

Hinton, H. E. (1945), *A Monograph of the Beetles Associated with Stored Products*, I (London: The Trustees of the British Museum).

Hodge, K. C. and Newton, G. W. A. (1979), 'Radiocarbon dating', in A. R. David (ed.), *The Manchester Museum Mummy Project: Multidisciplinary Research on Ancient Egyptian Mummified Remains* (Manchester: Manchester University Press), 137–47.

Hosey, G. R. (1981), 'Annual foods of the roe deer (*Capreolus capreolus*) in the south of England', *Journal of Zoology* 194, 276–78.

Isherwood, I., Jarvis, H. and Fawcitt, R. A. (1979), 'Radiology of the Manchester mummies', in A. R. David (ed.), *The Manchester Museum Mummy Project: Multidisciplinary Research on Ancient Egyptian Mummified Remains* (Manchester: Manchester University Press), 25–64.

Kaestle, F. A. and Horsburgh, K. A. (2002), 'Ancient DNA in anthropology: methods, applications, and ethics', *Yearbook of Physical Anthropology* 45, 92–130.

Kemp, B. J. (ed.) (1984), *Amarna Reports*, I (London: Egypt Exploration Society).

Kemp, B. M. and Smith, D. G. (2005), 'Use of bleach to eliminate contaminating DNA from the surface of bones and teeth', *Forensic Science International* 154, 53–61.

Mulvey, T. (1964), 'The development of the electron microscope: AEI's contribution', *AEI Engineering* (January/February), 1–11.

Neave, R. A. H. (1979), 'The reconstruction of the heads and faces of three ancient Egyptian mummies', in A. R. David (ed.), *The Manchester Museum Mummy Project: Multidisciplinary Research on Ancient Egyptian Mummified Remains* (Manchester: Manchester University Press), 149–57.

Prag, J. and Neave, R. (1997), *'Making Faces': Using Forensic and Archaeological Evidence* (London: British Museum Press).

Price, C. (2013), 'New light under old wrappings (1): reinvestigating Asru', *Egypt at the Manchester Museum* (blog), egyptmanchester.wordpress.com (last accessed 15 December 2014).

Rothwell, N. (2012), 'Foreword', in D. Logunov and N. Merriman (eds.), *The Manchester Museum: Window to the World.* (London: Third Millennium), 6.

Schweitzer, M. H. (2014), 'Blood from stone: mounting evidence from dinosaur bones shows that, contrary to common belief, organic materials can sometimes survive in fossils for millions of years', *Scientific American* 23 (2), 104–11.

Tapp, E. (1979a), 'Disease in the Manchester mummies', in A. R. David (ed.), *The Manchester Museum Mummy Project: Multidisciplinary Research on Ancient Egyptian Mummified Remains* (Manchester: Manchester University Press), 95–102.

Tapp, E. (1979b), 'The unwrapping of a mummy', in A. R. David (ed.), *The Manchester Museum Mummy Project: Multidisciplinary Research on Ancient Egyptian Mummified Remains* (Manchester: Manchester University Press), 83–93.

Tapp, E., Curry, A. and Anfield, C. (1975), 'Sand pneumoconiosis in an Egyptian mummy', *British Medical Journal* 2 (5965), 276.

Taylor, J. H. and Antoine, D. (2014), *Ancient Lives, New Discoveries: Eight Mummies, Eight Stories* (London: British Museum Press).

Wild, J. P. (1979), 'The textiles from the mummy 1770', in A. R. David (ed.), *The Manchester Museum Mummy Project: Multidisciplinary Research on Ancient Egyptian Mummified Remains* (Manchester: Manchester University Press), 133–6.

22

Slices of mummy: a thin perspective

John Denton

My first introduction

It was in 1973 at the University of Manchester Medical School, where I was a relatively young pathology technician, that I was introduced to Rosalie David for the first time. Her passion for the multi-faceted complex investigation of Egyptological remains was apparent from the beginning. In 1975 the team formed by Rosalie David came together in one of our seminar rooms to undertake the unwrapping of mummy 1770, one of the rare scientific studies of a relatively intact Egyptian mummy. The preparation of the project had taken about three years and involved many different disciplines that were currently used for the radiological, chemical, dental, microscopic and pathological investigations of hospital patients. In addition, examinations of the wrappings and body tissues were undertaken by new and cutting-edge scientific techniques such as carbon-14 dating. It is testament to the persuasiveness and vigour of Rosalie David that this international group of individuals came together with a common aim. Information gained from this scientific examination would pave the way for the opening of the field of biomedical Egyptology; Rosalie would become the first professor of the subject and subsequently leader of the KNH Centre for Biomedical Egyptology at the University of Manchester. It was at the investigation of mummy 1770 that I met Alan Curry, an electron microscopist (I had just started to learn the relatively new techniques of electron microscopy, but in another department) who was to become a lifelong scientific mentor and friend (see Curry in Chapter 21 above). It was Alan who told me of the young TV personality David Attenborough, who was also watching the unwrapping.

At the time of the unwrapping of mummy 1770, I, as a mineralised tissue histology technician, was asked: 'could a few samples from the mummy be histologically sectioned using your calcified tissue techniques?' Quite simply this

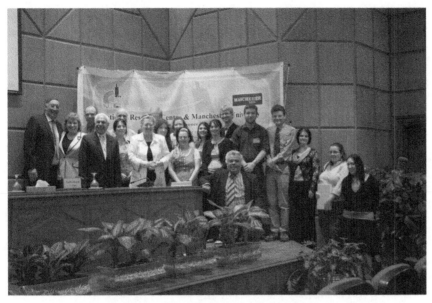

22.1 A meeting at the Egyptian National Research Centre, Cairo, in 2007 with Rosalie David, the president of the centre and MSc students. (Photograph by the author.)

proved to be near impossible, and with no meaningful results I abandoned the trial. Many years later I was asked to give a lecture on histological techniques to some MSc students studying biomedical Egyptology, where an interest in the scientific study of Egyptian remains was reignited. This was to become a major research interest of mine, and I was eventually invited to become module supervisor for histological techniques, supervising many MSc and PhD students. There were annual trips to Egypt and the Egyptian National Research Centre, where our students presented results of their histological examination of ancient remains of human, animal and vegetable tissues. Figure 22.1 shows a meeting at the Egyptian National Research Centre in 2007 with Rosalie David and the president of the centre with our MSc students.

Histology is also known as microscopic anatomy. The word 'anatomy' comes from the Greek 'ana', meaning 'up' or 'through', and 'tome', meaning 'a cutting'. Anatomy was once a 'cutting up' because the structure of the body was originally learned through dissecting it with knives. The word 'histology' came from the Greek 'histo-', meaning tissue, and 'logos', treatise. Therefore histology is a treatise about the tissues and cells of the body. When applied to mummified tissues it is generally known as palaeo-histology, a term first used by Moodie in 1920. However, while modern-day histology is used as a diagnostic tool, very different information is sought from the histological examination of the ancient tissues. In addition, it is sometimes possible to diagnose diseases and assess the nutritional status of the individual from whom the tissue was taken.

Essentially, histology is the preparation of thin (5 μm) sections of tissue, which are then mounted on glass slides. Following staining with coloured dyes, which identify different tissue components in different colours or shades of a colour, the section is encapsulated within a coverslip by a setting liquid. This liquid has the same refractive index of glass, providing a coloured transparent section that is thin enough to be examined by a transmitted light microscope.

Ancient tissues have many intrinsic problems that must be taken into consideration before histological techniques can be applied. They are brown, crisp, often contaminated with sand, oxidised and putrefied: in simple terms a histological nightmare. The universal problem is that the tissue is desiccated and crisp, unlike contemporary tissues, which are wet and soft. In this desiccated condition it is impossible to section using conventional techniques that would be applied to modern-day surgical tissues. In order to allow subsequent processing and in particular sectioning, it is necessary to soften the mummified tissues by rehydrating them. This rehydration step has two main purposes; firstly, it will allow the tissue to regain its normal hydrated architectural and cell structural form, and secondly, it will, following embedding, permit sectioning.

Czermack (1852) was the first person to attempt the histological examination of mummified tissue when he teased out tissue in a sodium hydroxide solution and microscopically examined the resulting fibres. It was not until Ruffer (1909: 1005–6) that the first true tissue rehydrating protocols were devised. He used an alkaline sodium carbonate solution to soften the tissue and formalin or an alcoholic solution to then harden the tissue prior to processing. Sandison (1955) further refined the technique originally described by Ruffer. Some twenty-six years later Turner and Holtom (1981) used a commercially available laundry fabric softener, Comfort® (Lever Bros), to soften pieces of mummified tissues. One of the problems with using commercially available materials is that the manufacturer often changes the formulation of the product and so standardisation of the technique is impossible. Comfort® in particular has the problem that as it is designed for laundry it contains optical brighteners to give a 'cleaner wash'. These optical brighteners also attach to the mummified tissues, changing staining patterns and causing undesirable changes to subsequent immuno-fluorescent examination. Mekota and Vermehren (2005) give a comprehensive review of the subject and evaluate the many attempts to refine the original rehydration techniques. Currie (2002), working from basic scientific principles, devised a solution of 1 per cent sodium laureth sulphate (a detergent) in formol saline for the rehydration of tissues. All rehydration solutions must have the capacity to kill or at least to inactivate bacterial and fungal organisms that would lead to putrefaction of the mummy tissues during the process. This technique is now my 'gold standard' for the preparation of ancient histology specimens.[1]

Bacteria and fungi

When mummified tissues are histologically examined, it is often the case that micro-organisms such as bacteria and fungi can be seen in the section. They are generally present as a result of the continuing putrefaction of the tissues. These micro-organisms are best seen in the toluidine blue staining reaction, where all of the tissue stains a shade of blue but the bacteria stain the darkest. Pathogenic bacteria that have caused an abscess in the individual before death usually produce a pus-filled cavity in the tissues which would typically be full of bacteria and would then leave evidence of a cavity in mummified tissues. These contrast with bacteria that are starting to invade the tissues as part of the putrefaction process, where they use the route of least resistance, which is normally along and between fibres.

Fungi of various types are also often seen in ancient tissues as a result of poor storage of the specimen. Histology allows researchers to identify, on morphological grounds, the fungus and to assess the effects of the organism on the tissue. One of the more problematic fungi that are encountered is *Serpula lacrymans*, or as it is more commonly known 'dry rot fungus'. Researchers normally rely on the control of fungi and bacteria by limiting the humidity in the air surrounding the exhibit. Unfortunately, dry rot fungus is adept at getting round this by producing its own water as a metabolic by-product, thus allowing further growth. So even producing a dry environment does not inhibit the growth of the fungus, and the fungus proceeds to use the soft tissues and bone as a food source, causing severe damage to the tissues. In Figure 22.2 the destructive power of the fungi is demonstrated by the foamy fungal mass eroding the bone trabeculae to form a scalloped edge on the bone, effectively dissolving the bone.

When is liver not liver?

It is often the case that tissues are typed solely on the anatomical site from which they were removed and not on specific pathological identification criteria. The identification of tissue can be problematic, as seen in a case of tissue removed

---

1   For a more in-depth description of the methodology for the preparation of mummified tissues see Denton 2008: 71–82.

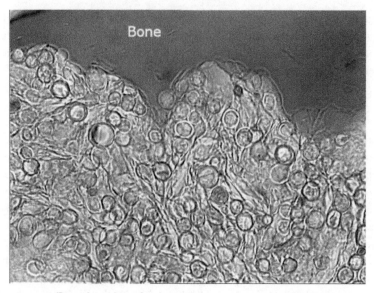

22.2 Fungal erosion of trabecular bone. (Created by the author.)

from a canopic jar, the contents of which were to be examined by a masters student using DNA techniques. The tissue had been catalogued and visually identified as a sample of liver. However, in order to microscopically examine the tissue to determine the extent of its preservation, a portion of it was processed and examined by histological techniques. Much to the surprise of the researcher the sample supposed to be liver was in fact a leaf. This finding illustrates the point that even though the tissue has a visual identification it cannot necessarily be assumed to be the correct one. If this tissue had not been correctly identified and had been used for more sophisticated analytical or molecular techniques it would not only have produced erroneous results but would have wasted rare archaeological material.

Lung disease

Like modern man, the ancient Egyptians lived in a polluted world and suffered lung diseases caused by the inhalation of organic and inorganic particles. Deposits of this type are accumulated throughout life when the individual is breathing air containing sand and other particles. The composition of the deposit is a reflection of the pattern of particulate inhalation throughout the individual's life and is nearly always a mixture. It is common to find sand in lungs from the inhabitants of desert areas, and soot derived from burning fats for lighting in a confined space such as a tomb, a mine or even the home.

The term 'hut lung' is now used to describe the condition (Mukhopadhyay *et al.* 2013). Chemical and crystallographic identification of the dust and smoke particles that an individual inhaled as part of their daily working life can give information as to their occupation (Montgomerie 2012). All ancient Egyptian lung specimens known to have been examined contain large deposits of soot and silica, which must have caused a certain amount of mortality and morbidity among the population (Gold *et al.* 2000: 310–17).

Bone and pregnancy

Bone is not a dead tissue but a dynamic calcified tissue that responds to external physical stresses and internal metabolic challenges. Bone is continuously being reshaped in a process called remodelling. In this process, cells called osteoclasts resorb bone tissues whereas cells called osteoblasts deposit new bone tissue. Normal trabecular bone has an ordered layered structure (lamellar bone), whereas bone that is laid down during times of metabolic stress has a random structure resembling loosely woven felt.

Bone in many ways contains a record of the life events and nutritional status of an individual. This is particularly illustrated in women during pregnancy, where the nutritional needs of the foetus are met in part by the destruction of the maternal skeleton (Shahtaheri *et al.* 1999). Bone remodelling during pregnancy is further exacerbated during lactation and possible further pregnancies, which put extra demands on the already weakened maternal skeleton (Salari and Abdallahi 2014). This pattern is well demonstrated in a sample of trabecular bone which was donated by Arthur Aufderheide following his excavations at the Dakhleh Oasis in 1998. The skeletal remains were labelled as being of a woman of approximately thirty years of age at the time of death. Histological examination of the bone demonstrated an episode of bone resorption where the existing bone has been removed, leaving a characteristic scalloped edge to the bone, followed then by the rapid apposition of immature woven bone on top of this resorption line, in an effort to repair the bone volume. At a later date resorption of bone occurred again, involving the original lamellar bone and the newer woven bone. The process then stopped, as there was no attempt at cellular repair of the bone. Many systemic diseases of bone cause resorption and apposition of bone but very few are episodic. However, one explanation for this bone pattern would be a case of two pregnancies, lactation, and then the rapid death of the mother, possibly during the second birth (Salari and Abdallahi 2014). Evidence for this is demonstrated in Figure 22.3, where the original lamellar bone is in the central area of the section and the first line of resorption is indicated as ES, the subsequent area of woven bone apposition is on the surface of this area, indicated as WB, and the final line of resorption is indicated

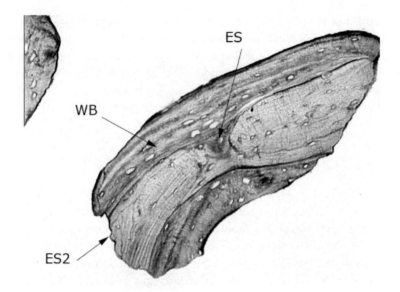

22.3 Histological section of lamellar bone during pregnancy. (Created by the author.)

as ES2. This example demonstrates resorption through both original lamellar bone and the more recent woven bone. There is then no evidence of the further activity of the bone which would normally be expected, possibly indicating the death of the mother.

Skin disease

Preservation of tissues is optimally achieved by rapid desiccation, normally at the extremities, of thin exposed structures, exposed skin and protruding thin structures such as the ears. One of the more interesting examples of disease in ancient tissues was the surprise finding of what appears to be a classical example of haemorrhagic smallpox in the skin specimen of a mummy (Rao 1972: 2–28). The specimen was described as being taken from the mummy of a child who was believed to be approximately three years old at the time of death. Following histological examination it was noted that there was a remarkable degree of skin preservation, comparable to that of a modern-day specimen. Although it is difficult to be certain, the small body size and the exposure of the skin of the child to the air, possibly associated with low environmental humidity, were factors which helped in the rapid desiccation of the skin that resulted in such excellent preservation (Plate 8). The preservation is so exceptional that even individual red blood cells (E) can be seen in the dome of the haemorrhagic skin vesicle.

The child had very pigmented skin, as shown by the heavy deposit of melanin in the basal layer (M).

Excellent preservation can also be demonstrated in an ear sample obtained from a mummified cat of unknown provenance which was donated to the KNH Centre. When it was histologically sectioned it was shown that there was excellent cellular preservation, even to the presence of cell nuclei in the central cartilage band running along the ear (cell nuclei are normally one of the first casualties of degradation processes). As with the skin sample previously described, a combination of circumstances had led to the rapid desiccation of the tissues, a process helped by the thinness of the ear tissues. By examining and identifying the different types of tissue that make up the ear it can be seen that there is a large band of cartilage running through the centre (Figure 22.4), as indicated by the somewhat paler and more cellular tissue, whereas the skin can be seen at the surface. Cartilage of this thickness would give the ears a great degree of stiffness, and from this it can be assumed that the ears of the cat were quite stiff and erect in life.

Another type of 'ear' that can be examined by histology is an ear of wheat. The seed capsule of cereal is designed to resist dehydration and remain in a viable condition for a long period of time, normally being harvested when dry. It is because of this dried state that the seed is often very well preserved and has

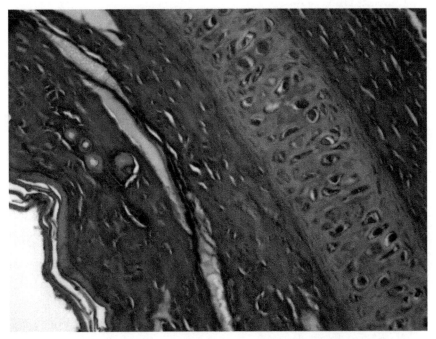

22.4 Histological cross-section of the ear of a cat. (Created by the author.)

resisted attack by microbial agents (Samuel 1997: 6). Histology of the seed allows the comparison between the types of wheat grown in ancient Egypt and the more modern crops grown today. The morphology of the wheat seed and the starch contents have excellent preservation even after 2,500 years have passed (Wasef 2005).

The technique of histology is probably the oldest scientific technique that is used for the investigation of ancient human, animal and plant remains; it is, however, the only technique that can identify specific tissues at a cellular level and allows the pathological diagnosis of disease states. It is one of the greatest credits to Rosalie David that this technique was included in the battery of techniques that were used by the individual investigators whom she so successfully bought together in her mummy team.

References

Currie, K. (2002), 'Ancient Egyptian skin, a comparative histological investigation' (MSc dissertation, University of Manchester).

Czermack, J. (1852), 'Beschreibung und mikroskopische Untersuchung zweier ägyptischer Mumien', *Sonderberichte Akademie Wissenschaft Wien* 9, 427–69.

Denton, J. (2008), 'Slices of mummy – a histologist's perspective', in R. David (ed.), *Egyptian Mummies and Modern Science* (Cambridge and New York: Cambridge University Press), 71–82.

Gold, J. A., Jagirdar, J., Hay, J. G., Addrizzo-Harris, D. J., Naidich, D. P. and Rom, W. N. (2000), 'Hut lung: a domestically acquired particulate lung disease,' *Medicine* (Baltimore) 5, 310–17.

Mekota, A. M. and Vermehren, M. (2005), 'Determination of optimal rehydration, fixation and staining methods for histological and immunohistochemical analysis of mummified soft tissues', *Biotechnique and Histochemistry* 80 (1), 7–13.

Montgomerie, R. D. (2012), 'Structural and elemental composition of inhaled particles in ancient Egyptian mummified lungs' (PhD thesis, University of Manchester).

Mukhopadhyay, S., Gujral, M., Abraham, J. L., Scaizetti, E. M. and Iannuzzi, M. C. (2013), 'A case of hut lung: scanning electron microscopy with energy dispersive X-ray spectroscopy analysis of a domestically acquired form of pneumoconiosis', *Chest* 141 (1), 323–7.

Rao, A. R. (1972), *Smallpox* (Bombay: Kothari Book Depot).

Ruffer, M. A. (1909), 'Note on the histology of Egyptian mummies', *British Medical Journal* 1 (2521), 1005–6.

Salari, P. and Abdallahi, M. (2014), 'The influence of pregnancy and lactation on maternal bone health: a systemic review', *Journal of Family and Reproductive Health* 5, 135–48.

Samuel, D. (1997), 'Cereal foods and nutrition in ancient Egypt', *Nutrition* 13, 6.

Sandison, A. T. (1955), 'The histological examination of mummified material', *Stain Technology* 30 (6), 277–83.

Shahtaheri, S. M, Aaron, J. E., Johnson, D. R. and Purdie, D. W. (1999), 'Changes in trabecular bone architecture in women during pregnancy', *British Journal of Obstetrics and Gynaecology* 106, 432–8.

Turner, P. J. and Holtom, D. B. (1981), 'The use of a fabric softener in the reconstitution of mummified tissue prior to paraffin wax sectioning for light microscopical examination', *Stain Technology* 56 (1), 35–8.

Wasef, S. (2005), 'Comparison between Ancient and Contemporary Pomegranate and Wheat Seeds' (MSc dissertation, University of Manchester).

23

Life and death in the desert: a bioarchaeological study of human remains from the Dakhleh Oasis, Egypt

Tosha L. Dupras, Lana J. Williams, Sandra M. Wheeler and Peter G. Sheldrick

The Dakhleh Oasis is one of five oases in the Western Desert of Egypt (25°31′N, 28°57′E), and is located approximately 550 km south-south-west of Cairo (Figure 23.1). This area of Egypt has been under archaeological scrutiny by the Dakhleh Oasis Project (DOP) since the initial surveys of 1978–79 (Mills 1979). Since its inception, one of the main objectives of the DOP has been to understand how humans adapted to such a physically challenging environment (Mills 1982: 94). The ancient village of Kellis (Figure 23.1, inset) has garnered particular attention, as it was believed to be an important administrative centre during the Romano-Christian Period (Hope 2001: 44). One way to understand human adaptation to such an environment is to study the remains of the people who occupied Kellis.

The dead from Kellis were buried in many locations – within the township, in the north and south tomb structures, and in two cemeteries designated as the West Cemetery (Kellis 1 cemetery or K1) and the East Cemetery (Kellis 2 cemetery or K2). The arid conditions, the low acidity of the soil in the Western Desert, and particular mortuary practices have created ideal conditions for the exceptional preservation of archaeological materials and human tissues. Here we focus on the information gleaned from the bioarchaeological investigations conducted on the individuals from the Kellis 2 cemetery.

The Kellis 2 cemetery is located on a broad plateau east of the ancient town of Kellis. The cemetery extends for at least 150 m east–west and 60 m north–south, and the number of graves in the visible extent of the cemetery is estimated to be between 3,000 and 4,000, assuming that the density of the burials in the excavated portion reflects the density of graves in the cemetery as a whole (Molto 2002: 243). Archaeological evidence from the associated ancient village of Kellis suggests occupation from 50 to 360 AD (Hope 2001: 48–55); however, numerous radiocarbon dates from the Kellis 2 cemetery indicate use

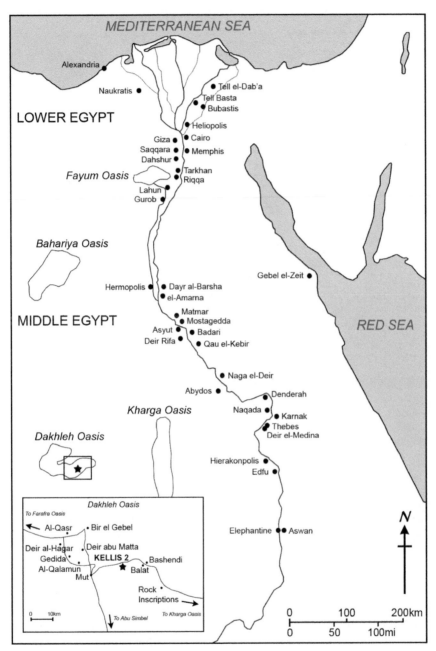

23.1 Map showing the location of the Dakhleh Oasis in Egypt and the location of the Kellis 2 cemetery. (Created by the author.)

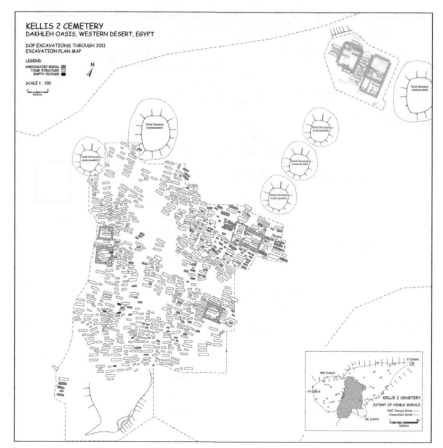

23.2 Excavation plan of the Kellis 2 cemetery in the Dakhleh Oasis, Egypt.
(Created by the author.)

between 100 and 450 AD (Molto 2002: 243; Stewart, Molto and Reimer 2003: 376). Systematic excavations commenced in 1992 and, to date, have recovered the remains of 770 individuals (Figure 23.2).

The cemetery is characterised by the presence of mud-brick enclosures, signifying mausolea, and low mud-brick mastaba-like superstructures, and it is densely filled with simple rectangular pit graves dug into the hard-packed red Nubian clay (Birrell 1999: 38). It is hypothesised that individuals interred in mausolea are related to one another either genetically or through marriage, with other potential family members buried in an accretionary fashion outwards from each mausoleum. Haddow's (2012: 213) research on dental non-metric traits and the non-metric skeletal trait studies by Molto (2002: 253) and Kron (2007: 81) have identified potential kin group burial

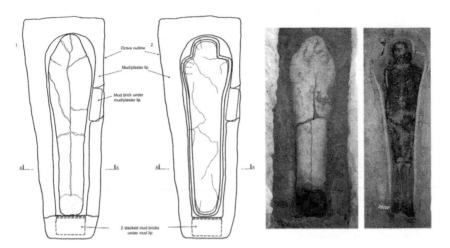

23.3 Illustration and photographic example of an anthropomorphic pottery coffin.
(Created by the author.)

clusters, potentially indicating a kin structure for at least that part of the cemetery. With few exceptions, individuals are interred in single burials, some in ceramic coffins (Plate 9A), some with mud-brick superstructures (Plate 9B) and substructures, and others with burial inclusions such as botanicals (Plates 9A and 9F), ceramics (Plate 9E) and jewellery (Plate 9D) (Wheeler 2009: 54–61). On rare occasions individuals are also buried in pottery coffins (Figure 23.3). Most individuals are wrapped in a burial shroud (Plate 9B), and all are placed in an extended position with the head facing west, indicating a Christian-style burial (Birrell 1999: 40; Bowen 2003: 167). While adults appear to have been shrouded in purposefully made burial linen textiles, most children and infants appear to be wrapped in adult clothing such as tunics, or in pieces of used linen textiles (Livingstone 2012: 323). The state of natural preservation varies with each individual, and while some individuals still present with preserved soft tissue and hair, others are completely skeletonised. Although these are not intentionally mummified as seen in previous Egyptian periods (and as is documented in the Kellis 1 cemetery: Aufderheide *et al.* 1999; Aufderheide, Cartmell and Zlonis 2003; Aufderheide *et al.* 2004; Aufderheide 2009), there appears to have been some attempt at mortuary treatment beyond natural preservation (Williams *et al.* 2013). A mixture of botanical physical remains and oils, myrrh resin and clay was placed directly on the body, in between linens or on top of linens on several individuals, most notably on children.

Table 23.1   Demographic profile of skeletal remains from the Kellis 2 cemetery for 724 individuals

	Total Kellis 2 sample	
Sex (adult)	**N**	**%**
Male	105	14.5
Female	153	21.1
Adult (unknown sex)	3	0.4
Age category	**N**	**%**
Foetal–birth	106	14.6
Birth–12 months	178	24.5
1–4 years	102	14.2
5–10 years	47	6.5
11–15 years	22	3.1
Juveniles of unknown age	8	1.1
16–35 years (young adult)	128	17.6
36–50 years (middle adult)	79	10.9
51+ years (old adult)	51	7.1
Adults of unknown age	3	0.4
Total juvenile	463	64
Total adult	261	36
Total	**724**	**100**

Analysis of the life cycle

At Kellis 2, the unique mortuary landscape and the inclusion of all individuals, no matter what their age (Tocheri *et al.* 2005: 338) or pathological condition (e.g. Mathews 2008; Cope and Dupras 2011), has allowed for an examination of individuals at all stages of the life cycle. Analysis of 724 individuals (out of 770 excavated) indicates that 64 per cent of the Kellis 2 population are juvenile and 36 per cent are adult (59 per cent female, 40 per cent male, 1 per cent unknown sex) (Table 23.1). Multiple methods, including DNA and stable isotope analyses, palaeodemographic reconstruction, differential diagnoses of pathological conditions, and growth and development studies, are combined to provide a better understanding of life and death in the community of ancient Kellis and the Dakhleh Oasis during the Romano-Christian Period.

Pregnancy and birthing practices

Not unexpectedly in an archaeological population, foetal, infant and childhood mortality at Kellis was high. The proportion of foetuses represented in the sample (n = 106, 14.6 per cent) may appear unusual in an archaeological sample; however, this is due to exceptional preservation and the inclusion of all individuals in the cemetery, rather than practices such as infanticide. Sharman's (2007: 94–5) study of fertility based on the Kellis 2 demographic profile suggests that the total fertility rate was probably seven to eight births per woman to keep the population growing, however, the infant mortality rate (death before the age of one) was approximately 24 per cent presuming a population growth rate of 1.48 per cent per year. This rate, in comparison to those of other archaeological populations, is relatively low. It is likely, however, that the Kellis population was able to remain demographically stable through immigration to the oasis (Dupras and Schwarcz 2001). Before the establishment of the Kellis 2 cemetery, inclusion of foetal remains in burial locations such as the Kellis 1 cemetery was rare (Aufderheide *et al.* 1999: 201). The adoption of Christian burial practices (Marlow 2001; Bowen 2003: 167; 2012: 352) ensured that every individual, regardless of age and pathological condition, was included in the cemetery. Thus, demographically, most of the information regarding pregnancy outcomes derives from the Kellis 2 cemetery. Tocheri *et al.* (2005: 337) examined a sample of foetuses from the Kellis 2 population and found that the foetal age distribution does not differ from the natural expected mortality distribution of a pre-industrial population. Practices such as infanticide can be eliminated as a contributing factor to the mortality distribution, and because each gestational age category is well represented, this suggests that all premature stillbirths and neonatal deaths received similar burial rites. The age distribution of the Kellis 2 foetal remains suggests that emerging Christian concepts, such as the 'soul' and the 'afterlife', were being applied to everyone, including foetuses of all gestational ages, and thus all individuals were deemed appropriate for inclusion in communal burial spaces.

The configuration of graves in the Kellis 2 cemetery is notable, with a defined accretionary pattern of grave orientation (Figure 23.2) (e.g. Abd Elsalam 2011). Of the graves recorded, 98 per cent were orientated at an angle between 63° and 117° east of north, corresponding to the orientation of the rising sun along the horizon throughout the year (Williams 2008: 51–6). By combining the grave orientation with stable isotope analyses of short-term tissues such as hair and nails, it was determined that the majority of foetuses, newborns and women of child-bearing age were dying at a specific time of the year, in particular March and April (Williams 2008: 57–65).

The age at death for foetuses and newborns was also used as a starting point for determining the month of conception, by counting back gestational weeks. The results from this analysis indicate that the majority of conceptions were occurring in the months of July and August (Williams 2008). These months correlate with the timing of Roman-Egyptian fertility festivals in Dakhleh (Kaper 2001: 73–6). In addition, the months of fewest conceptions, December and January, correlate with the timing of early Christian behavioural and sexual prohibitions throughout the Advent season (e.g. Brown 1990). This timing of the birth process suggests a spiritual and social influence for conception and may also contribute to the demographic pattern seen in the Kellis 2 cemetery, as seasonal timing of childbirth can contribute to a greater risk of mortality for mother and infant.

Given the high number of females of childbearing age, and the number of late-term foetuses and young infants in the cemetery, it is likely that pregnancy and childbirth were dangerous, and many would have died through complications during this time (Dupras *et al.* 2014: 46). The presence of certain skeletal traumas in foetuses and infants indicates that the birth process was dangerous and was probably assisted by someone, potentially a midwife. Greenstick fractures on the sternal ends of ribs and healed fractures of first cervical vertebra in foetal and infant remains indicate birth trauma. Additional traumas such as healed fractures of the lateral clavicles, a healed fracture of a proximal humerus and four cases of humerus varus (Molto 2000; Dupras *et al.* 2014: 51) have also been noted as possible results of birth trauma.

Infancy and childhood

Weaning patterns at Kellis have been reported by Dupras (1999: 247) and Dupras, Schwarcz and Fairgrieve (2001) through the use of stable carbon and nitrogen isotope analyses on a cross-sectional sample of juveniles. The nitrogen data show that the $\delta^{15}N$ values increased to a peak value at six months of age, indicating an exclusive dependence on breast milk until approximately six months of age. Nitrogen values then begin a steady decrease until approximately three years, indicating that the weaning process had ceased by this time and that children would no longer be reliant on breast milk as part of their diet.

The stable carbon isotope values also show enrichment during the first year of life, and Dupras, Schwarcz and Fairgrieve (2001: 208) suggest that the enrichment may be due to the types of complementary foods that were introduced around six months of age. The presence of pearl millet (*Pennisetum glaucum*) in Kellis, and complementary isotope enrichment in cow and goat remains, suggests that millet may have been present in the diet of these infants (Thanheiser, Kahlheber and Dupras in press). Ancient literary sources such as Galen and Soranus suggested that mothers should introduce complementary foods at six months of age and that gruel or pap mixtures made with cow or goat milk were favoured (Dupras, Schwarcz and Fairgrieve 2001: 210). Given this evidence, it is possible that infants from Kellis were fed complementary foods that included pearl millet or that they drank milk from cows or goats that were fed pearl millet. Stable isotope analyses therefore indicate that the infants from the Kellis 2 cemetery were breastfed exclusively for the first six months of life, with a long transitional feeding period, and weaned completely by three years of age. Dental pathology data, particularly an increase in the rate of dental caries by the age of four, also support this (Shkrum 2008: 95–8). Further longitudinal research conducted by Dupras and Tocheri (2007: 71) on enamel stable oxygen isotopes supports this interpretation of weaning practices at Kellis.

In Kellis it appears that if an individual could survive past the infancy stage (and through the weaning period), he or she stood a good chance of surviving through to adulthood. Many children, however, still died during or soon after infancy. It is likely that, for the most part, children died quickly of acute ill-nesses that we now take for granted as rare, such as tetanus, diphtheria, polio, whooping cough and other serious respiratory infections, and gastroenteritis – diseases that modern humans have all but conquered in the developed world with proper immunisation and sanitation. However, acute illnesses do not leave specific pathological conditions on bones or teeth, so it is difficult to provide a definitive cause of death for these children. Nevertheless, there are a few indi-viduals who presented with congenital conditions that were likely to be lethal, such as neural tube defects (e.g. Cope 2008; Mathews 2008), osteogenesis imper-fecta (Cope and Dupras 2011), and skeletal trauma. Two individuals, one a child of approximately three years of age showing numerous healed, healing, and fresh non-accidental fractures (Wheeler et al. 2013; Figure 23.4a), and another, a juvenile of approximately eleven years of age showing numerous peri-mortem fractures (Wheeler, Dupras and Williams 2014), were the only cases of severe trauma in children that could be linked to a cause of death. Another notable pathological condition linked to cause of death in a child, in this case aged three to five years at death, is cancer, probably lymphocytic leukaemia (Molto 2002: 249). The significant number of lytic lesions and skeletal destruction indicates that this child would have had to have significant care.

Other children who showed skeletal indicators of stress survived through their early years but probably later succumbed to acute illness that left no skel-etal pathological indicators. Wheeler (2009, 2011), in her analysis of 239 infants and children, used a suite of skeletal and dental indicators of non-specific stress (cribra orbitalia, enamel hypoplasia, osteoperiostosis) and trauma to measure the overall well-being of the Kellis 2 juveniles (Figure 23.4b). These analyses revealed moderate levels of stress, low prevalence of trauma and overall improvement in health from pre-Roman times. Juveniles exhibiting cribra orbitalia showed similar mortality patterns on the basis of grave orienta-tion to individuals exhibiting no skeletal lesions, suggesting that all juveniles were equally affected by adverse environmental pressures during particular seasons.

Wheeler (2009, 2011) also assessed skeletal growth using diaphyseal lengths and the rate of growth towards adult size for juveniles from birth to the age of

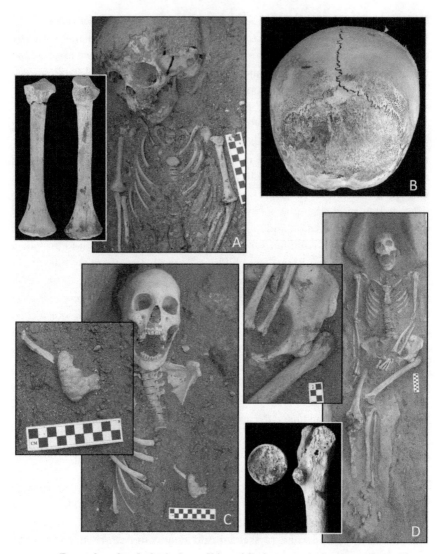

23.4 Examples of pathological conditions (all photographs by the author): (a)
Three-year-old child with intentional fractures of the proximal humeri. (b) Young
child with porotic hyperostosis on the parietals and occipital. (c) Adult with staghorn
kidney stone. (d) Adult female with severe fracture of the left proximal femur.

twelve years. The Kellis 2 data were compared with data from contemporaneous Wadi Halfa (Nubia) groups, as well as a modern sample from the USA.
Unsurprisingly, the Kellis 2 juveniles were found to be significantly smaller for
their age than their modern counterparts, but achieved adult size at similar
rates. Compared with the archaeological sample, Kellis 2 juveniles were similar

in absolute size, but were slightly accelerated in their rate of growth towards adult size, suggesting that they were at a slight advantage over their Nubian counterparts in growth attained for age. No relationships were found between skeletal growth and the number of physiological stressors exhibited, suggesting that the effects of cumulative stressors and ill health did not significantly impact patterns of growth in the children at Kellis 2.

In her analysis of the dental health of the juveniles at Kellis, Shkrum (2008) found significant differences in the prevalence of dental disease in various age cohorts. Caries were present in both deciduous and permanent teeth, occurring more frequently in the first and second deciduous and permanent molars (Shkrum 2008: 56). The total prevalence of juveniles with deciduous and permanent caries was 38.5 per cent and 23.7 per cent respectively. Shkrum (2008: 61, 71) also found evidence of calculus and periapical abscessing, particularly in older children, suggesting that dental health contributed to the overall pattern of morbidity and mortality seen in the Kellis 2 juvenile population.

Mortality, or probability of dying, was lowest for males and females between the ages of ten and fifteen (Sharman 2007), as would be expected given the typical pattern of human mortality in pre-industrial populations (Howell 1976; Wood et al. 2002). This is supported by our findings in the Kellis 2 cemetery, as only twenty-two individuals (3.1 per cent) have been classified in the eleven-to-fifteen-year-old cohort. This represents the smallest age cohort in the Kellis 2 cemetery sample (see Table 23.1).

Adulthood

Adults make up approximately 36 per cent (N = 261) of the total sample at Kellis 2, with 105 males (14.5 per cent), 153 (21.1 per cent) females and three individuals whose sex could not be determined. While one would expect a more even distribution between adult males and females, there are many reasons why adult males might be underrepresented in the demographic structure of the population. Preliminary stable oxygen isotope results (Dupras and Schwarcz 2001: 1204; Groff 2015) indicate that adult males migrated between the Dakhleh Oasis and the Nile valley, perhaps as part of the caravan to move goods in and out of the oasis, as soldiers, or to secure employment. This migratory pattern may have resulted in male individuals dying and being buried outside the oasis. In addition, there are a disproportionate number of adult females of childbearing age in the cemetery, and we hypothesise that many of them died during childbirth.

Non-metric dental traits (Haddow 2012: 213) and non-metric skeletal traits (Molto 2001; Molto et al. 2003) suggest that individuals buried in the Kellis 2 cemetery were genetically homogenous, and perhaps inbred. Parr (2002), however, found genetic evidence of thirteen mitochondrial DNA lineages, suggesting a pattern of patrilocal residence. Although it is very difficult to compare these two forms of evidence, and Y-chromosome DNA analysis has yet to be conducted, stable isotope analysis (e.g. Dupras and Schwarcz 2001) has indicated a movement of individuals between the Dakhleh Oasis and the Nile valley. The oasis was located on a well-known caravan route during this period and produced goods (e.g. dates, olives, wine and alum) that were sought after in greater Egypt and beyond (Hope, Kucera and Smith 2009).

Estimates of stature show that males from the Kellis 2 cemetery were approximately 166 cm tall on average, while the average female stature was 156 cm. These figures are similar to those for other contemporaneous populations in the oases of Egypt (e.g. Dunand *et al.* 2005: 109). Bleuze and colleagues (2014b: 225–7) demonstrated that adult body proportions (intralimb differences) were achieved during childhood growth, and that juvenile growth was under significant selective pressures from the particular climatic factors of the oasis. Further metric studies of individuals from the Kellis 2 cemetery demonstrate the unique effect of the desert environment on body shape and limb proportions (Bleuze *et al.* 2014a: 500–3), and highlight the complicated relationship between human growth and development in such an ecozone. Adult skeletal remains showed similar body shape to populations in high-latitude locations, while demonstrating limb proportions similar to those of low-to-mid-latitude populations.

Archaeological excavations of Kellis have indicated that for the most part, the occupants of Kellis lived an agrarian lifestyle. In addition to botanical analyses from Kellis (Thanheiser 1999; Thanheiser, Kahlheber and Dupras in press) and faunal analyses (Churcher 1983, 1993), the discovery of the Kellis Agricultural Account Book (Bagnall 1997) has allowed for the determination of what food items would have been grown and raised in the oasis, and what would have been potentially consumed. This evidence, in combination with stable isotopic analyses (Dupras 1999; Williams 2008; Williams, White and Longstaffe 2011), has shown that the inhabitants of Kellis ate mainly C_3 plants such as grains including wheat and barley, vegetables and fruit, and protein sources including cattle, pigs, goats, sheep and chickens. Millet, a C_4 plant, was also consumed on a seasonal basis. Isotopic evidence indicates a sexual division in the consumption of protein, with males consuming more protein and females consuming more carbohydrates (Dupras 1999: 246).

The skeletal remains of the adults who lived in Kellis show typical signs of occupational stress linked to farming and other types of physical activity. In his study of 135 adult skeletons from Kellis 2, Robin (2011) found a high prevalence of osteoarthritis in the hip and knee joints. While males and females showed similar rates of osteoarthritis in their knee joints, males showed significantly more osteoarthritic changes in their hip joints, suggesting a link with adult male occupations, such as farming, or perhaps mobility. Similar osteoarthritic characteristics in the knee joints indicate that both males and females were engaging in activities that involved repetitive kneeling or squatting behaviours, perhaps related to farming activities among males and textile weaving among females. Our observations have also indicated that osteoarthritic changes to the cervical vertebra were more common in adult females, while osteoarthritic changes to the lower lumbar spinal region were more common in males. This is probably again linked to repetitive occupation-related activities, such as females carrying things on their heads and males using farming implements such as the short-handled hoe. Both activities can still be observed in the modern oasis population.

In addition to occupational stress, many adults also showed the effects of living in a harsh desert environment. While individuals buried in the Kellis 2 cemetery were not artificially mummified like those in the Kellis 1 cemetery (e.g. Aufderheide 1999), we can only assume that individuals buried in the Kellis 2 cemetery would have suffered from some of the same diseases linked to the environment that can only be diagnosed from soft tissues. Diseases such as sand pneumoconiosis (Cook 1994: 267; Cook and Sheldrick 2001: 104), emphysema and anthracosis (black lung disease), and parasitic infections such as *Enterobius vermicularis* (pinworm), *Schistosoma haematobium* (schistosomiasis) and *Ascaris lumbricoides* (giant roundworm) have been diagnosed in mummified individuals from Kellis 1 (Aufderheide, Cartmell and Zlonis 2003; Aufderheide 2009; Zimmerman and Aufderheide 2010). Vascular and degenerative changes linked to diet, such as atherosclerosis, are also present, and one case of cirrhosis of the liver has been noted as a possible result of overindulgence in alcohol (Zimmerman and Aufderheide 2010: 18; Branson 2013: 56). Given that the individuals buried in Kellis 2 lived in the same environment, with sand, smoke and similar dietary choices, it can be assumed that similar diseases would have been present in this population. Skeletal evidence of environmental hardships has been noted in the Kellis 2 population with the discovery of four cases of significant kidney stones (Figure 23.4c). The presence of kidney stones indicates chronic dehydration, which is not surprising given the lack of precipitation and arid conditions of the oasis. One case of an ossified aortic artery indicating atherosclerosis is also present in the Kellis 2 population.

While many adults show pathologic conditions that were probably associated with their cause of death, many did not. Like many other Egyptian populations, the adult inhabitants of Kellis showed severe dental pathology linked to their environment. Severe wear and attrition, dental calculus, periodontal disease, caries and advanced dental abscesses are common in almost every individual. These conditions were probably caused by the chronic ingestion of grit and sand in food. We hypothesise that many individuals died from systemic infection caused by dental abscesses. Other pathological conditions in the adult population include metabolic or haematologic diseases such as cribra orbitalia, porotic hyperostosis and osteoporosis, joint disease such as ankylosing spondylitis, neoplasias (benign and malignant), congenital disorders such as spina bifida occulta, and trauma. In a preliminary report on the bioarchaeology of the Kellis 2 sample, Molto (2002: 244) reports a skeletal trauma rate of 35 per cent in males and 30 per cent in females. While not significantly different between males and females, the rate of trauma in adults is significantly higher than that observed in juveniles (Wheeler 2009). When age and type of trauma are considered, however, significant patterns are noted. Males show significantly more trauma than females in age cohorts under sixty, while trauma increases significantly in females over the age of sixty, probably because of the link between osteoporosis and fractured femora (Molto 2002: 244). Another significant difference has been noted between accidental and intentional trauma, with only males displaying intentional trauma, probably linked to interpersonal violence and not organised conflict (Molto 2002: 249).

Infectious disease was also present in the population at Kellis 2, as both tuberculosis and leprosy have been identified. Leprosy has been diagnosed in eight individuals, and notably almost all of them were young adult males in their twenties. Interestingly, their graves were not segregated but interspersed throughout the cemetery, possibly suggesting that individuals affected with leprosy were not stigmatised but accepted into the community. Although Molto (2002: 250) has suggested that leprosy may have been endemic in the oasis, stable isotope evidence suggests that several of these individuals spent part of their youth in the Nile valley region, and then migrated to the oasis not long before their deaths (Dupras and Schwarcz 2001; Groff 2015). Similarly, pathologic changes associated with tuberculosis have been diagnosed in three individuals at Kellis (Molto 2002: 250). Analyses of ancient DNA have confirmed the morphological analyses of both leprosy and tuberculosis diagnoses (Donoghue *et al.* 2005).

Of the 724 skeletons from the Kellis 2 cemetery, only fifty-one (7 per cent) lived beyond the age of fifty years, not an uncommon finding for archaeological populations. Of these fifty-one individuals, forty-two were female: women were again proportionally overrepresented, but this is not surprising given the life expectancy of males. The presence of osteoporosis in the majority of these adult females indicates the loss of calcium and bone tissue resulting from the decline of oestrogen after menopause. Seven (17 per cent) of these adult females showed fractures of the femoral neck (Figure 23.4d), a prevalence rate reflected in modern clinical sources for adult females in industrial nations. One adult female displayed a peri-mortem fracture, while two others showed complete healing, suggesting that there was knowledge and experience in the treatment for this injury. Four individuals showed evidence of walking with unhealed and unstable fractures.

Summary

The exceptional preservation and environment demonstrated at the archaeological site of Kellis and its surrounding cemeteries have allowed for unprecedented bioarchaeological analyses of human remains. All stages of the life cycle, from foetus to old age, are represented in the Kellis 2 cemetery, allowing for the reconstruction of individual life histories and a clearer understanding of how individuals lived and died in the oasis. Not surprisingly, foetuses, infants and children make up the majority of the skeletal sample from the Kellis 2 cemetery. Analyses of individuals in these age categories have revealed that infants were breastfed exclusively for six months, and then weaned until approximately three years of age. Most juveniles probably died from acute conditions that did not affect their skeletal structures, and thus it remains impossible to determine their cause of death. Those that do show skeletal indicators of stress illustrate the 'osteological paradox' (Wood *et al.* 1992) that although their skeletons indicate that they suffered from physiological stress, they were strong enough to survive through it, only to die later from another affliction.

While teenagers make up a very small part of the Kellis 2 population, adult females make up a larger proportion than adult males. Many adult females of childbearing age probably died during the process of childbirth. Adult males may be underrepresented in the demographic profile because of their migratory patterns and the possibility that they died elsewhere and their bodies were not returned to Kellis for burial. Those individuals who did survive into old age were mainly females, and most display the classic characteristics of menopause-related osteoporosis and bone fracture. Many of the pathological conditions associated with adult skeletal remains reflect the environment in which the inhabitants of Kellis lived. The presence of kidney stones indicates chronic dehydration and emphasises the arid environment of the Dakhleh Oasis. Ossified arteries associated with atherosclerosis speak to the diet of the individuals. Osteoarthritis in both adult males and females indicates the repetitive motions associated with an agrarian lifestyle and the effects of old age. The presence of infectious diseases such as tuberculosis and leprosy indicates that these individuals were living with long-term chronic pain and illness. In addition, the fact that these individuals were not buried in segregated locations in the cemetery may also indicate that the population in Kellis was accepting of individuals with disfiguring maladies.

Although we present only a glimpse into the bioarchaeological analyses conducted on the skeletal remains from the Kellis 2 cemetery, it is clear that individuals living in Kellis dealt with a unique environment. The isolated location, lack of precipitation, arid conditions, fluctuating hot and cold desert temperatures and sandy environment required that the inhabitants of the Dakhleh Oasis had to adapt in order to survive. Bioarchaeological investigations allow us to consider questions of behaviour and lifestyle, population history, identity, biological relatedness and quality of life through the integration of biological and archaeological data. This approach emphasises multiple lines of enquiry to provide important information about the people who lived and died in Kellis.

Acknowledgements

The authors would like to thank the Egyptian Ministry of State for Antiquities for their continued support of our mission. We would like to extend thanks to all the members of the Dakhleh Oasis Project (DOP) and the DOP Bioarchaeology Team, who helped to make this research possible. We would also like to thank the editors for the chance to participate in this important volume. This research was funded in part by a standard Social Science and Humanities Research Council grant (#50-1603-0500) awarded to Dr El Molto, the Department of Anthropology at the University of Central Florida, the Department of Anthropology at Western University, London, Canada, and the Institute for the Study of the Ancient World at New York University.

References

Abd Elsalam, H. (2011), 'Using Geographic Information Systems (GIS) in Spatial Analysis of Mortuary Practices in the Kellis 2 Cemetery, Dakhleh Oasis, Egypt' (MA thesis, University of Central Florida).

Aufderheide, A. C. (2009), 'Reflections about bizarre mummification practices on mummies at Egypt's Dakhleh Oasis: a review', *Anthropologischer Anzeiger* 67, 385–90.

Aufderheide, A. C., Cartmell, L. and Zlonis, M. (2003), 'Bio-anthropological features of human mummies from the Kellis 1 cemetery: the Database for Mummification Methods', in G. E. Bowen and C. A. Hope (eds.), *The Oasis Papers*, III: *Proceedings of the Third International Conference of the Dakhleh Oasis Project* (Oxford: Oxbow Books), 137–51.

Aufderheide, A. C., Cartmell, L., Zlonis, M. and Sheldrick, P. (2004), 'Mummification practices at Kellis site in Egypt's Dakhleh Oasis', *Journal of the Society for the Study of Egyptian Antiquities* 31, 63–77.

Aufderheide, A. C., Zlonis, M., Cartmell, L. L., Zimmerman, M. R., Sheldrick, P., Cook, M. and Molto, J. E. (1999), 'Human mummification practices at Ismant el-Kharab', *Journal of Egyptian Archaeology* 85, 197–210.

Bagnall, R. (1997), *The Kellis Agricultural Account Book* (Oxford: Oxbow Books).

Birrell, M. (1999), 'Excavations in the cemeteries of Ismant el-Kharab', in C. A. Hope and A. J. Mills (eds.), *Dakhleh Oasis Project: Preliminary Reports on the 1992–1993 to 1993–1994 Field Seasons* (Oxford: Oxbow Books), 29–41.

Bleuze, M. M., Wheeler, S. M., Dupras, T. L., Williams, L. J. and Molto, J. E. (2014a), 'An exploration of adult body shape and limb proportions at Kellis 2, Dakhleh Oasis, Egypt', *American Journal of Physical Anthropology* 153, 496–505.

Bleuze, M. M., Wheeler, S. M., Williams, L. J. and Dupras, T. L. (2014b), 'Ontogenetic changes in intralimb proportions in a Romano-Christian Period sample from the Dakhleh Oasis, Egypt', *American Journal of Human Biology* 26, 221–8.

Bowen, G. E. (2003), 'Some observations on Christian burial practices at Kellis', in G. E. Bowen and C. A. Hope (eds.), *The Oasis Papers*, III: *Proceedings of the Third International Conference of the Dakhleh Oasis Project* (Oxford: Oxbow Books), 167–82.

Bowen, G. E. (2012), 'Child, infant and foetal burials of the Late Roman Period at Ismant el-Kharab, ancient Kellis, Dakhleh Oasis', in M.-D. Nenna (ed.), *L'enfant et la mort dans l'antiquité*, II: *Types de tombes et traitment du corps des enfants dans l'antiquité Gréco-romaine* (Alexandria: Centre d'Études Alexandrines), 351–72.

Branson, J. (2013), 'Evaluation of a Field Histology Technique and its Use in Histological Analyses of Mummified Tissues from Dakhleh Oasis, Egypt' (MA thesis, University of Central Florida).

Brown, P. (1990), *The Body and Society: Men, Women and Sexual Renunciation in Early Christianity* (New York: Columbia University Press).

Churcher, C. S. (1983), 'Dakhleh Oasis Project palaeontology: interim report on the 1988 field season', *Journal of the Society for the Study of Egyptian Antiquities* 13, 178–87.

Churcher, C. S. (1993), 'Roman-Byzantine and Neolithic diets in the Dakhleh Oasis', *Bulletin of the Canadian Mediterranean Institute* 8, 1–2.

Cook, M. A. (1994), 'The mummies of Dakhleh', in A. Herring and L. Chan (eds.), *Strength in Diversity: A Reader in Physical Anthropology* (Toronto: Canadian Scholars Press), 259–77.

Cook, M. and Sheldrick P. (2001), 'Microns, microbes, microscopes and molecules', in C. A. Marlow and A. J. Mills (eds.), *The Oasis Papers*, I: *Proceedings of the First International Symposium of the Dakhleh Oasis Project* (Oxford: Oxbow Books), 101–4.

Cope, D. J. (2008), 'Bent Bones: The Pathological Assessment of Two Fetal Skeletons from the Dakhleh Oasis, Egypt' (MA thesis, University of Central Florida).

Cope, D. J. and Dupras, T. L. (2011), 'Osteogenesis imperfecta in the archeological record: an example from the Dakhleh Oasis, Egypt', *International Journal of Paleopathology* 1, 188–99.

Donoghue, H. D., Marcsik, A., Matheson, C., Vernon, K., Nuorala, E., Molto J. E., Greenblatt, C. L. and Spigelman, M. (2005), 'Co-infection of *Mycobacterium tuberculosis* and *Mycobacterium leprae* in human archaeological samples: a possible explanation for the historical decline of leprosy', *Proceedings of the Royal Society B* 272, 389–94.

Dunand, F., Heim, J.-L., Henein, N. and Lichtenberg, R. (2005), *La nécropole de Douch, Oasis de Kharga*, II: *Tombes 73 à 92* (Cairo: Institut Français d'Archéologie Orientale).

Dupras, T. L. (1999), 'Dining in the Dakhleh Oasis, Egypt: Determination of Diet from Documents and Stable Isotope Analysis' (PhD dissertation, McMaster University).

Dupras, T. L. and Schwarcz, H. P. (2001), 'Strangers in a strange land: stable isotope evidence for human migration in the Dakhleh Oasis, Egypt', *Journal of Archaeological Science* 28, 1199–208.

Dupras, T. L., Schwarcz, H. P. and Fairgrieve, S. I. (2001), 'Infant feeding and weaning practices in Roman Egypt', *American Journal of Physical Anthropology* 115, 204–12.

Dupras, T. L. and Tocheri, M. W. (2007), 'Reconstructing infant weaning histories at Roman Period Kellis, Egypt using stable isotope analysis of dentition', *American Journal of Physical Anthropology* 134, 63–74.

Dupras, T. L., Wheeler, S. M., Williams, L. and Sheldrick, P. (2014) 'Birth in ancient Egypt: timing, trauma, and triumph? Evidence from the Dakhleh Oasis', in S. Ikram, J. Kaiser and R. Walker (eds.), *Egyptian Bioarchaeology: Humans, Animals and the Environment* (Leiden: Sidestone Press), 41–53.

Groff, A. T. (2015), 'Evaluating Migratory Aspects of Adults from Kellis 2 Cemetery, Dakhleh Oasis, Egypt, Through Oxygen Isotope Analysis to Address Social Organization and Disease Stigma' (PhD dissertation, University of Florida).

Haddow, S. D. (2012) 'Dental Morphological Analysis of Roman Era Burials from the Dakhleh Oasis, Egypt' (PhD dissertation, University College London).

Hope, C. A. (2001), 'Observations on the dating of the occupation at Ismant el-Kharab', in C. A. Marlow and A. J. Mills (eds.), *The Oasis Papers*, I: *Proceedings of the First International Symposium of the Dakhleh Oasis Project* (Oxford: Oxbow Books), 43–59.

Hope, C. A., Kucera, P. and Smith, J. (2009), 'Alum exploitation at Qasr el-Dakhleh in the Dakhleh Oasis', in S. Ikram and A. Dodson (eds.), *Beyond the Horizon: Studies in Egyptian Art and History in Honour of Barry J. Kemp*, I (Cairo: The American University of Cairo Press), 165–79.

Howell, N. (1976), 'Toward a uniformitarian theory of human paleodemography', in R. H. Ward and K. M. Weiss (eds.), *The Demographic Evolution of Human Populations* (New York: Academic Press), 25–40.

Kaper, O. E. (2001), 'Local perceptions of the fertility of the Dakhleh Oasis in the Roman Period', in C. A. Marlow and A. J. Mills (eds.), *The Oasis Papers*, I: *Proceedings of the First International Symposium of the Dakhleh Oasis Project* (Oxford: Oxbow Books), 70–9.

Kron, H. (2007), 'The Efficacy of GIS for Spatial Analysis of Mortuary Data based on Morphogenetic Traits in the Kellis 2 Cemetery, Dakhleh Oasis, Egypt' (MA thesis, University of Western Ontario).

Livingstone, R. (2012), 'Five Roman-Period tunics from Kellis', in R. S. Bagnall, P. Davoli and C. A. Hope (eds.), *The Oasis Papers*, VI: *Proceedings of the Sixth International Conference of the Dakhleh Oasis Project* (Oxford: Oxbow Books), 317–25.

Marlow, C. A. (2001), 'Miscarriages and infant burials in the Dakhleh cemeteries: an archaeological examination of status', in C. A. Marlow and A. J. Mills (eds.), *The Oasis Papers*, I: *Proceedings of the First International Symposiumof the Dakhleh Oasis Project* (Oxford: Oxbow Books), 105–10.

Mathews, S. (2008), 'Diagnosing Anencephaly in Archaeology: A Comparative Analysis of Nine Clinical Specimens from the Smithsonian Institution National Museum of Natural History, and One from the Archaeological Site of Kellis 2 Cemetery in Dakhleh Oasis, Egypt' (MA thesis, University of Central Florida).

Mills, A. J. (1979), 'Dakhleh Oasis project: reports on the first season of survey, October–December 1978', *Journal of the Society for the Study of Egyptian Antiquities* 9, 163–85.

Mills, A. J. (1982), 'The Dakhleh Oasis project: reports on the fourth season of survey, October 1981–January 1982', *Journal of the Society for the Study of Egyptian Antiquities* 12, 93–101.

Molto, J. E. (2000), 'Humerus varus deformity in Roman Period burials from Kellis 2, Dakhleh, Egypt', *American Journal of Physical Anthropology* 113, 103–9.

Molto, J. E. (2001), 'The skeletal biology and paleoepidemiology of populations from Ein Tirghi and Kellis, Dakhleh, Egypt', in C. A. Marlow and A. J. Mills (eds.), *The Oasis Papers*, I: *Proceedings of the First International Symposium of the Dakhleh Oasis Project* (Oxford: Oxbow Books), 88–100.

Molto, J. E. (2002), 'Bio-archaeological research at Kellis 2: an overview', in C. A. Hope and G. E. Bowen (eds.), *Dakhleh Oasis Project: Preliminary Reports on the 1994–1995 to 1998–1999 Field Seasons* (Oxford: Oxbow Books), 239–55.

Molto, J. E., Sheldrick, P., Cerroni, A. and Haddow, S. (2003), 'Late Period human skeletal remains from Areas D/6 and D/7 and North Tomb 1 at Kellis', in: G. E. Bowen and C. A. Hope (eds.), *The Oasis Papers*, III: *Proceedings of the Third International Conference of the Dakhleh Oasis Project* (Oxford: Oxbow Books), 345–63.

Parr, R. L. (2002), 'Mitochondrial DNA sequence analysis of skeletal remains from the Kellis 2 Cemetery', in C. A. Hope and G. A. Bowen (eds.), *Dakhleh Oasis Project: Preliminary Reports on the 1994–1995 to 1998–1999 Field Seasons* (Oxford: Oxbow Books), 257–61.

Robin, J. (2011), 'A Paleopathological Assessment of Osteoarthritis in the Lower Appendicular Joints of Individuals from the Kellis 2 Cemetery in the Dakhleh Oasis, Egypt' (MA thesis, University of Central Florida).

Sharman, J. (2007), 'Modeling Fertility and Demography in a Roman Period Population Sample from Kellis 2, Dakhleh Oasis, Egypt' (MA thesis, University of Western Ontario).

Shkrum, S. (2008), 'The Paleoepidemiology of Oral Health in the Children from Kellis 2, Dakhleh, Egypt' (MA thesis, University of Western Ontario).

Stewart, J. D., Molto, J. E. and Reimer, P. J. (2003), 'The chronology of Kellis 2: the interpretative significance of radiocarbon dating of human remains', in G. E. Bowen and C. A. Hope (eds.), *The Oasis Papers*, III: *Proceedings of the Third International Conference of the Dakhleh Oasis Project* (Oxford: Oxbow Books), 373–8.

Thanheiser, U. (1999), 'Plant remains from Kellis: first results', in C. A. Hope and A. J. Mills (eds.), *Dakhleh Oasis Project: Preliminary Reports on the 1992–1993 and 1993–1994 Field Seasons* (Oxford: Oxbow Books), 89–94.

Thanheiser, U., Kahlheber, S. and Dupras, T. (in press), 'Pearl millet in the Dakhleh Oasis, Egypt', in U. Thanheiser (ed.), *Proceedings of the Seventh International Workshop for African Archaeobotany* (Vienna: Vienna University Press).

Tocheri, M. W., Dupras, T. L., Sheldrick, P. and Molto, J. E. (2005), 'Roman Period fetal skeletons from the east cemetery (Kellis 2) of Kellis, Egypt', *International Journal of Osteoarchaeology* 15, 326–41.

Wheeler, S. M. (2009), 'Bioarchaeology of Infancy and Childhood at the Kellis 2 Cemetery, Dakhleh Oasis, Egypt' (PhD dissertation, University of Western Ontario).

Wheeler, S. M. (2011), 'Nutritional and disease stress of juveniles from the Dakhleh Oasis, Egypt', *International Journal of Osteoarchaeology* 22, 219–34.

Wheeler, S. M., Dupras, T. L. and Williams, L. (2014), 'Broken body: a case of multiple skeletal fractures in a juvenile from ancient Egypt', poster presented at the 41st Annual Meeting of the Paleopathology Association, Calgary, Alberta, Canada.

Wheeler, S. M., Williams, L., Beauchesne, P. and Dupras, T. L. (2013), 'Shattered lives and broken childhoods: evidence of physical child abuse in ancient Egypt', *International Journal of Paleopathology* 3, 71–82.

Williams, L. (2008), 'Investigating Seasonality of Death at Kellis 2 Cemetery Using Solar Alignment and Isotopic Analysis of Mummified Tissues' (PhD dissertation, University of Western Ontario).

Williams, L. J., White, C. D. and Longstaffe, F. J. (2011), 'Improving stable isotope interpretations made from human hair through reduction of growth cycle error', *American Journal of Physical Anthropology* 145, 125–36.

Williams, L., Dupras, T. L. Wheeler, S. and Sheldrick, P. (2013), 'Mortuary mixtures: botanicals used in body treatment within the Kellis 2 cemetery, Dakhleh Oasis, Egypt', paper presented at the 'Bioarchaeology in Egypt' conference, Cairo, Egypt.

Wood, J. W., Holman, D. J., O'Connor, K. A., and Ferrell, R. J. (2002), 'Mortality models for paleodemography', in: R. D. Hoppa and J. W. Vaupel (eds.), *Paleodemography – Age Distributions from Skeletal Samples* (Cambridge: Cambridge University Press), 129–68.

Wood, J. W., Milner, G. R., Harpending, H. C. and Weiss, K. M. (1992), 'The osteological aradox: Problems of inferring prehistoric health from skeletal samples', *Current Anthropology* 33, 343–70.

Zimmerman, M. R. and Aufderheide, A. C. (2010), 'Seven mummies of the Dakhleh Oasis, Egypt: seventeen diagnoses', *Paleopathology Newsletter* 150, 16–23.

24

An investigation into the evidence of age-related osteoporosis in three Egyptian mummies

Mervyn Harris

Osteoporosis can be defined as a systemic skeletal disease characterised by low bone density, micro-architectural deterioration of bone tissue and low-trauma fragility fractures. Prolonged immobilisation of a limb can result in a localised osteoporosis, whereas in instances of metabolic bone disease, the complete skeleton is affected (Legrand *et al.* 2000: 13–19). The condition normally affects females far more than males, and in females the onset commonly occurs at the time of the menopause. It can also be seen in elderly male and female individuals, and in conditions such as malignant disease (Mundy 1999: 208).

As the average lifespan (i.e. average age at death) of the population in ancient Egypt was short, in the region of thirty-five years (Filer 1995: 225; Toivari-Viitalia 2001), would the onset of the menopause and conditions such as osteoporosis have occurred at an earlier age than in modern-day populations? This chapter examines full body radiographs of the three adult mummies from different collections (the British Museum, the World Museum in Liverpool and the Rijksmuseum van Oudheden in Leiden) that were previously examined during the 1960s (Gray 1967; Gray and Slow 1968) and which appear to demonstrate radiographic evidence of osteoporosis. By looking for radiographic skeletal markers of ageing, this chapter seeks to determine whether the condition occurred at a younger age in ancient Egypt than in present-day individuals.

There are two types of osteoporosis. The first is post-menopausal osteoporosis, which is the result of a decrease in oestrogen levels accompanying the menopause and accounts for approximately 95 per cent of all cases. The second type is age-related osteoporosis, which is secondary to the ageing process. This is a result of the deterioration of physical systems with age (hormonal and musculo-skeletal), and the condition is also referred to as senile osteoporosis (Mundy 1999: 208).

Hip fractures are a common characteristic of age-related osteoporosis, often resulting from a fall (Dequeker *et al.* 1997: 881). Obese people may be orientated to impact the ground nearer to the hip than other people, protective responses may fail with increasing age, and local soft tissues may absorb less energy (Cummings and Nevitt 1989: 107), all of which add to the likelihood of fracture occurring in bones weakened by osteoporosis. In the USA today, 54 per cent of post-menopausal white women are osteopaenic (having lower than normal bone density) and 38 per cent are osteoporotic (having a bone density lower than that which is considered to be osteopaenic) (Jordan and Cooper 2002: 795). In modern clinical practice, diagnosis is usually made by dual-energy X-ray absorptiometry (DXA). In the case of ancient Egyptian mummies, DXA is problematic because of the absence of hydrated soft tissue. Attempts have been made to overcome the problem in the case of dry bone specimens by immersing the specimens being studied in water (Lees *et al.* 1993: 675), but obviously immersion of a mummy in water would be likely to cause damage to the specimen. Haigh (2000: 1365) employed DXA to determine bone density in ancient Egyptian femora from the Elliot Smith collection, formerly in the Manchester Museum, by using bags of dry rice to simulate soft tissue.

The specimens cited in this chapter are fully wrapped mummies, in some cases still lying within their anthropoid coffins. The radiographs are archived in the British Museum, and copies of them also exist in the KNH Centre for Biomedical Egyptology at the University of Manchester. Details of the radiographic equipment and settings used in the original study have, unfortunately, been lost with the passage of time. Diagnosis of low bone density was made solely from the radiographic evidence present. Spinal osteopaenia is detectable on conventional radiographs only after a loss of at least 20 to 40 per cent of bone mass has occurred (Grampp, Steiner and Imhof 1997: S11). Osteoporosis is equally difficult to detect from plain film radiographs, and an individual must lose between 30 and 50 per cent of bone mass before it can be detected by this method (Harris and Haeney 1969: 193). It is clear, therefore, that there is no definitive dividing line which would allow a clear distinction between diagnoses of osteopaenia and osteoporosis to be made from plain film radiographs. Variations in film exposure and developing technique can also impart a false appearance of low bone density; therefore, diagnosis of age-related osteoporosis based on radiographic appearance alone is unreliable and one must also look for additional specific skeletal markers such as radiographic indicators of ageing.

Radiographic appearance

Trabecular bone resorption in the axial skeleton causes thinning and loss of the transverse trabeculae, and this is accompanied by preservation of the primary trabeculae or those that are aligned with the axis of stress. Reinforced primary trabeculae produce a striated appearance in osteoporotic bones, which occasionally helps in distinguishing osteoporosis from osteomalacia (soft bones, often caused by a lack of vitamin D), in which the trabeculae may have an indistinct appearance. The loss of trabecular bone mass also emphasises the cortical outline. In the peripheral skeleton, bone loss is often seen initially at the ends of the long bones because of the predominance of cancellous bone in these regions. In the spine, loss of horizontal trabeculae and a decrease in the cortical thickness of the vertebrae, together with endplate opaqueness, are indicators of osteoporosis. A concave appearance of the vertebral body and anterior wedging (collapse of the anterior aspect of the vertebral body) are the typical radiographic appearances of vertebral body fractures seen in present-day cases of osteoporosis (Genant, Vogler and Block 1988).

Materials

Three mummies from the British Museum, Liverpool and Leiden collections demonstrated radiographic evidence of low bone density, as follows:

British Museum (BM) 24957 is the mummy of an elderly female, dated to the 26th Dynasty (664–525 BC), possibly from Thebes.

Liverpool, World Museum 11 is the mummy of a very elderly individual listed as male, tentatively attributed to the Late Period (664–332 BC) and is also considered to have originated from Thebes.

Leiden, Rijksmuseum van Oudheden 17 is the mummy of an elderly adult, listed as being of uncertain sex and attributed to the 21st Dynasty (1069–664 BC).

Results

BM 24957

The radiographic appearance of the skull suggests a lower than normal bone density. Thinning of the mandibular cortex is evident and there is significant resorption of the maxillary and mandibular alveolar bone (Figure 24.1a), indicative of chronic periodontal disease, which is commonly associated with poor oral hygiene and advanced age. Although the occlusal areas of the upper and lower teeth are partially obscured, there is evidence to suggest significant occlusal wear, another indicator of age. The circular radiolucent area visible on the left side of the mandible is evidence of a chronic periapical infection.

The thoracic cavity is partly obscured by radiopaque material but cortical thinning and radiolucency are evident in all of the ribs. Post-mortem displacement of the cervical vertebrae C5 and C6 is noted (Figure 24.1b). Osteophytosis (evidence of degenerative osteoarthritis) is also evident in the lumbar region. The radiograph of the thorax demonstrates a number of radiopaque foreign bodies, suggestive of some form of packing but insufficiently radiopaque to be

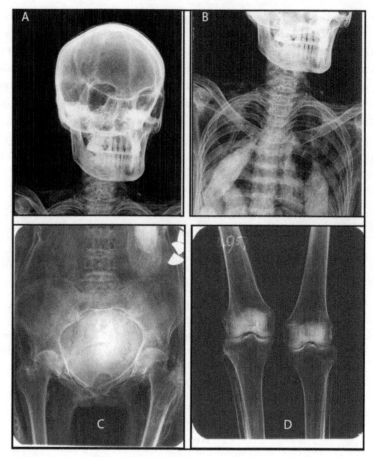

24.1 Four X-rays of BM 24957 (all images courtesy of the Trustees of the British
Museum): (a) Skull demonstrating generalised appearance of osteopaenia.
(b) Thoracic cavity with generalised appearance of thinning of the cortices
and bone fragility, typical of osteopaenia. (c) Female pelvis with both femora.
(d) Tibiae and fibulae with radiographic appearance of decreased bone density
and thinning of the cortices.

suggestive of artefacts such as amulets. The mid-thoracic vertebrae are partially
obscured by packing material but the upper thoracic vertebrae, T1, T2 and
T3, demonstrate a loss of trabecular bone mass and an emphasis of the cortical outline. The radiograph is insufficiently clear to positively determine a loss
of transverse trabeculae (Figure 24.1b). The pelvic morphology appears to be
female. No evidence of degenerative arthritic disease is noted in the hip joints
and knees. The radiographic appearance of both femora is paler and more
radiolucent than one would normally expect to see in a radiograph of adult
femora with normal bone density. The cortices of the femora are also thinner

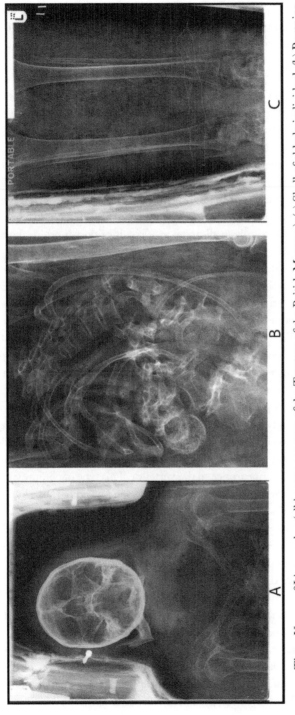

24.2 Three X-rays of Liverpool 11 (all images courtesy of the Trustees of the British Museum): (a) Skull of elderly individual. (b) Remains of thorax in very poor condition. (c) Both tibiae and fibulae demonstrating pale radiographic appearance and thinning of the cortices.

than one would expect to see in normal adults (Figure 24.1c). In addition, both tibiae have the radiographic appearance of low bone density, and the cortices are thinner than normal for an adult individual (Figure 24.1d).

Liverpool 11

This mummy is in very poor condition with a large number of post-mortem fractures, possibly a result of the brittle nature of the bones. The skull is edentulous, apart from the possible presence of four lower incisor teeth, although definitive confirmation of this is difficult because of the projection of the radiograph, which superimposed the occipital area of the skull onto the anterior portion of the mandible. The mandible is disarticulated, and remodelling of the maxillary and mandibular bone indicates that tooth loss occurred a number of years before death, another common indictor of advanced age (Figure 24.2A).

The thoracic cavity is in disarray as a result of post-mortem damage. Both humeri have the radiographic appearance of decreased bone density, and the cortices are thinner than one would expect to see in a normal adult (Figure 24.2B). The thoracic vertebrae are completely displaced from their anatomical position but it is possible to identify abnormal radiolucency of the vertebral bodies, loss of trabecular bone mass with a prominent striated trabecular pattern and a prominent cortical outline. Because the appearance of abnormal radiolucency of the vertebral bodies can be caused by incorrect radiographic exposure, or faulty developing technique, this characteristic cannot be relied on as a definitive radiographic indicator of low bone density. However, features such as loss of trabecular bone, a prominent striated trabecular pattern and a prominent cortical outline are radiographic features commonly seen in cases of osteoporosis in living patients. Also present are two vertebral body fractures, one moderate and the other severe in which the anterior part of the vertebral body is compressed, giving a triangular appearance to the vertebra. This type of compression fracture is also typical of the vertebral body fractures seen on radiographs and computed tomography (CT) scans of modern-day patients suffering from spinal osteoporosis. These fractures are the result of compression forces on a weakened vertebral body caused by the weight of an individual moving in an upright position. Such damage is unlikely to have occurred post-mortem, when the body is horizontal and immobile and there is no vertical load on the vertebral body. The large numbers of fractures seen in numerous other bones of this skeleton appear to have occurred randomly and demonstrate no evidence of healing. They must therefore have occurred immediately before, or after, death. This type of extensive random and indiscriminate damage, in the absence of any evidence of any healing, is more likely to be the result of post-mortem damage. Both tibiae and fibulae demonstrate the pale radiographic appearance of decreased bone density together with thinning of the cortices (Figure 24.2C).

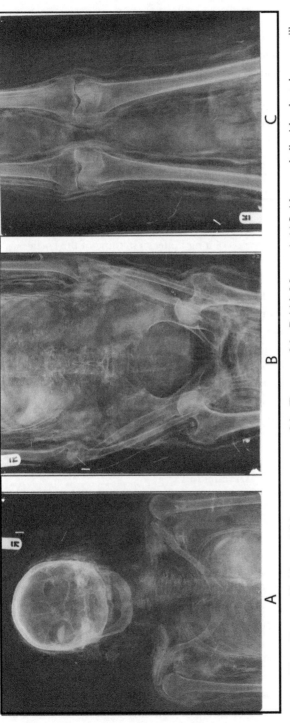

24.3 Three X-rays of Leiden 17 (all images courtesy of the Trustees of the British Museum): (a) Leiden 17: skull with edentulous maxilla and mandible. Extensive bone remodelling of the mandibular and maxillary alveolar ridges indicate tooth loss many years before death. Elliptical radiopaque inclusion in the left eye socket is probably a prosthetic eye placed as part of the funerary process. The upper part of the thoracic cavity, also visible, is partially obscured by radiopaque packing material. A large radiolucent area is present at the head of the right humerus and radius appeared to be radiographically paler, suggesting that these bones had a less than normal bone mineral density. (b) Leiden 17: lower part of the thoracic cavity and abdominal area with the thorax partially obscured by radiopaque packing material. Both humerii and radii appeared radiographically paler, suggesting a bone mineral density less than that seen in radiographs of an adult with a normal bone mineral density. Slight post-mortem disarticulation of the left hip joint is noted. Osteophytosis is suggested at L_3–L_4 although packing material present prevents a definitive diagnosis. (c) Leiden 17: radiograph of the left and right femora and tibia. The radiograph is upside down. The femoral and tibial cortices both on the right and left appear to be of normal thickness. Packing material is visible between both legs.

Leiden 17

This is the mummy of an elderly adult. The maxilla and mandible are edentulous with evidence of extensive remodelling, indicative of tooth loss many
years before death and possibly suggestive of advanced age. The presence of an
elliptical radiopaque inclusion in the left eye socket can, perhaps, be attributed
to a prosthetic eye placed as part of the embalming process (Figure 24.3A).

The thoracic cavity is partially obscured by radiopaque packing material,
and therefore detailed interpretation is not possible other than that the general
appearance suggests a lower than normal bone density (Figure 24.3B). The
humeri, ulnae and radii are less dense radiographically than one would expect
to see in a normal adult skeleton. There is also a large radiolucent area visible
at the head of the right humerus. This is a feature frequently identified in cases
of osteoporosis and is due to the depletion of large numbers of trabeculae,
which are normally seen at the ends of long bones. Thinning of the cortices is
also evident (Figure 24.3B). Parts of the femora, tibiae and fibulae visible on the
radiograph appear more radiolucent than one would expect in a normal adult;
all of these features suggest a decreased bone mineral density (Figure 24.3C).

Post-mortem disarticulation of the left hip joint is evident on the radiograph,
and there is no visible evidence of osteoarthritic changes. No evidence of arthritic
changes is evident in the right hip. Visual examination of the radiographs
indicates osteophytosis (outgrowths of bony tissue associated with degenerative
joints) in the lumbar vertebrae L3 and L4, which is indicative of degenerative
osteoarthritis in this region. Post-mortem displacement of the cervical vertebrae
makes accurate assessment of this region impossible, but there is no obvious
evidence of arthritic changes.

Discussion

The dental conditions of Liverpool 11 and Leiden 17 suggest that these individuals were elderly. The poorly preserved condition of Liverpool 11 makes
it impossible to obtain further radiographic information regarding the age of
that individual from, for example, evidence of degenerative osteoarthritis. The
bones are in disarray but the radiolucent appearance of all of the bones, abnormal thinning of the cortices, striated trabecular pattern of the vertebral bodies
and vertebral body fractures are all features of osteoporosis that are noted on
radiographs and CT scans of living patients. The upper and lower jaws of
Liverpool 11 are edentulous except for the lower central and lateral incisors,
suggesting that this was an elderly individual (in approximately the late fourth
or fifth decade). The extensive remodeling of the maxilla and mandible indicate
tooth loss a number of years before death, again suggestive of advanced age.

The upper and lower jaws of Leiden 17 are edentulous, and the degree of remodelling indicates that the teeth were lost a considerable number of years before death, suggesting that this was also an elderly individual (in the late fourth or the fifth decade). The radiographic appearance of the entire skeleton is one of low bone density.

In the case of BM 24957, the radiographic appearance of the teeth shows significant wear on the occlusal surfaces of the molar teeth. However, attrition alone is not the sole cause of loss of tooth tissue. The chewing over a long period of time of fibrous food which has been contaminated by inorganic particles also contributes significantly to loss of hard tooth tissue (Forshaw 2009: 422). This process would not have occurred quickly, rather taking many years to reach the stage seen in the radiographs. This, combined with the degree of upper and lower alveolar resorption present, suggests that the dentition is that of an individual in their late fourth or early fifth decade, or perhaps beyond. In the mandible, cortical thinning is evident together with post-mortem displacement of cervical vertebrae C5 and C6.

The thoracic vertebrae T1, T2 and T3 demonstrate a definite loss of trabecular bone mass and emphasis of the cortices, features which are seen in present-day cases of osteopaenia and osteoporosis. Cervical and lumbar osteophytosis is another indicator which suggests that the individual was not young.

From the information discussed above, it is clear that the radiographs of the mummies in this study indicate that all of the individuals were in at least their late fourth decade or older. As mentioned previously, average lifespan in ancient Egypt is generally estimated to have been in the region of the mid-thirties, although the elite survived longer, probably because of better nutrition and a less ardous lifestyle (David and Garner 2003: 153). Ramesses II and the 6th Dynasty pharaoh Pepy II are reputed to have lived into their nineties, although the latest known regnal date of Pepy II is that of the thirty-third census, suggesting a reign of fifty to seventy years (Grimal 1992: 89). Bagnall and Frier (1994: 75s91) estimated the average life expectancy in Roman Egypt as being twenty-two and a half years for women and twenty-four years for men. Although there are differing opinions regarding the average life expectancy in ancient Egypt, the average age was lower in comparison with modern Western populations, although the elite classes could expect to live longer.

In present-day populations, post-menopausal osteoporosis does not normally occur before the fifth decade. It is mainly a result of the reduction in oestrogen levels which normally occur at the time of the menopause and can be compared with the more gradual decline in testosterone levels seen amongst males (Ortner 2005: 410). In a study of bone loss in three ancient Nubian skeletal populations, it was found that osteoporosis occurred earlier among females than in modern Western counterparts (Dewey, Armelagos and Bartley 1969: 13), although this finding may be due to underestimating the age at death, which is not uncommon when analysing ancient skeletons. The bone loss among females was assessed as occurring around the sixth decade, a decade earlier than similar bone loss among females from a modern population. The reason suggested for the earlier bone loss among the ancient Nubian population was insufficient calcium intake and prolonged and frequent periods of lactation (Dewey, Armelagos and Bartley 1969: 410; Ortner 2003: 13). Pregnancy and lactation in conditions of reduced calorie intake have also been attributed to the significant decline in bone mineral density found among young medieval women (Turner-Walker, Syversen and Mays 2001: 263). Some modern studies support the importance of calcium intake in the maintenance of bone density (Heaney 2007). Other authors have suggested that the female skeleton demineralises during lactation to provide calcium for milk and that prolonged lactation does have a significant effect on bone mineral density (Woodrow et al. 2006: 4010; Dursun et al. 2006: 651). Women living through the Dutch famine of 1944–45 experienced a slight decrease in the age of onset of the menopause (Elias et al. 2003: 399). Other authors have taken the opposite view (Karlsson, Ahlborg and Karlsson 2005: 290). It would seem therefore, that the role of prolonged lactation and osteopaenia is unclear.

A study of seventy-four Old Kingdom skeletons from Giza found that osteoporosis was more frequent in male workers than in adult males of higher status, and this was attributed to factors such as workload, physical stress and poor diet among the workers. Throughout the study, however, evidence of osteoporosis was found among female skeletons considered to be younger than those of their male counterparts demonstrating evidence of the disease (Zaki et al. 2009: 85). A study of osteoporotic bone loss among two prehistoric Indian populations found that rates of bone loss were not related to dietary variation, protein intake or periods of reduced food intake (Perzigian 1973: 87). Did osteoporosis occur much earlier in antiquity? It would appear that there are conflicting theories regarding the causes of early-onset menopause, and in antiquity, the age of menopausal onset may have been a little earlier than the modern-day average in Egypt of 46.7 years (Sallam, Galal and Rashed 2006). However, the radiographic evidence from the mummified remains of the individuals described in this chapter appears to suggest that all the individuals exceeded the average life expectancy of ancient Egyptian populations described by others.

Conclusion

Although osteoporosis among ancient Egyptian remains is well documented (Dequeker et al. 1997; Sallam, Galal and Rashed 2006; Zaki et al. 2009), sufficient evidence from skeletal and mummified remains has not been found which would scientifically prove that post-menopausal or age-related osteoporosis occurred at a significantly earlier age than in present-day populations. The skeletal evidence from the small number of mummies presented in this chapter would suggest that osteoporosis, either post-menopausal or age-related, occurred in these individuals no earlier than the fourth or fifth decade of life and would have been something more likely to affect the elite classes who lived, on average, longer than the average individual of the time. It is possible, however, that females from the lesser elite groups may have had a diet less rich in calcium than the elite classes, which could have contributed to the earlier onset of osteoporosis, although prolonged periods of lactation may have been common to both.

Acknowledgements

The author is grateful to Dr J. Taylor of the Department of Egypt and Sudan, British Museum, London, for allowing access to the radiographs from the various collections cited, and to Mr T. O'Mahoney of the KNH Centre for Biomedical Egyptology, University of Manchester, for his invaluable IT assistance in the manipulation of the images used in this chapter.

References

Bagnall, R. S. and Frier, B. W. (1994), *The Demography of Roman Egypt* (Cambridge: Cambridge University Press).

Cummings, S. R and Nevitt, M. C. (1989), 'A Hypothesis: the causes of hip fractures', *Journal of Gerontology*, 44, 107–11.

David, A. R. and Garner, V. (2003), 'Asru, an ancient Egyptian temple chantress: modern spectrometric studies as part of the Manchester Egyptian Mummy Research Project', *Molecular and Structural Archaeology: Cosmetic and Therapeutic Chemicals, NATO Science Series* 117, 153–62.

Dequeker, J., Ortner, D. J., Stix, A. I., Cheng, X.-G., Brys, P. and Boonen, S. (1997), 'Hip fracture and osteoporosis in a XIIth Dynasty female skeleton from Lisht, Upper Egypt', *Journal of Bone Mineral Research* 12, 881–8.

Dewey, J., Armelagos, G. and Bartley, M. (1969), 'Femoral cortical involution in three Nubian archaeological populations', *Human Biology* 41, 13–28.

Dursun, N., Akin, S., Dursun, E., Sade, I., and Korkusuz, F. (2006), 'Influence of duration of total breast-feeding on bone mineral density in a Turkish population: does the priority of risk factors differ from society to society?', *International Journal of Osteoporosis* 17 (5), 651–5.

Elias, S. J., Van Noord, P. A. H., Peeters, P. H. M., den Tonkelaar, I. and Grobbee, D. E. (2003), 'Caloric restriction reduces age at menopause: the effect of the 1944–1945 Dutch famine', *Menopause* 10, 399–405.

Filer, J. (1995), *Disease* (London: British Museum Press).

Forshaw, R. J. (2009), 'Dental health and disease in ancient Egypt', *British Dental Journal* 206, 421–4.

Genant, H. K., Vogler, B. and Block, J. E (1988), 'Radiology of osteoporosis', in B. L. Riggs and L. J. Melton (eds.), *Osteoporosis: Etiology, Diagnosis and Management* (New York: Raven Press), 181–220.

Grampp, S., Steiner, E. and Imhof, H. (1997), 'Radiological diagnosis of osteoporosis', *European Radiology* 7 (supplement 2) S11–S19.

Gray, P. H. K. (1967), 'The radiography of ancient Egyptian mummies', *Medical Radiography and Photography* 43, 34–44.

Gray, P. H. K. and Slow, D. (1968), *Egyptian Mummies in the City of Liverpool* (Liverpool: Liverpool Corporation).

Grimal, N. (1992), *A History of Ancient Egypt* (Oxford: Blackwell Publishing).

Haigh, C. (2000), 'Estimating osteological health in ancient Egyptian bone via applications of modern radiological technology', *Assemblage: The Sheffield Graduate Student Journal of Archaeology* 5, 1365–81.

Harris, W. H. and Haeney, R. P. (1969), 'Skeletal renewal and metabolic bone disease', *New England Journal of Medicine*, 280 (4) 193–302.

Heaney, R. P. (2007), 'Bone health', *American Journal of Clinical Nutrition* 85, 3005–35.

Jordan, K. M. and Cooper, C. (2002), 'Epidemiology of osteoporosis', *Best Practice and Research Clinical Rheumatology* 16, 795–806.

Karlsson, M. K., Ahlborg, H. G. and Karlsson, C. (2005), 'Pregnancy and lactation are not risk factors for osteoporosis or fractures', *Lakartidningen* 102, 290–3.

Lees, B., Stevenson, J. C., Molleson, T. and Arnett, T. R. (1993), 'Differences in proximal femur bone density over two centuries', *The Lancet* 341 (13), 673–6.

Legrand, E., Chappard, D., Pascaretti, C., Duquenne, M., Krebs, S., Rohmer, V., Basl, M.-F. and Audran, M. (2000), 'Trabecular bone microarchitecture, bone mineral density and vertebral fractures in male osteoporosis', *Journal of Bone and Mineral Research* 15, 13–19.

Mundy, G. R. (1999), *Bone Remodelling and its Disorders* (London: Martin Dunitz).

Ortner, D. J. (2003), *Identification of Pathological Conditions in Human Skeletal Remains* (London: Academic Press).

Perzigian, A. J. (1973), 'Osteoporotic bone loss in two prehistoric Indian populations', *American Journal of Physical Anthropology* 39, 87–95.

Sallam, H., Galal, A. and Rashed, A. (2006), 'Menopause in Egypt: past and present perspectives', *Climacteric* 9, 421–9.

Toivari-Viitala J. (2001), *Women at Deir el-Medina: A Study of the Status and Roles of the Female Inhabitants in the Workmen's Community during the Ramesside Period* (Leiden: Instituut voor het Nabije Oosten).

Turner-Walker, G, Syversen, U. and Mays, S. (2001), 'The archaeology of osteoporosis', *European Journal of Archaeology* 4, 263–9.

Woodrow, J., Sharpe, C. J., Fudge, N. J., Hoff, A. O., Gagel, R. F. and Kovacs, C. S. (2006), 'Calcitonin plays a critical role in regulating skeletal mineral metabolism during lactation', *Endocrinology* 147 (9), 4010–21.

Zaki, M. E., Hussein, F. H. and El Shafy El Bana, R. A. (2009), 'Osteoporosis among ancient Egyptians', *International Journal of Osteoarchaeology* 19, 78–89.

25

The International Ancient Egyptian Mummy Tissue Bank

Patricia Lambert-Zazulak

The concept of tissue banking is well established, and has many applications in the medical field. Good examples are tissues stored for transplant surgery and also blood and blood product banking, all of which have contributed in many ways to modern medicine and research. Tissues are collected, stored, studied and distributed in a variety of ways appropriate to their uses, and each type of tissue bank has its own scientific and ethical considerations, which are complementary to each other in that tissue bank's mission. We can look at tissue banking generally as primarily a medical and research concept, with the aim of advancing the treatment of and research into diseases in modern times.

So what part can ancient Egyptian mummies play in this concept? What kinds of scientific study can be applied to their tissues, what kinds of knowledge does this give us; and what are the many archaeological, practical and ethical issues involved in collecting and studying ancient Egyptian mummy tissue in this way? Museums and allied institutions, such as university research departments, act as repositories for many types of artefact, and are a primary resource for collecting information on those objects and applying that knowledge in various fields. Museums, universities, research institutes and learned societies have historically sometimes created 'libraries' of samples from collections, both ancient and modern, such as animal tissues, insects, plants and other materials such as stone samples taken from particular types of stone artefacts, or samples of textiles. These primary resources, and the records held relating to them, can then be accessed by researchers from anywhere in the world and can substantially add to knowledge, not least by creating a meeting point for the interrelation of different areas of scholarly expertise.

Egyptian mummies, in terms of scientific research, can not only illuminate the health, diet, occupations, medical and embalming practices of the past, but may also contribute to our understanding of modern-day diseases. While some tissue banking already existed before the establishment of the International Ancient Egyptian Mummy Tissue Bank, mainly for South American mummies located within America (Krajick 2005), this concept had never before been attempted formally, on an international scale, for Egyptian mummies located outside Egypt. So what first gave rise to the idea to apply the concept of international tissue banking to Egyptian mummies, and what is new and unique about this?

The inception of the International Ancient Mummy Tissue Bank at Manchester

The idea to set up such a tissue bank was first suggested in 1996 in the context of the worldwide Schistosomiasis Research Project, which was a study designed by Medical Service Corporation International in the USA, in cooperation with the Egyptian Ministry of Health. The Schistosomiasis Research Project involved collecting statistics on the present-day incidence of the parasitic disease schistosomiasis or bilharzia worldwide. Because of the preserved nature of the tissue in the mummies from ancient Egypt, it was suggested that it might be possible to look at the incidence of the disease in ancient times and compare the data with the present-day statistics (Contis and David 1996).

The President of Medical Service Corporation International, Dr George Contis, therefore met with Professor Rosalie David, then Keeper of Egyptology at the Manchester Museum, director of the Manchester mummy research team and later Director of the KNH Centre for Biomedical Egyptology at the University of Manchester. Also present at the meeting was Mr Tristram Besterman (then Director of the Manchester Museum), who supported the vision that the museum could provide the most appropriate environmental storage conditions and record-keeping facilities for such a new and unique collection as well as formulating much of the background for the ethical and legal framework of the tissue bank's administration. External financial support for this large undertaking has been provided by a Leverhulme Trust research grant, the Kay Hinckley Charitable Trust and the North West Museum Service.

Schistosomiasis in Egypt

Schistosomiasis is a parasitic helminth disease contracted from the Nile river environment (Sturrock 2001: 9). The mature schistosome worms release many eggs into the host's bloodstream, and in *Schistosoma haematobium* they lodge in the urinary bladder thereby giving rise to blood in the urine (haematuria) and eventually cancers in the bladder (Rowling 1967). Haematuria may be mentioned some fifty times in the ancient Egyptian medical papyri (Nunn 1996: 63). In *Schistosoma mansoni* the eggs lodge in the blood vessels around the rectum, and Papyrus Chester Beatty VI, a specialised work on proctology (Jonckheere 1947), may refer to the symptoms caused by this species of the parasite. Bilharz (1853; translated in Warren 1973: 11–23) first identified the schistosome worm in two contemporary cadavers that he had dissected in Egypt. Ruffer (1910) went on to identify the calcified eggs in two ancient Egyptian mummies. Napoleon's army (Nunn 1996: 69), and the British Royal Army Medical Corps (Leiper 1915), all had to contend with schistosomiasis during their time in Egypt, where it was likened to male menstruation (Hoeppli 1973). The characteristic abdominal shape which occurs in chronic schistosomiasis may be shown in some art-works from ancient Egypt (Loebl 1995: 1–4; Ghalioungui 1962), while some texts (Erman 1978: 67–72) and artworks record the ancient Egyptians' daily activities in the Nile river environment where they became exposed to the disease. (See Rutherford in Chapter 16 above for further information relating to schistosomiasis.)

So the initial impetus to create the tissue bank was to help provide a means by which a palaeo-epidemiological picture of schistosomiasis in antiquity could emerge (Rutherford 1997, 2002, 2008), and then this information could be compared with the modern-day incidence of the disease, and perhaps lead to the identification of any evolutionary or adaptive changes that may have taken place in the parasite itself or in the human immune system's response to it. This type of study could then provide a model for future similar large-scale studies of other endemic diseases (Lambert-Zazulak 2000), such as malaria.

Background study for the creation of the tissue bank

In order to create the tissue bank, samples had to be obtained, non-destructively, from the maximum number of individual mummies now outside Egypt, as mummies within the Egyptian border could only be studied within the country (Besterman and David 1996). This is a complex and long-term process, and the two main aspects of background study that need to be understood before undertaking such a project are the mummification process itself on the one hand and the history of the collecting and distribution of Egyptian mummies outside Egypt on the other.

The mummification process has a profound effect on the tissues available for study today, both in terms of which tissues are preserved and in terms of their condition. Ancient Egyptian mummification was essentially a religious ritual, using practical methods to create a permanent, stable image of the deceased from their organic remains. The mummy was then recognisable to the spirit of that individual to visit and to ensure a continued existence in the afterlife.

By studying the gross anatomy of mummies, we can see evidence of the embalmers' procedures which demonstrate the ancient Egyptians' knowledge of human anatomy, along with their beliefs about the afterlife (Lambert-Zazulak 1997). Thus many aspects of learning and faith were brought together in the special methods of treating the human body in order to make an everlasting image (Smith 1906; Faulkner 1985: 152). However, the method of embalming the body has to be taken into consideration when conducting a modern scientific study as the process results in differential preservation of the body tissues and can affect the substances found within and upon the mummy.

The distribution of Egyptian mummies today

From the time of the individuals' deaths onwards, Egyptian mummies have been on a long and eventful journey, throughout the whole history of their existence. This journey continues today, and it is one of the ongoing tasks of the International Ancient Egyptian Mummy Tissue Bank to locate Egyptian mummies now outside Egypt, and where possible to document the history of their travels for the tissue bank's records.

Historically, mummies were used for a variety of purposes, such as in the drug *mumia* (Budge 1890: 13; Dawson 1927; Spielmann 1932), fuel and fertiliser. Animal mummies, in particular, were exported in large quantities for use as a fertiliser. A Renaissance-period pigment called 'mummy brown' was used for painting; there are even records of mummy wrappings being used to make paper, and the flesh was utilised as fish bait (Wortham 1971: 16, 44–6, 93–5; Jarcho 1981; Woodcock 1996; Germer 1997: 95–115; Ikram and Dodson 1998: 61–102).

The collecting of mummies tells a colourful story, which reflects the interests and resources of the collectors and even the fashions of the time. Mummies could be obtained on the open market from dealers supplying the demand for both antiquities and the raw materials for many different purposes. In addition, planned excavations were funded by museums and private art collectors, seeking the best specimens for display. Most usually, their interest focused on the accoutrements of the mummy, rather than on the human remains themselves: indeed there was one famous incident of a museum acquiring the arm of a mummy, which it then discarded after removing the bracelets (Spencer 1988: 34–5). Private collectors sought whole or partial mummies as souvenirs of their travels abroad in the age of the popularity of the grand tour for the wealthy, and this accounts for many of the separate heads, hands and feet available for study today.

The gatherings of such collectors often became the bases of museum collections, and met with a variety of fates. The stable climate of Egypt was a major factor in the concept of mummification, the religion which mythologised it and in the creation, stabilisation and indefinite preservation of intentionally embalmed Egyptian mummies. Once they were removed from this hot, dry environment, the seasonal changes and increased humidity of European countries frequently resulted in decomposition setting in (Leca 1980: 241). The condition of the human remains today is therefore dependent not only on the natural environment of Egypt and activities of tomb robbers in antiquity, followed by collection, transportation and storage in more recent centuries, but also on the motives and results of the work of the early investigators, keepers and conservators.

Locating sources of samples for the International Ancient Egyptian Mummy Tissue Bank

The sources of tissue may include whole mummies, mummy parts, material found in canopic jars and also samples of the drug *mumia* (Lambert-Zazulak, Rutherford and David 2003). In order to locate these potential sources of tissue, extensive searches were conducted, by post and telephone, covering over 8,000 possible locations, based on directories of museums, universities, research institutes, medical schools, learned societies, grand houses, public schools and so on, all and any of which may house human remains from ancient Egypt (Lambert-Zazulak 2000). The remains may have reached their present locations via routes which included study from many perspectives, such as medicine, anthropology, ethnology, phrenology, ancient history, art, archaeology, language, classics, theology, Bible studies, eugenics, pharmacology and even the history of circuses and showmanship.

The resulting response to the tissue bank's initial survey was huge, and remains were located as far apart and in such unexpected places as Iceland and India. Collections varied from very large groups of hundreds of individuals excavated prior to the creation of Lake Nasser (Van Gerven 1981) to just a single finger, probably collected for its ring. Canopic jars were found in art collections; and anatomical curiosities, such as a polydactylous foot or an ancient healed bone fracture, were found in collections for the history of medicine. Some mummies were also found which had passed through the care of some unusual places such as castles, libraries, monasteries, a morticians' college and even a lido.

Collecting samples for the tissue bank

Once remains are located, and the permission of their keepers is given for tissue sampling to proceed, the tissue bank seeks deposits of approximately one to two grams of dried tissue from each individual, which may be bone, teeth, soft tissue such as skin, brain, muscle or viscera, and hair. The tissue bank itself is kept under secure, optimum temperature- and humidity-controlled conditions (Lambert-Zazulak, Rutherford and David 2003).

Tissue is collected only when it is not detrimental to the preservation of the specimen, for example if there is already an open area in the body, where there is a severed area of a separate limb or head or by endoscopy from the internal parts of the mummy (Tapp, Stanworth and Wildsmith 1984). Samples are left intact, as they often include various different tissue types, and this macroscopic appearance helps researchers to identify the area of a sample which may be the most appropriate for their particular study. Such a procedure also helps to conserve the sample.

The scientific study of mummy tissue

A key element of the modern approach to mummy investigation is conservation, and the development of increasingly sophisticated diagnostic techniques applicable to the remains is a part of this process. In the case of small tissue samples often obtained by virtually non-destructive endoscopy, then studies utilising histology, chemical analysis, pharmacology, virology, spectrometry, pathology, serology, DNA, immunology, carbon dating, stable isotopes and the analysis of embalming substances and processes are all modern-day methods which can be applied in both forensic science and the investigation of mummies. Indeed, some of the techniques first developed on mummy tissue, such as the fingerprinting of dehydrated remains, have subsequently found applications in the forensic field (Fletcher and Neave 1984: 135–49). Another key element is accessible central record-keeping and information storage, so that nothing will be lost for future generations of researchers.

The concept of the International Ancient Egyptian Mummy Tissue Bank has a crucial role in fulfilling these objectives. It is important for the conservation of ancient human remains that they be disturbed as little as possible, and therefore the storage of tissue in the tissue bank will mean that a mummy needs to be X-rayed, be endoscoped and have tissue samples taken only once in order for the tissue to be available in the tissue bank and carefully selected for future work.

The central recording of the results of the investigations can obviate the need for the repetition of tests requiring more tissue samples, and the data can be made available worldwide. This has the potential to bring together investigators for the study of Egyptian mummies on a larger scale than ever before.

Previously the largest investigation of ancient Egyptian human remains was that carried out by the anatomists Elliot Smith and Wood Jones in the early years of the twentieth century on the mummified and skeletal remains of some 6,000 individuals in Nubia in Upper Egypt, which were being removed as part of the programme to raise the dam at Aswan (Smith and Jones 1910). The bodies represented a long period of history, and the statistical value of the work on the gross anatomy of these individuals can now be obtained at the ultrastructural and molecular level by the study of large numbers of small tissue samples brought together by the tissue bank.

The administration of the samples in the tissue bank

Each specimen is allocated a unique identification code, which stays with it at all stages. Manchester has a materials transfer agreement with each depositor of tissue, which states that the tissue is transferred to the bank for a renewable period of ten years, and that it can be loaned on approved application for use in well-planned and documented scientific research projects.

Researchers using material from the tissue bank for investigation sign a researcher's agreement, allowing them to borrow the tissue for one year, after which it is returned to the tissue bank, and this may include permanent preparations such as histological blocks and microscope slides. The researchers in due course report their results for the tissue bank's administration, and any publications record the tissue sample's reference code and an acknowledgement of its depositor. Similarly, the materials transfer agreement states that the bank will report to the depositors on the research conducted on the samples they have deposited with the bank (Lambert-Zazulak, Rutherford and David 2003).

The tissue bank's mission is to collect samples from several thousand mummies, and it currently holds samples which have come from depositing institutions in the UK, Australia, the USA, Chile, Greece, Germany and Canada. The bank also contains some samples from mummies originating in Sudan, South America and the Canary Islands.

The tissue bank's records

Occasionally remains cannot be biopsied, as for example in the case of those now located in the American south-west, where there may be an agreement with local tribes that all human remains in museum collections will not be sampled; or where the remains are inaccessible due to thick and tight wrappings. Nevertheless they may still be photographed, X-rayed and recorded, thus still contributing valuable information on the ancient Egyptian population for the tissue bank's records.

A particular strength of locating and collecting tissue on this scale is the statistical and palaeo-epidemiological potential, highlighted by the current work on schistosomiasis, which may be applied to other diseases in the future. The records produced and continually added to at Manchester represent, as far as can be ascertained, the largest centralised record anywhere in the world for the locations of ancient Egyptian human remains outside Egypt (Lambert-Zazulak 2000).

Current use of the tissue bank

Professor Andrew Chamberlain, Director of the KNH Centre for Biomedical Egyptology at the University of Manchester, describes the work presently being carried out on the tissue bank samples:

> The Tissue Bank is currently being used by doctoral and post-doctoral researchers in several research projects. For example, small samples of skin, cartilage and hair are being studied in an investigation of dietary effects on the stable isotope composition of proteins. Some specimens in the tissue bank have been stored as wax-embedded samples, and a selection of these are currently being analysed to determine whether detectable traces of ancient DNA can be recovered from this type of preserved tissue. (Andrew Chamberlain, personal communication, 2014)

Conclusion

Mummy research is a field that must take a very long-term view. The mummies of the ancient Egyptian people have existed for many centuries, and have seen historical trends in attitudes towards them and beliefs about them come and go. They have passed through many hands and conditions of burial, excavation, collection, storage, conservation, investigation and record-keeping over time. Much may still await discovery. The ancient expectation of eternity is answered today with the respectful and ethical treatment of the human remains, in fields of research in which the preservation of the remains, and indeed of our knowledge about them, is uppermost.

Acknowledgements

This chapter is an edited version of a paper first presented by the author within a lecture to the Egypt Exploration Society Northern Branch (Lambert-Zazulak 2002), and as part of a lecture to postgraduate students at the University of Manchester (Lambert-Zazulak 2004).

I am grateful to the late Professor Arthur Aufderheide, Tristram Bestermen Frank Bradley, Professor Andrew Chamberlain, Dr George Contis, Professor Rosalie David, the late John Davies, John Denton, the late Dr George Fildes, Roy Garner, Dr Jacqueline Hobbs, Dr David Lambert, Dr Michael Loze, Dr Susan Martin, the late Dr Desmond Norton, Dr Patricia Rutherford,

Dr Edmund Tapp, Angela Thomas, Leigh Travis, Dr Karen Vowles, Alison Walster, Angela White and Ken Wildsmith. I should also like to thank all of the tissue bank's depositors, many of whom have granted the author access to their collections and records in order to carry out sampling, photography and documentation; and especially Professor Dennis Van Gerven for permitting the author and Dr David Lambert several days' access to work on the large collection at the University of Colorado at Boulder.

References

Besterman, T. and A. R. David (1996), 'Letters: Mummy's the word', *New Scientist* 2060, 52.

Bilharz, T. M. (1853), 'A study of human helminthography, derived from information by letter from Dr Bilharz in Cairo, along with remarks by Prof. Th. v. Siebold in Breslaw', *Zeitschrift für wissenschaftliche Zoologie* 4: 53–71.

Budge, E. A. W. (1890), *Prefatory Remarks Made on Egyptian Mummies on the Occasion of Unrolling the Mummy of Bak-ran* (London: Harrison and Sons).

Contis, G. and David, A. R. (1996), 'The epidemiology of bilharzia in ancient Egypt: 5000 years of schistosomiasis', *Parasitology Today* 2 (11), 253–5.

Dawson, W. R. (1927), 'Mummy as a drug', *Proceedings of the Royal Society of Medicine* 21 (1), 34–9.

Erman, A. (1978), *The Ancient Egyptians: A Sourcebook of their Writings*, trans. A. M. Blackman (Gloucester, MA: Peter Smith). First published 1927; German original 1923.

Faulkner, R. O. (trans.) (1985), *The Ancient Egyptian Book of the Dead*, ed. C. Andrews (London: Book Club Associates).

Fletcher, T. A. and. Neave, R. A. H (1984), 'Faces and fingerprints', in A. R. David and E. Tapp (eds.), *Evidence Embalmed: Modern Medicine and the Mummies of Ancient Egypt* (Manchester: Manchester University Press), 135–49.

Germer, R. (1997), *Mummies: Life after Death in Ancient Egypt* (Munich and New York: Prestel-Verlag).

Ghalioungui, P. (1962), 'Some body swellings illustrated in two tombs of the Ancient Empire and their possible relation to aaa', *Zeitschrift für ägyptische Sprache und Altertumskunde* 87, 108–14.

Hoeppli, R. (1973), 'Morphological changes in human schistosomiasis and certain analogues in ancient Egyptian sculpture', *Acta Tropica* (Basel) 30, 1–11.

Ikram, S. and Dodson, A. (1998), *The Mummy in Ancient Egypt: Equipping the Dead for Eternity* (London: Thames and Hudson).

Jarcho, S. (1981), 'Some historical problems connected with the study of Egyptian mummies', *Bulletin de l'Institut d'Egypte* (Cairo) 58–9 (1976–77, 1977–78), 106–21.

Jonckheere, F. (1947), *Le Papyrus Medical Chester Beatty* (Brussels: Fondation Égyptologique Reine Élisabeth).

Krajick, K. (2005), 'The mummy doctor (Arthur Aufderheide)', *The New Yorker* 81 (13), 66–75.

Lambert-Zazulak, P. I. (1997), 'The Concept of Healing in the Ancient Egyptian Context' (PhD dissertation, University of Manchester).

Lambert-Zazulak, P. I. (2000), 'The International Ancient Egyptian Mummy Tissue Bank at the Manchester Museum', *Antiquity* 74, 44–8.

Lambert-Zazulak, P. I. (2002), 'The International Egyptian Mummy Tissue Bank: a resource for scientific study', lecture, Egypt Exploration Society Northern Branch, University of Manchester, 19 March.

Lambert-Zazulak, P. I. (2004), 'The International Ancient Egyptian Mummy Tissue Bank', lecture, School of Biological Sciences, University of Manchester, 15 November.

Lambert-Zazulak, P. I., Rutherford, P. and David, A. R. (2003), 'The International Ancient Egyptian Mummy Tissue Bank at the Manchester Museum as a resource for the palaeoepidemiological study of schistosomiasis', *World Archaeology* 35 (2), 223–40.

Leca, A.-P. (1980), *The Cult of the Immortal. Mummies and the Ancient Egyptian Way of Death*, trans. L. Asmal (London: Souvenir Press).

Leiper, R. T. (1915), 'Report on the results of the bilharzia mission in Egypt 1915', *Journal of the Royal Army Medical Corps* 15, 1–55.

Loebl, W. Y. (1995), 'A case of Symmers' fibrosis of the liver during the Eighteenth Dynasty?', in S. Campbell and A. Green (eds.), *The Archaeology of Death in the Ancient Near East* (Oxford: Oxbow Books), 1–4.

Nunn, J. F. (1996), *Ancient Egyptian Medicine* (London: British Museum Press).

Pettit, C. and. Fildes, G. (1984), 'Organising the information: the international mummy database', in A. R. David and E. Tapp (eds.), *Evidence Embalmed: Modern Medicine and the Mummies of Ancient Egypt* (Manchester: Manchester University Press), 150–7.

Pettit, C and Fildes, G. (1986), 'The international mummy database', in A. R. David (ed.), *Science in Egyptology: Proceedings of the 'Science in Egyptology' Symposia* (Manchester: Manchester University Press), 175–82.

Rowling, J. T. (1967), 'Urology in Egypt', in D. R. Brothwell and A. T. Sandison (eds.), *Diseases in Antiquity* (Springfield, IL: Charles C. Thomas), 532–7.

Ruffer, M. A. (1910), 'Note on the presence of "Bilharzia haematobia" in Egyptian mummies of the Twentieth Dynasty (1250–1000 BC)', *British Medical Journal* 1 (2557), 16.

Rutherford, P. (1997), 'The Diagnosis of Schistosomiasis by Means of Immunocytochemistry upon Appropriately Prepared Modern and Ancient Mummified Tissue' (MSc dissertation, University of Manchester).

Rutherford, P. (2002), 'Schistosomiasis: The Dynamics of Investigating a Parasitic Disease in Ancient Egyptian Tissue' (PhD dissertation, University of Manchester).

Rutherford, P. (2008), 'The use of immunocytochemistry to diagnose disease in mummies', in R. David (ed.), *Egyptian Mummies and Modern Science* (Cambridge and New York: Cambridge University Press), 99–115.

Smith, G. E. (1906), 'Contribution to the study of mummification in Egypt', *Mémoires présentés à l'Institut égyptien* 5 (1), 1–53.

Smith, G. E. and Jones, F. W. (eds.) (1910), *The Archaeological Survey of Nubia Report for 1907–1908*, II: *Report on the Human Remains* (Cairo: National Printing Department).

Spencer, A. J. (1988), *Death in Ancient Egypt* (London: Penguin Books).

Spielmann, P. E. (1932), 'To what extent did the ancient Egyptians employ bitumen for embalming?', *Journal of Egyptian Archaeology* 18, 177–80.

Starkey, P. and Starkey, J. (eds.) (1998), *Travellers in Egypt* (London: I. B. Tauris).

Sturrock, R. F. (2001), 'The schistosomes and their intermediate hosts', in A. A. F. Mahmoud (ed.), *Schistosomiasis* (London: Imperial College Press), 7–84.

Tapp, E., Stanworth, P. and Wildsmith, K. (1984), 'The endoscope in mummy research', in A. R. David and E. Tapp (eds.), *Evidence Embalmed: Modern Medicine and the Mummies of Ancient Egypt* (Manchester: Manchester University Press), 65–77.

Van Gerven, D. P. (1981), 'Nubia's last Christians: the cemeteries of Kulub Narti', *Archaeology* 34 (3), 22–9.

Warren, K. S. (1973), *Schistosomiasis: The Evolution of a Medical Literature: Selected Abstracts and Citations 1852–1972* (Cambridge, MA: Massachusetts Institute of Technology).

Woodcock, S. (1996), 'Body colour: the misuse of mummy', *The Conservator* 20: 87–94.

Wortham, J. D. (1971), *British Egyptology 1549–1906* (Newton Abbot: David and Charles).

26

The enigma of the Red Shroud mummies

Robert D. Loynes

It is generally accepted that details of embalming and mummification practices changed over time and also conventionally accepted that in the Roman Period (*c*.30 BC–AD 395) less attention was paid to the embalming process and more to the outer appearance of the 'finished article' (Ikram and Dodson 1998: 129; David 2002: 337; Aufderheide 2003: 248).

Roman Period human mummies are numerous and found in many museums and some of these mummies are described as Portrait mummies. However, within this cohort there are at least three distinct styles of wrapping, referred to as Rhombic wrapped, Red Shroud and Stucco mummies (Corcoran and Svoboda 2010: 11). The experience of the writer is that the Rhombic wrapped mummies are the most common and the Red Shroud mummies the least common of these styles.

The opportunity to examine computed tomography (CT) scans of the Red Shroud mummies in the Manchester Museum and a mummy in the Antikenmuseum Basel und Sammlung Ludwig, Basel, resulted in it becoming apparent that there may have been differences in the approach to the details of mummification techniques used within this small group. The search for references to these mummies resulted in the information shown in Table 26.1 below indicating the known Red Shroud mummies, their current locations and their provenances in Egypt.[1]

---

1 The 'mummy' from Hildesheim is, in fact, only an empty shroud. Part of another Red Shroud and its portrait panel belonging to Isadora are in the John Paul Getty Museum in Malibu. These, along with the two mummies from Cairo (which have not been CT scanned), are not considered in the following discussions. The mummy of Artemidorus, in the British Museum (EA 21810), was CT-scanned in 1997 and reported by Filer (1998: 21–4). Neither digital nor analogue image files are available

Of the twelve 'mummies' documented in Table 26.1, nine have been sub-jected to CT scans and have image files available for contemporary analysis. Variation in the format and content of the image files influences the usefulness of each of these CT scan files. However, the majority of the files are in the Dicom format,[2] and these have been analysed using Osirix software.[3] In one case the files are incomplete and cover the individual areas of the head, the upper thorax and the pelvis. Despite this, a significant amount of information was obtained. In this respect, it should be noted that the CT scan files of the mummy in the Ny Carlsberg Glyptotek Copenhagen, were in Mimics format and had to be analysed using Mimics software.[4]

Clearly, the defining feature of these mummies is that they have a painted portrait and a shroud coloured with red pigment (Plate 10). The pigment used in the cases of mummies from Brooklyn, Copenhagen, Cambridge, Basel, Malibu and Urbana has been analysed and shown to contain red lead with a trace of tin. This has been taken to indicate the same origin of the chemical used in these particular cases – namely Rio Tinto in Spain – having been used, previously, in the cupellation of silver and subsequently exported to Egypt (Corocoran and Svoboda 2010: 104). It has, therefore, been postulated that these mummies were probably all prepared in the same embalming workshop.

The work of Corcoran and Svoboda, together with that of Wisseman (2003), Julie Dawson (personal communication, 2014) and Wrapson (2006, 2007), rep-resents the corpus of work on Red Shroud mummies to date. The focus of their work has been on individual mummies and the analysis of the shrouds them-selves. This study will explore the CT findings of the mummies and compare the embalming techniques within the group and with a randomly selected group of Roman Period mummies without Red Shrouds (see Tables 26.2 and 26.3).

The head is the first area of the body to be considered. Excerebration had been performed on all of the 'non-Red Shroud' mummies considered, except for one mummy from the Faiyum and the youngest child mummy from Hawara. In adults this was always via the ethmoidal, trans-nasal route, but in the children a variety of routes were employed including the ethmoid, sphenoid, trans-nasal/trans-orbital and trans-foraminal routes. The eyes were always left in situ. In two of the three cases from Thebes the globes were opened and

for re-examination today. However, Filer's description is useful in revealing certain aspects that will be considered in this chapter.

2   Dicom is a standard for handling, storing, printing and transmitting information in medical imaging. It includes a file format definition and a network communications protocol.

3   Osirix v 5.8.5. 64 bit from Pixmeo SARL, CH1233, Bernex, Switzerland (2013).

4   Mimics Research [64 bit] v 9.0.0.231 from Materalise UK Ltd, AMP Technology Centre, Sheffield S60 5WG, UK (2014).

packed. Treatment of the mouth varied somewhat with no obvious pattern being evident (Table 26.4).

In contrast, there were only two mummies from the Red Shroud group where excerebration was evident – a child from Hawara via a sphenoidal, transnasal route and an adult from El Hibeh via the trans-foraminal route. In only two cases from this group were the eyes removed. Resin was used to pack the mouth in one case from El Hibeh and a metal plate placed over the tongue in a child from Hawara (Table 26.5).

When treatment of the trunk is considered, it becomes apparent that in the non-Red Shroud group there is a distinct pattern, with those mummies from Thebes having approaches from both a left-flank incision and the perineum. This subgroup does, however, represent a distinct pattern of wrapping, with the limbs wrapped separately and the face wrappings painted with outlines of the facial features. These three mummies are very similar to three described by Raven and Taconis (2005: 191–203). It could be argued that these 'Free Limb mummies' should be regarded as another distinct subgroup from the Roman Period. The majority of the Hawara group were not eviscerated, and only one demonstrates a perineal evisceration. Those from an unknown origin had left-flank incisions, with one of this number exhibiting an additional perineal route. It is possible, therefore, that they represent further examples from Thebes (Table 26.6).

In the Red Shroud group there was no evidence of evisceration in the majority of the mummies. However, an incomplete evisceration had been carried out in two of the three mummies from El Hibeh. In one of these cases the viscera were returned to the body as canopic packages, this technique being accompanied by the use of a granular packing material within the abdomen (Table 26.7).

Another aspect of Roman Period mummification that is frequently detected is the deformity and compression of the rib cage (Loynes 2014: 542–8; Figure 26.1). In the non-Red Shroud group (see Table 26.8), chest compression accompanied by either costo-vertebral dislocation or fracture of ribs is evident in three of six children and five of six adults that were assessed.

In the Red Shroud group (Table 26.9) only one child was assessed and it demonstrated compression of the chest. In the adults this was present in six out of seven mummies. The outlier here is Demitris from the Brooklyn Museum. In this case there was no chest compression, but there was displacement of the right fourth and sixth ribs from their original position. Therefore, it can be seen that with regard to the technique of chest compression, there was no significant difference between the Red Shroud group and Roman Period mummies without Red Shrouds.

As the process of preparing a mummy essentially consists of two stages, namely preparation and preservation of the body followed by wrapping, consideration of the wrapping technique is appropriate. It reveals that, in the non-Red

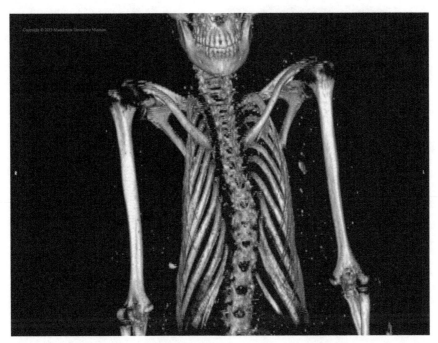

26.1 3D reconstruction showing the compressed rib cage in mummy MM 11630. (Courtesy of Manchester Museum, University of Manchester.)

Shroud group, 'stiffeners' were used in the form of pericules of palm fronds. This occurred in two cases. Both were children, one from Hawara and one from an unknown origin. In two other cases (one adult and one child) a wooden board was used (Table 26.10).

These results contrast sharply with the Red Shroud group, where a wooden board (two in one case) was placed posterior to the body in seven of the cases (Table 26.11). In two of these cases the upper end of the board (at the level of the head and shoulders) was shaped (Figure 26.2). This practice was found in mummies from Hawara, the Faiyum and El Hibeh. In all cases the body was wrapped before placement of the board and then, subsequently, further layers of wrapping were applied (Table 26.11).

One of the peculiarities of Red Shroud mummies is the inclusion of objects within the wrappings, a practice not found in other Roman Period mummies (Table 26.11). In a middle-aged mummy from the Faiyum a first cervical vertebra that had become detached from the body was included in the bandaging over the upper abdomen. The most unusual inclusion that was discovered was that of an ibis placed within the wrappings in two of the mummies from El Hibeh (Figure 26.3). In both cases a single ibis was found on the anterior abdominal wall, between the arms. In one of these mummies a further ibis

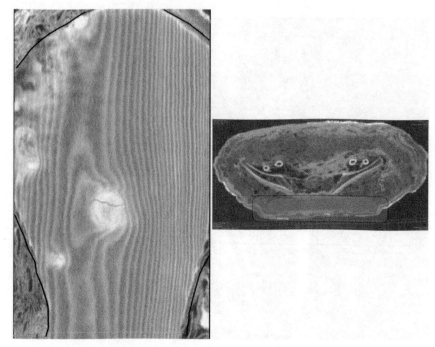

26.2 Coronal and axial views of mummy 1989.06.0001A showing the posterior board with shaped head and shoulder portion. (Courtesy of Spurlock Museum, Urbana, USA.)

was found between the thighs, and in the other mummy a coiled-up necklace had been included within the wrappings anterior to the right side of the upper thorax. The significance of the inclusion of an ibis is unknown but may relate to the god Thoth (sometimes represented as an ibis) or possibly to his role as a scribe. This may indicate that the deceased was associated with the worship of Thoth, was a scribe or otherwise associated with the cult of the sacred ibis.

The subject of skeletal trauma displayed in the Red Shroud mummies needs to be addressed as it is a feature that occurs more frequently in this group than in other groups of mummies. For example, in a collection of mummies dated from eras other than the Roman Period there were instances of fractures in two of forty-three mummies (Loynes 2014: 464). These were of the distal limbs and did not involve the skull. In the group of Roman Period mummies without Red Shrouds there were two fractures of the limbs in fourteen mummies. Again there were no fractures of the skull. In the Red Shroud mummies there were four fractures of the occiput plus one (possibly) old separation of a posterior skull suture. This was from a cohort of nine mummies as shown in Table 26.12. In one of these (Artemidorus, MM 1775 in Manchester) there were also fractures of

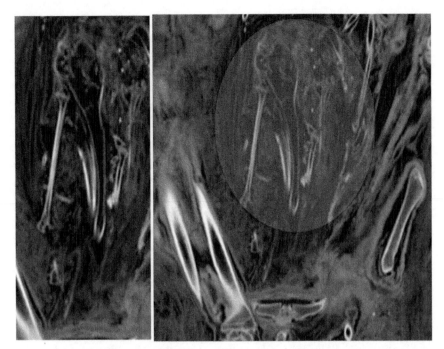

26.3 Coronal view of mummy 91.AP. 6 (Herakleides) showing an ibis within wrappings, lying between the arms. (Courtesy of the John Paul Getty Museum, Malibu, USA.)

the facial and limb bones as well as the spine and pelvis. In another case there was no fracture of the skull but fractures of the pelvis, but these may have been pre- or post-mortem.

It can be seen that this group of mummies, a subgroup of the Roman portrait mummies, have more than the red shroud that distinguishes them from others. The vast majority have one or two wooden boards running posteriorly from head to heel, enclosed in separate bandaging which has been added to the previously bandaged body and limbs.

The inclusion of an ibis within the mummy seems to be unique to this group, and in both cases this was performed in mummies found (and possibly prepared) in El Hibeh. It is also interesting to note that in both cases a further inclusion was made. In one case this was a second ibis and in the other a coiled necklace. Excerebration was performed in the majority of non-Red Shroud mummies but was performed on only two occasions in the Red Shroud group. Furthermore, the mouth was packed in many fewer cases of the Red Shroud group.

The method of evisceration was similar in the groups of mummies that originated from Hawara and the Faiyum. In the non-Red Shroud group a different approach to evisceration was taken in the mummies from Thebes (both perineal and abdominal routes being used), as it was in the Red Shroud group from El Hibeh (where a perineal route was used in two of three mummies).

The incidence of occipital fractures (new or old) in five of the Red Shroud group is suspicious of a high incidence of head injury that may have been significant in the deaths of these people. Furthermore, the occurrence of only occipital-region bony trauma to the skull is itself a distinct pattern. This trauma would, most likely, have been caused by a blow to the area just above or at the junction of the head and the neck. This could well indicate a deliberate act rather than a random occurrence, which tends to militate against clumsy post-mortem handling and points more towards a deliberate pre-mortem act. The use of an imported pigment to produce the rare Red Shroud finish to these mummies may indicate high status. This would be at odds with any concept of criminal execution, where the subsequent treatment of the bodies would have been unlikely to follow a high-status route. The actual scenario of the deaths of these individuals remains a mystery, the solution of which may be helped by the analysis of further mummies from this group, if such mummies do exist.

Having established that there are several differences between the Red Shroud group and other Roman Period mummies it is interesting to look within the group to understand whether or not there is sufficient evidence to support the concept of them all being prepared in one workshop. Certainly the fact that some mummies came from Hawara, some from the wider Faiyum and some from El Hibeh (only fifty miles south-east of the Faiyum) does not exclude the possibility of a single workshop. Although the majority underwent no form of excerebration, the use of a trans-nasal route in a child from Hawara and the use of the somewhat unusual technique of the trans-foraminal route in a young adult from El Hibeh does tend to weaken the argument. Different approaches to mouth and eye packing further add to this weakness. When considering evisceration, the different approach used in El Hibeh (the perineal route) stands out, as does the return of viscera in packages to the body and the use of some intra-corporeal packing. A final inconsistency within the group is the use, in two cases, of an inclusion – namely an ibis (or two) within the wrappings. However, care must be taken in the interpretation of these facts. One explanation may be that more than one workshop was involved. An alternative theory is that the same workshop may have varied its technique from one time in history to another, while maintaining its 'signature' feature of applying a Red Shroud at the conclusion of the process. It is also possible that although the body to be mummified was 'processed' in one workshop, different practitioners could have been involved in the various stages of mummification. These different practitioners may have been allied to the workshop or could have been 'journeymen', visiting a single workshop when requested. The small size of the group makes interpretation difficult, and drawing firm conclusions has its risks. If more Red Shroud mummies are discovered, either in Egypt or in museums outside Egypt, the increased size of the cohort will make interpretations more robust.

Tables

Abbreviations

CP	canopic packages
des.	desiccated
FM	foramen magnum
gran.	granular
L	left
MA	middle aged
per.	perineum
rem.	removed
rem. lin. pack	removed and linen pack inserted
TN/TO	trans-nasal/trans-orbital
YA	young adult

Table 26.1   Red Shroud mummies

Name	Location, accession no.	Origin
Artemidorus	Manchester Museum, MM 1775	Hawara
Unnamed	Manchester Museum, MM 1767	Faiyum
Artemidorus	British Museum, EA 21810	Hawara
Unnamed	Antikenmuseum Basel und Sammlung Ludwig, Basel, BSAe 1030	El Hibeh
Demetris	Brooklyn Museum, 11.600	Hawara
Unnamed	Egyptian Museum, Cairo, 33219	El Hibeh
Unnamed	Egyptian Museum, Cairo, 33220	El Hibeh
Unnamed	Ny Carlsberg Glyptotek, Copenhagen, AE IN 1426	Hawara
Unnamed	Fitzwilliam Museum, Cambridge, E 63.1903	El Hibeh
Herakleides	John Paul Getty Museum, Malibu, 91.AP.6	?El Hibeh
Unnamed	Roemer-und-Pelizaeus-Museum, Hildesheim, L-SN1	Unknown
Unnamed	Spurlock Museum, Urbana 1989.06.0001A	Faiyum

Sources: Corcoran and Svoboda 2010; J. Dawson, personal communication, 2004.

Table 26.2   Red Shroud mummies, arranged by provenance

Name	Location, accession no.	Origin
Unnamed	Manchester Museum, MM 1767	Faiyum
Unnamed	Spurlock Museum, Urbana 1989.06.0001A	Faiyum
Artemidorus	Manchester Museum, MM 1775	Hawara
Artemidorus	British Museum, EA 21810	Hawara
Demetris	Brooklyn Museum, 11.600	Hawara
Unnamed	Ny Carlsberg Glyptotek, Copenhagen, AE IN 1426	Hawara
Unnamed	Antikenmuseum Basel und Sammlung Ludwig, Basel, BSAe 1030	El Hibeh
Unnamed	Fitzwilliam Museum, Cambridge, E 63.1903	El Hibeh
Herakleides	John Paul Getty Museum, Malibu, 91.AP.6	El Hibeh

Table 26.3   Roman Period mummies without Red Shrouds

Location, accession no.	Origin
Birmingham Museum and Art Gallery, 1894A15	unknown
Manchester Museum, MM 1768	Faiyum
World Museum, Liverpool, 13.10.11.25	Hawara
World Museum, Liverpool, M13997a	Thebes
World Museum, Liverpool, M14048	Thebes
Naturhistorisches Museum, Altdorf, child	unknown
Manchester Museum, 11630	Hawara
Museum Burghalde, Lenzburg, K10351	unknown
Manchester Museum, MM 1766	Hawara
Manchester Museum, MM 1769	Hawara
Manchester Museum MM 9319	Hawara
Manchester Museum, MM 2109	Hawara
British Museum, EA 22108	Hawara
British Museum, EA 6704	Thebes

Table 26.4   Non-Red Shroud mummies: treatment of the head

Location, accession no.	Origin	Excerebration	Eyes	Mouth	Age
Manchester Museum, MM 1768	Faiyum	none	des.	resin	YA
Manchester Museum, MM 9319	Hawara	none	des.	none	2 yrs
Manchester Museum, MM 2109	Hawara	ethmoid	des.	none	2–3 yrs
British Museum, EA 22108	Hawara	sphenoid	des.	none	2–3 yrs

Location, accession no.	Origin	Excerebration	Eyes	Mouth	Age
World Museum, Liverpool, 13.10.11.25	Hawara	FM	des.	plate	5 yrs
Manchester Museum, MM 1769	Hawara	TN/TO	des.	linen	6 yrs
Manchester Museum, 11630	Hawara	ethmoid	des.	linen	YA
Manchester Museum, MM 1766	Hawara	ethmoid	des.	linen	YA
World Museum, Liverpool, M13997a	Thebes	ethmoid	linen	resin	YA
World Museum, Liverpool, M14048	Thebes	ethmoid	des.	none	YA
British Museum, EA 6704	Thebes	ethmoid	linen/resin	linen/resin/gran.	MA
Naturhistorisches Museum, Altdorf, child	Unknown	ethmoid	linen	none	3–4 yrs
Museum Burghalde, Lenzburg, K10351	Unknown	ethmoid	des.	resin	3–6 yrs
Birmingham Museum and Art Gallery, 1894A15	Unknown	ethmoid	des.	none	YA

Table 26.5   Red Shroud mummies: treatment of the head

Location, accession no.	Origin	Excerebration	Eyes	Mouth	Age
Manchester Museum, MM 1767	Faiyum	none	rem. lin. pack	none	MA
Spurlock Museum, Urbana, 1989.06. 0001A	Faiyum	none	des.	none	2 yrs
Manchester Museum, MM 1775	Hawara	sphenoid	des	plate	MA
British Museum, EA 21810	Hawara	?	?	?	YA
Brooklyn Museum, 11.600	Hawara	none	des.	none	MA
Ny Carlsberg Glyptotek, Copenhagen, AE IN 1426	Hawara	none	des.	none	YA
Antikenmuseum Basel und Sammlung Ludwig, Basel, BSAe 1030	El Hibeh	none	des.	none	YA
Fitzwilliam Museum, Cambridge, E 63.1903	El Hibeh	FM	rem.	none	YA
John Paul Getty Museum, Malibu, 91.AP.6	El Hibeh	none	des.	resin	YA

Table 26.6   Non-Red Shroud mummies: treatment of the trunk

Location, accession no.	Evisceration route	Evisceration complete	Returned viscera	Packing material	Origin	Age
Manchester Museum, MM 1768	disrupted	disrupted	disrupted	disrupted	Faiyum	YA
Manchester Museum, MM 9319	none	none	none	none	Hawara	2 yrs
Manchester Museum, MM 2109	none	none	none	none	Hawara	2–3 yrs
British Museum, EA 22108	none	none	none	none	Hawara	2–3 yrs
World Museum, Liverpool, 13.10.11.25	none	none	none	none	Hawara	5 yrs
Manchester Museum, MM 1769	none	none	none	none	Hawara	6 yrs
Manchester Museum, 11630	none	none	none	none	Hawara	YA
Manchester Museum, MM 1766	per.	incomplete	none	none	Hawara	YA
World Museum, Liverpool, M13997a	L. flank + per.	complete	CP	resin	Thebes	YA
World Museum, Liverpool, M14048	L. flank + per.	complete	CP	resin	Thebes	YA
British Museum, EA 6704	L. flank + per.	complete	CP	resin	Thebes	MA
Naturhistorischses Museum, Altdorf, child	L. flank + per.	complete	CP	linen	unknown	3–4 yrs
Museum Burghalde, Lenzburg, K10351	L. flank	complete	none	linen	unknown	3–6 yrs
Birmingham Museum and Art Gallery, 1894A15	L. flank	complete	loose + CP	linen	unknown	YA

Table 26.7   Red Shroud mummies: treatment of the trunk

Location, accession no.	Evisceration route	Evisceration complete	Returned viscera	Packing material	Origin	Age
Manchester Museum, MM 1767	none	none	none	none	Faiyum	MA
Spurlock Museum, Urbana, 1989.06.0001A	none	none	none	none	Faiyum	5–6 yrs

Manchester Museum, MM 1775	none	none	none	none	Hawara MA
British Museum, EA 21810	?	?	?	?	Hawara YA
Brooklyn Museum, 11.600	none	none	none	none	Hawara MA
Ny Carlsberg Glyptotek, Copenhagen, AE IN 1426	none	none	none	none	Hawara YA
Naturhistorisches Museum, Basel, BSAe 1030	per	incomplete	CP	granular	El Hibeh YA
Fitzwilliam Museum, Cambridge, E 63.1903	per.	incomplete	none	none	El Hibeh YA
John Paul Getty Museum, Malibu, 91.AP.6	none	none	none	none	El Hibeh YA

Table 26.8   Non-Red Shroud mummies: chest compression

Location, accession no.	Chest compression	Costo-vertebral joint dislocation	Rib fracture	Origin	Age
Manchester Museum, MM 1768	disrupted	disrupted	disrupted	Faiyum	YA
Manchester Museum, MM 9319	no	no	no	Hawara	2 yrs
Manchester Museum, MM 2109	yes	bilateral	no	Hawara	2–3 yrs
British Museum, EA 22108	?	?	?	Hawara	2–3 yrs
World Museum, Liverpool, 13.10.11.25	yes	no	no	Hawara	5 yrs
Manchester Museum, MM 1769	yes	bilateral	no	Hawara	6 yrs
Manchester Museum, 11630	yes	bilateral	no	Hawara	YA
Manchester Museum, MM 1766	yes	bilateral	no	Hawara	YA
World Museum, Liverpool, M13997a	yes	no	yes	Thebes	YA

World Museum, Liverpool, M14048	yes	bilateral	yes	Thebes	YA
British Museum, EA 6704	no	no	no	Thebes	MA
Naturhistorisches Museum, Altdorf, child	no	no	no	unknown	3–4 yrs
Museum Burghalde, Lenzburg, K10351	no	no	no	unknown	3–6 yrs
Birmingham Museum and Art Gallery, 1894A15	yes	bilateral	no	unknown	YA

Table 26.9 Red Shroud mummies: chest compression

Location, accession no.	Chest compression	Costo-vertebral joint dislocation	Rib fracture	Origin	Age
Manchester Museum, MM 1767	yes	bilateral	no	Faiyum	MA
Spurlock Museum, Urbana, 1989.06.0001A	yes	bilateral	no	Faiyum	5–6 yrs
Manchester Museum, MM 1775	yes	right	yes	Hawara	MA
British Museum, EA 21810	?	?	?	Hawara	YA
Brooklyn Museum, 11.600	no	no	no	Hawara	MA
Ny Carlsberg Glyptotek, Copenhagen, AE IN 1426	yes	bilateral	no	Hawara	YA
Antikenmuseum Basel und Sammlung Ludwig, Basel, BSAe 1030	yes	bilateral	bilateral	El Hibeh	YA
Fitzwilliam Museum, Cambridge, E 63.1903	yes	bilateral	no	El Hibeh	YA
John Paul Getty Museum, Malibu, 91.AP.6	yes	bilateral	yes	El Hibeh	YA

Table 26.10   Non-Red Shroud mummies: wrapping inclusions

Location, accession no.	Board	Board separate from body	Inclusion	Limbs wrapped separately	Origin	Age
Manchester Museum, MM 1768	2	yes	none	no	Faiyum	YA
Manchester Museum, MM 9319	pericules	yes	none	no	Hawara	2 yrs
Manchester Museum, MM 2109	none	none	none	no	Hawara	2–3 yrs
British Museum, EA 22108	none	none	none	no	Hawara	2–3 yrs
World Museum, Liverpool, 13.10.11.25	1	yes	none	no	Hawara	5 yrs
Manchester Museum, MM 1769	none	none	none	yes	Hawara	6 yrs
Manchester Museum, MM 11630	none	none	none	yes	Hawara	YA
Manchester Museum, MM 1766	none	none	none	no	Hawara	YA
World Museum, Liverpool, M13997a	none	none	none	yes	Thebes	YA
World Museum, Liverpool, M14048	none	none	none	yes	Thebes	YA
British Museum, EA 6704	none	none	none	yes	Thebes	MA
Naturhistorisches Museum, Altdorf, child	none	none	none	yes	unknown	3–4 yrs
Museum Burghalde, Lenzburg, K10351	pericules	no	none	no	unknown	3–6 yrs
Birmingham Museum and Art Gallery, 1894A15	none	none	none	yes	unknown	YA

Table 26.11   Red Shroud mummies: wrapping inclusions

Location, accession no.	Board	Board separate from body	Inclusion	Limbs wrapped separately	Origin	Age
Manchester Museum, MM 1767	none	none	C1 vertebra	no	Faiyum	MA

Spurlock Museum, Urbana, 1989.06.0001A	1 shaped	yes	none	no	Faiyum	5–6 yrs
Manchester Museum, MM 1775	1	yes	none	no	Hawara	MA
British Museum, EA 21810	?	?	?	?	Hawara	YA
Brooklyn Museum, 11.600	1 shaped	yes	none	no	Hawara	MA
Ny Carlsberg Glyptotek, Copenhagen, AE IN 1426	1	yes	none	no	Hawara	YA
Antikenmuseum Basel und Sammlung Ludwig, Basel, BSAe 1030	1	yes	2 ibis	no	El Hibeh	YA
Fitzwilliam Museum, Cambridge, E 63.1903	2	yes	none	no	El Hibeh	YA
John Paul Getty Museum, Malibu, 91.AP.6	1	yes	1 ibis + necklace	no	El Hibeh	YA

Table 26.12   Red Shroud mummies: incidence of trauma

Location, accession no.	Skull fracture	Other fracture	Origin	Age
Manchester Museum, MM 1767	no	no	Faiyum	MA
Spurlock Museum, Urbana, 1989.06.0001A	yes	no	Faiyum	5–6 yrs
Manchester Museum, MM 1775	yes	yes	Hawara	MA
British Museum, EA 21810	yes	no	Hawara	YA
Brooklyn Museum, 11.600	no	no	Hawara	MA
Ny Carlsberg Glyptotek, Copenhagen, AE IN 1426	yes	no	Hawara	YA
Antikenmuseum Basel und Sammlung Ludwig, Basel, BSAe 1030	no	yes	El Hibeh	YA
Fitzwilliam Museum, Cambridge, E 63.1903	no	no	El Hibeh	YA
John Paul Getty Museum, Malibu, 91.AP.6	old	no	El Hibeh	YA

Acknowledgements

Thanks are due to everyone who cooperated by supplying data in the form of Dicom files and other media. These include: Dr Campbell Price, Curator of Egypt and Sudan, Manchester Museum; Dr John H. Taylor, Assistant Keeper in the Department of Ancient Egypt and Sudan at the British Museum; funerary archaeology at the British Museum; Dr Joyce Filer, London; Professor Frank Ruhli, Director of the Institute of Evolutionary Medicine, University of Zurich; Dr Andre.Wiese, Conservateur: Égypte, Antikenmuseum Basel und Sammlung Ludwig, Basel; Dr Edward Bleiberg, Curator, Egyptian, Classical, and Ancient Near Eastern Art, Managing Curator, Ancient Egyptian, African, and Asian Art, Brooklyn Museum, New York; Professor Niels Lynnerup, Head of the Forensic Anthropology Unit at the Department of Forensic Medicine, University of Copenhagen; Dr Chiara Villa, Laboratory of Biological Anthropology, Department of Forensic Medicine, University of Copenhagen; Dr Mogens Jorgensen, Curator, Egyptian Collection, the Near East and Palmyrene Collection, Ny Carlsberg Glyptotek, Copenhagen; Dr Julie Dawson, Senior Assistant Keeper (Conservation), the Fitzwilliam Museum, Cambridge; Professor Lorelei Corcoran, Director, Institute of Egyptian Art and Archaeology, The University of Memphis; Marie Svoboda, Associate Conservator Antiquities Conservation, the John Paul Getty Museum, Malibu; Antje Spiekermann, Registrar at Roemer und Pelizaeus-Museum, Hildesheim; Jessica Followell, Assistant Registrar, Documentary Multimedia Collection, the Spurlock Museum, Urbana, Illinois; and Daniel Daryaie of Mimics for supplying free software to make possible the analysis of the images of one mummy.

References

Aufderheide, A. C. (2003), *The Scientific Study of Mummies* (Cambridge: Cambridge University Press).

Corcoran, L. H. and Svoboda, M. (2010), *Herakleides. A Portrait Mummy from Roman Egypt* (Los Angeles: Getty Publications).

David, A. R. (2002), *Religion and Magic in Ancient Egypt* (London: Penguin).

Filer, J. (1998), 'Revealing the face of Artemidorus', *Minerva* 9 (4), 21–4.

Ikram, S. and Dodson, A. (1998), *The Mummy in Ancient Egypt: Equipping the Dead for Eternity* (London: Thames and Hudson).

Loynes, R. (2014), 'Prepared for Eternity: A Study of Embalming Techniques in Ancient Egypt Using Computerized Tomography Scans of Mummies' (PhD thesis, University of Manchester).

Raven, M. J. and Taconis, W. K. (2005), *Egyptian Mummies: Radiological Atlas of the Collections in the National Museum of Antiquities in Leiden* (Turnhout: Brepols).

Wisseman, S. (2003), *The Virtual Mummy* (Illinois: University of Illinois Press).

Wrapson, L. (2006), 'The technical study and conservation of four 2nd century AD Romano-Egyptian portraits at the Fitzwilliam Museum in Cambridge, UK'. Preprints of ICOM-CC Icon and Portrait International Conference, Maryut 2006.

Wrapson, L. (2007), 'A technical study of the Red-Shroud mummy from El Hibeh, Fitzwilliam Museum, Cambridge', poster presented at the conference 'Decorated Surfaces on Ancient Egyptian Objects: Technology, Deterioration and Conservation', Cambridge, 2007.

27

The evolution of imaging ancient Egyptian animal mummies at the University of Manchester, 1972–2014

Lidija M. McKnight and Stephanie Atherton-Woolham

The Manchester Museum Mummy Project, established by Professor Rosalie David in 1972, pioneered the study of ancient Egyptian mummified remains using a multi-disciplinary approach. As Keeper of the Manchester Museum's Egyptology collection, David set out to understand the lives of the mummified individuals, whose remains became part of the collection following its establishment as the Manchester Natural History Society in 1821 (David 1979b: vii).

Since the foundation of the Manchester Museum Mummy Project, the University of Manchester has continued to study mummified remains by way of the same multi-disciplinary approach. In the first stages human mummies formed the basis of the project, with little research dedicated to the animal mummies beyond basic cataloguing. Since 2000, however, work by the authors has raised the profile of animal mummy research; in particular those dedicated as votive offerings (Ikram 2005: 9–14; McKnight and Atherton-Woolham 2015). In 2010, funding was secured through the KNH Charitable Trust to continue this early work, leading to the formation of the Ancient Egyptian Animal Bio Bank (McKnight *et al.* 2011). The award of a Research Project Grant from the Leverhulme Trust (RPG-2013-143) in September 2013 further made possible the non-invasive investigation of mummified non-human remains using clinical imaging modalities.

This chapter highlights the role of the University of Manchester in imaging mummified remains, from the humble beginnings in the 1970s to the technology in current use. It has a particular focus on how the study of animal mummies capitalised on advances in imaging science, which, in turn, enabled the potential of the techniques to be documented.

The imaging history of the Manchester Museum collection

The Manchester Museum is both Britain's largest university-owned museum and houses one of the largest Egyptology collections in the country. The museum contains twenty complete human mummies, numerous isolated mummified human body parts and forty-six animal mummies.

Seventeen human mummies, body parts and thirty animal mummies from the collection were studied using plain film radiography (XR) at the Department of Neuroradiology, Manchester Royal Infirmary, in 1972.[1] Computed tomography (CT) was conducted on two human mummies, Khary and Asru, from the collection. The results formed the basis of the catalogue of the collection (David 1979a: 13–15). Unfortunately, the original radiographs of the animal mummies from 1972 no longer survive, making comparison with more recent images impossible.

In 2001, thirty-nine animal mummies in the Manchester collection were studied using XR at the Manchester Royal Infirmary (Owen 2001);[2] fifteen were restudied between 2011 and 2012 using digital radiography (DR).[3] This technique obviated the use of radiographic film; instead the data were recorded in an electronic format to produce a digital image directly from the image receptor (Chhem and Brothwell 2008: 26). In addition, CT was employed for the first time on the animal mummy collection in 2011.[4] The radiographic investigation on the collection was completed in 2015 using the established 'Manchester Methodology'.

The Manchester Methodology

Multi-disciplinary research began at Manchester over four decades ago (David 1979a and 2008, McKnight 2010, McKnight and Atherton-Woolham 2015) and has made possible the formulation of a best-practice methodology. The methodology, which can be applied to human and animal mummies, incorporates multiple imaging modalities, including macroscopic, photographic and radiographic (presently DR and CT), the combination of which enables the maximum amount of information to be gained efficiently. In addition, archival

---

1   Elema Schonander Mimer III unit with a focal spot size of 0.3 mm, Kodak Industrex C film and high-speed controlled film processing (Isherwood, Jarvis and Fawcitt 1979: 25).
2   Philips Medical System (Best, Netherlands), focal spot of 0.6 mm, 57 kV, 1 mAs.
3   Siemens Medical System (Germany), YSIO Fluorospot Compact and Philips Eleve Digital Diagnostic, 57 kV, 1 mAs.
4   General Electric (Milwaukee, USA), LightSpeed 64-row spiral MDCT and Siemens Medical System (Germany) Somatom Definition 128-row MDCT, 0.625 mm slice thickness.

information relating to provenance and acquisition provides archaeological context, in terms of both the mummies' find-spot and their post-excavation history.

Macroscopic, photographic and archival investigation of animal mummies

Macroscopic techniques describe the condition of the mummified remains and decorative methods used in their construction. Such information is recorded photographically using a digital single-lens reflex camera (SLR);[5] and a pro-forma document, copies of which are sent to the holding institutions. This establishes a dated 'snapshot' of the condition of each mummy bundle, which is useful for conservation risk assessments, future stabilisation, storage and display. Accurate dimensions are recorded and details pertaining to provenance and acquisition are obtained from archival sources, where available.

A variety of decoration and style was noted within the Manchester Museum's animal mummy collection: elaborate herringbone, square and rhomboid lozenge designs created from linen and decorative appliqué motifs, alongside painted, modelled and false facial features and accoutrements. As in many other collections, many of the mummy bundles lacked a secure find-spot reference. However, the collection does contain artefacts from excavations carried out by the Egypt Exploration Society and by the noted Egyptologist W. M. F. Petrie on behalf of the British School of Archaeology in Egypt, alongside donations from private benefactors such as the major museum donor Jesse Haworth and interested scholars and travellers (Price 2015). This varied acquisition history demonstrates the pivotal role that Manchester played in the discovery, excavation and subsequent curation of mummified animal material.

Radiographic (DR and CT) investigation

The use of multiple imaging modalities offers the most comprehensive view of the content of wrapped mummy bundles and maximises access to radiographic facilities. Therefore, DR is conducted in dual projections (anteroposterior and lateral with oblique projections as required) as a 'triage' method to assess the presence or absence of skeletal remains. CT is routinely applied and proved useful in cases where DR revealed interesting anomalies, but was unable to clarify their nature, and in highlighting mummy bundle construction methods.

Imaging techniques have limitations when dealing with mummified tissue, and the use of dual modalities can help to eliminate the problems associated

---

5   Canon EOS 350D.

with each method in isolation. DR provides excellent spatial and contrast resolution, although it is hampered by the superimposition and magnification of
structures, whereas CT eliminates superimposition and magnification but with
reduced spatial resolution (McKnight *et al.* 2015).

A selection from the Manchester Museum collection

As the Manchester collection was previously published in its entirety
(McKnight 2010), this chapter focuses on selected examples that demonstrate the merits of the Manchester Methodology implemented in their
study during 2011. The first mummy under discussion, a mummified hawk
(AEABB54, acc. no. 4295), was described as a complete mummy bundle
measuring 360 × 160 × 50 mm (Figure 27.1). No information regarding its
find-spot or collection accession details were available. The bundle exterior
conformed to a rhomboid lozenge pattern created from linen with a modelled head, although no attempt had been made to create facial features. The
mummy was imaged using DR and CT, the former of which confirmed the
presence of multiple individuals including a partial wing and partial leg of a
Falco tinnunculus (kestrel) and a partial wing of a smaller, unidentified avian
individual. CT highlighted several points, the first of which was the use of
linen rolls placed within the core, which provided support to the incomplete
skeletal remains identified using DR. The disarticulated nature of the content
created numerous air-filled voids within the mummy bundle visible in the
sagittal plane. In addition, radio-dense areas were highlighted, particularly
to the anterior aspect, with an average attenuation value of *c.*1385 Hounsfield
Units (HU). Two further radio-dense anomalies were highlighted: *c.*1790
HU, a value similar to metal, and 1246 HU (1.4 mm in the sagittal plane by
9.5 mm in the coronal), although the exact nature of these anomalies remains
unknown. The presence of an unidentifiable package measuring 25.2 mm
(coronal plane) by 1.5 mm (sagittal plane) was visible within the bundle. The
bundle core appeared to be wrapped in a loose layer of linen, prior to the
application of the linen layers which made up the rhomboid pattern visible
on the exterior.

The second mummy, an unwrapped feline head (AEABB60, acc. no. 12015)
from Beni Hasan, measured 120 × 65 × 85 mm (Figure 27.2). The ears were
desiccated and lay flattened against the cranium, a common scenario with
unwrapped mummified felines. DR identified five articulated cervical vertebrae and a complete dentition, with the individual being tentatively identified
as *Felis silvestris libyca* (African wildcat). CT demonstrated an anomaly in the
right orbital socket, which may represent packing, most probably linen soaked
in a resinous substance. Brain matter was visible in the cranial cavity. The

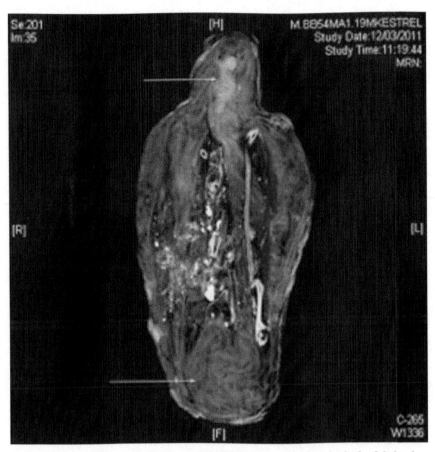

27.1 Sagittal reformat of mummy AEABB54 demonstrating the lack of skeletal integrity of the contents and the presence of air-filled voids. (Courtesy of the Ancient Egyptian Animal Bio Bank.)

oesophagus was clearly visible on the CT reformat, which demonstrated an excellent level of preservation.

Third was a mummified hawk (AEABB81, acc. no. 11293) acquired from the Robinow Collection (no. 71) in January 1959. The bundle, anthromorphic in form, has a modelled and gilded falcon head and breastplate, and measured 361 × 70 × 85 mm (Plate 11). A shroud of light linen covered the postcranial aspect of the mummy bundle. DR highlighted the complete absence of skeletal material, with reeds laid longitudinally to create the bundle length (Figure 27.3). There was evidence of a fracture through the bundle in the 'knee' region, and a false foot was added. CT demonstrated that the thickness of the wrappings varied between c.16.7 mm and 26 mm with loose layers visible at the distal end, applied in three distinct, concentric layers. The body

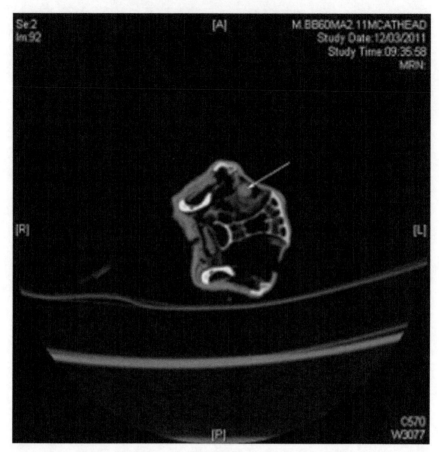

27.2 Coronal reformat of mummy AEABB60 with evidence of packing in the right orbit. (Courtesy of the Ancient Egyptian Animal Bio Bank.)

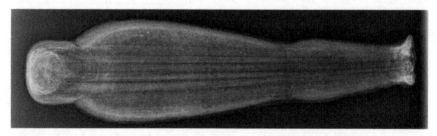

27.3 Anterior-posterior digital radiograph of mummy AEABB81 showing the apparent lack of skeletal material and evidence for the use of reeds appearing as linear structures to provide shape and rigidity to the bundle. (Courtesy of the Ancient Egyptian Animal Bio Bank.)

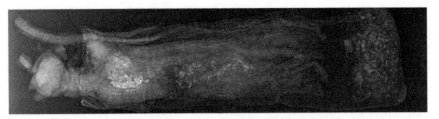

27.4 Lateral digital radiograph of mummy AEABB86 showing the bundle formed from linen with disarticulated skeletal remains. (Courtesy of the Ancient Egyptian Animal Bio Bank.)

displayed two distinct lines of small circular anomalies separated by a horizontal divider.

The final mummy was recorded as an unprovenanced, composite animal mummy (AEABB86, acc. no. EA16/2b), which measured 300 × 80 × 30 mm (Figure 27.4). It resembled a small 'sock-like' holder containing an item with individually wrapped limbs fashioned from linen and bound with thread, possibly intended to represent a feline. DR revealed a complete mummy bundle containing a mass of small, unidentifiable skeletal elements with visible growth plates that had settled at the base of the linen holder. A mass, which may represent cranial material, was visible in the mid-section of the bundle. The skeletal remains were thought to belong to a foetal or stillborn mammal, although identification beyond this was impossible. CT was unable to add further information because of the small size of the disarticulated skeletal elements.

The Manchester Museum's contribution to the study of animal mummies: current and future research

A primary aim of the Ancient Egyptian Animal Bio Bank was to make possible more thorough research through the compilation of a large data set; at the time of writing this chapter, this stood at 800 animal mummies from fifty-five museums across the UK, Europe and the USA. The use of this method was the primary causal factor in the research outcomes discussed below.

Assessment of suitable radiographic imaging techniques for animal mummies

The investigation of the Manchester Museum animal mummies employed forty years of advances in radiographic technology. It was therefore possible to document the potential of the methods, both individually and in tandem, on mummified animal material. In particular, the development of DR in a clinical setting allowed time- and cost-effective techniques to be employed in mummy studies:

a result which increased capabilities for comparable studies across museum collections. The use of CT furthered the understanding of the mummification materials and methods, although it is noted that the use of tandem radiography, DR in conjunction with CT (McKnight 2010), remains the optimum mode for study. The manipulation of digital imaging and communications in medicine (DICOM) data to produce high-resolution reformatted images and 3D printed models will allow increased accuracy of content identification in animal mummy bundles, a relatively new technique for this field which has relied, to date, on digital images alone.

However, clear limitations of clinical imaging pertain to the size of mummy bundles, in particular those which measured less than 5 cm² or were particularly flat in nature; and also those with severely fragmented content such as AEABB86 (acc. no. EA16/2b). Such examples demonstrated reduced spatial resolution, mainly because of the application of technology designed for clinical use. Initial results show that the use of micro-CT in the study of such examples will resolve this issue, alongside aiding the identification of anomalies highlighted through clinical imaging.

Re-evaluation of the assessment of true and pseudo-remains

Ongoing research and the continual implementation of the Manchester Methodology to mummified animal remains caused the stereotypical perspectives regarding their purpose to be redefined (McKnight and Atherton 2014: 109–10). Traditionally, animal mummies were defined as 'true', those containing a single complete, articulated individual, as would be expected of a mummy bundle; and 'pseudo', those containing either incomplete skeletal remains or unexpected non-skeletal materials (Moodie 1993; Owen 2001; Ikram 2005). The existence of pseudo-examples was taken as evidence of fraudulent behaviour by the embalmers (Ikram 2005: 14); in other words, incomplete remains were intended to deceptively appear as complete representations of the god in mummy form. For some animal cemetery sites, such as that at Saqqara where evidence for pilgrim activity is apparent, such practices may hold true. However, it is problematic to apply such regional evidence to animal cemeteries across Egypt. Therefore, reconsiderations were based on the following concepts: was an incomplete animal less effective as a devotional tool than a complete animal, and did purchasers have an understanding of the contents of their mummy, and thus what their purchase represented?

The study of such a large variety of animal mummies indicated that perhaps these mummies represented something less intentionally deceptive. The concept of 'fake mummies' did not exist *per se*; it was rather that those mummy bundles produced from portions of animals and associated materials, such as eggshell and reed, held sacred connotations, despite their incomplete nature (McKnight and Atherton 2014). In effect, the ratio of true to pseudo-mummies studied as part of the Ancient Egyptian Animal Bio Bank project under radiological examination was 3:1.

Public engagement

David's pioneering efforts to make Egyptology accessible to the public have left a considerable legacy. Public engagement, helping to raise awareness of this material and its study, is a crucial element of current research. The Manchester Museum's first touring exhibition in over twenty years, and the first on the scientific study of animal mummies in Britain, toured to Glasgow (May–September 2016) and Liverpool (September 2016 – February 2017), providing visitors with the opportunity to see many specimens, some of which have never been on public display. Developed around the Ancient Egyptian Animal Bio Bank research project, the exhibition aims to engage the general public with votive animal mummies and the role that British investigators, including current Manchester-based research, continue to play in the discovery, study and preservation of this material.

Acknowledgements

The authors would like to express thanks to the Manchester Museum curators and conservators who have, since 2001, actively encouraged the study of the collection; to Professor Judith Adams, clinical radiologist, and the radiographers at the Central Manchester Teaching Hospitals NHS Foundation Trust for their time, expertise and support over the years; and to the KNH Charitable Trust, the Leverhulme Trust and the Wellcome Trust for financial support. Finally, we owe a huge debt of gratitude to Professor Rosalie David for her immeasurable support of the animal project, among others, and for pioneering the multidisciplinary study of ancient Egyptian mummified remains at Manchester.

References

Chhem, R. K. and Brothwell, D. R. (2008), *Paleoradiology: Imaging Mummies and Fossils* (Berlin: Springer-Verlag).

David, A. R. (1979a), 'A catalogue of Egyptian human and animal mummified remains', in A. R. David (ed.), *The Manchester Museum Mummy Project: Multidisciplinary Research on Ancient Egyptian Mummified Remains* (Manchester: Manchester University Press), 1–17.

David, A. R. (1979b), *The Manchester Museum Mummy Project: Multidisciplinary Research on Ancient Egyptian Mummified Remains* (Manchester: Manchester University Press).

David, R. (ed.) (2008), *Egyptian Mummies and Modern Science* (Cambridge and New York: Cambridge University Press).

Ikram, S. (2005), *Divine Creatures: Animal Mummies in Ancient Egypt.* (Cairo: American University in Cairo Press).

Isherwood, I., Jarvis, H. and Fawcitt, R. A. (1979), 'Radiology of the Manchester mummies', in A. R. David (ed.), *The Manchester Museum Mummy Project: Multidisciplinary Research on Ancient Egyptian Mummified Remains* (Manchester: Manchester University Press), 25–64.

McKnight, L. M. (2010), *Imaging Applied to Animal Mummification in Ancient Egypt* (Oxford: Archaeopress).

McKnight, L. M. and Atherton, S. D. (2014), 'How to "pigeon-hole" your mummy: a proposed categorization system for ancient Egyptian animal remains based on radiographic evaluation', *Yearbook of Mummy Studies* 2 (Munich: Verlag Dr Friedrich Pfeil), 109–16.

McKnight, L. M. and Atherton-Woolham, S. D. (2015), *Gifts for the Gods: Ancient Egyptian Animal Mummies and the British* (Liverpool: Liverpool University Press).

McKnight, L. M., Atherton-Woolham, S. D. and Adams, J. E. (2015), 'Imaging of ancient Egyptian animal mummies', *Radiographics* 35, 2108-20.

McKnight, L. M., Atherton, S. D. and David, A. R. (2011), 'Introducing the Ancient Egyptian Animal Bio Bank at the KNH Centre for Biomedical Egyptology, University of Manchester', *Antiquity Project Gallery* 329, http://antiquity.ac.uk/projgall/mcknight329 (last accessed 12 August 2015).

Moodie, R. L. (1931), *Roentgenologic Studies of Egyptian and Peruvian Mummies* (Chicago: Field Museum of Natural History).

Owen, L. M. (2001), 'A Radiographic Investigation of the Ancient Egyptian Animal Mummies from the Manchester Museum' (MSc dissertation, University of Manchester).

Price, C. (2015), 'The mummies of Cottonopolis: the Manchester Museum Collection', in L. M. McKnight and S. D. Atherton-Woolham (eds.), *Gifts for the Gods: Ancient Egyptian Animal Mummies and the British* (Liverpool: Liverpool University Press), 59–63.

28

Eaten by maggots: the sorry tale of Mr Fuller's coffin

Robert G. Morkot

It is a pleasure, some forty years on, to offer this paper to Rosalie David, who was my first teacher in Egyptology, the first to enable me to have direct contact with Egyptian artefacts and the first to show me Egypt itself. Mummies excite the interest of the public, and Rosalie's renowned work on mummies has, over the years, attracted enormous interest not only in Manchester and the north-west of England but also much further afield. She has, in the best sense, been a populariser and public educator on the subject of ancient Egypt. As a teenager I benefited from the study days in Manchester which Rosalie organised shortly after she took up her post in the Manchester Museum; I was also one of the first cohort to take the University of Manchester Certificate in Egyptology, which continued with such success. It was through those classes that I learned the pleasure (and benefit) of 'adult education', which has played a significant role in my career. Rosalie encouraged me to spend the summer of 1975 as a volunteer in the Manchester Museum, where I gained first-hand experience of Egyptian objects (the foundation deposits of Queen Tawosret are etched vividly on my memory).

This chapter derives from two completely different lines of research which, as so frequently happens, ultimately became entwined. Arriving in Exeter, I was pleased to find that it been the home in later life of James Mangles, who with Charles Irby and Henry Beechey assisted Belzoni in the 'opening' of the Great Temple of Ramesses II at Abu Simbel in 1817 and was author of a stimulating travel narrative. Working on the Egyptian collection in the Royal Albert Memorial Museum (RAMM) I found that there was some Belzoni-related material, as well as a coffin and royal head of a statue with an acquisition date of 1819 which called for further research. For a long time it was usual to criticise and disparage early travellers and collectors, particularly Belzoni, as little more than pillagers: this view is now rightly challenged. I hope that this chapter demonstrates how it is possible, using such narratives, to propose contexts for early acquisitions and also shed some additional light on the important travel narratives of the period.

When the RAMM in Exeter was opened in 1868, the collections of the Devon and Exeter Institution were transferred to it. Among those were Egyptian arte-facts that had been acquired earlier in the century, including a mummy with its coffins and mummy board, and a granodiorite Egyptian royal head from a group statue of late 18th Dynasty date. The coffins had been given to the institution in 1819 and the minute books record that they had been acquired in Thebes by the Rev. Fitzherbert Fuller. The records also state that a blackened wooden shabti, said to be from the tomb of Sety I, was found among the bandages. This shabti has not been identified in the RAMM collection, and must surely have been intrusive.

The early date of acquisition makes the assemblage particularly interesting. By the time of the 'opening' of Egypt to Western Europe by the new pasha Muhammad Ali mummies had been familiar for several centuries: the use of *mumiya* in medicine has been extensively discussed, and from the seventeenth century there was an increasing interest in them from the antiquarian perspec-tive. The relatively few travellers who visited Egypt were generally confined to the Cairo region, but many of them visited and described the 'mummy pits' at Saqqara. Animal, bird and human mummies were brought back to Europe and were put on public display in the new museums of the mid-eighteenth century. The numbers of mummies, particularly human ones brought to the British Isles, increased enormously in the early nineteenth century, and by 1850 almost every significant natural history or philosophical society in Great Britain and Ireland had received a mummy by donation. By the mid-nineteenth century mummies had also entered European literature, changing into the generally malign pres-ences that continue to be a staple of Hollywood films (Luckhurst 2012).

While it is possible that Fitzherbert Fuller acquired his mummy without travelling to Egypt, it is far more likely that he did obtain it directly. As the date of presentation was 1819, Fuller's (presumed) travels in Egypt probably took place in 1817 or 1818 — years in which there were a large number of British travellers. Indeed, his presumed travels are circumscribed by events: he took his degree at Oxford in 1817, and presented the mummy in 1819, in which year he also became Perpetual Curate of the family livings of Crowhurst and Lingfield in Sussex. Given his association with Oxford and Sussex, the gift to the Devon and Exeter Institution also requires explanation. The RAMM records state that the coffin came from 'Said in Upper Egypt', Said actually being a common term at the time *for* Upper Egypt.

The name on the coffin and mummy board has generally been rendered as Iu-es-em or en-hesut-Mut, although there are a number of variant spellings (Ranke 1935–52, II: 261, 25). She was a *nbt pr* and *šm'yt n 'Imn*. The coffin is of a typical 21st Dynasty type, and an origin in one of the communal burials in the Theban necropolis therefore seems likely. Obviously, an acquisition date of around 1817 or 1818 raises the possibility that Belzoni may have been the provider.

Of other travellers in Egypt at this time, several published accounts of their journeys. One of the most celebrated is the series of letters of two naval captains, the Hon. Charles Irby and James Mangles. Their account was first published privately in 1823 and was later produced for popular consumption. It is important for a number of reasons: most notably, it contains a lengthy account of the first modern European entry into the temple of Ramesses II at Abu Simbel in Nubia. Irby and Mangles were also the first to give a brief description of the scene of towing a colossal statue in the tomb of Djehutyhetep at Bersha. They also provided the first plan and full account of the site of Petra, which they visited with William Bankes (of Kingston Lacy, Dorset) and Thomas Legh (of Lyme Park, Cheshire). The volume contains numerous additional asides which, combined with other narratives and sources, broaden our understanding of British travellers and workers in Egypt and the Near East between 1817 and 1819. The plans help us to place some museum artefacts precisely in their find-spots: notably the sphinxes and statues from Abu Simbel now in the British Museum.

Irby and Mangles (1823: 155) refer to a 'Mr. Fuller' as the travelling companion of a distinguished army officer, Colonel (later Sir) Joseph Straton. For their journey into Upper Egypt, Straton and Fuller joined with another officer, Captain Bennett, and the group is also mentioned in the narratives of Giovanni Belzoni (1820), and of Giovanni Finati (1830), who acted as their dragoman. Unfortunately, none of these accounts gives either the first name or initial of Mr Fuller, nor do any of the associated graffiti (De Keersmaecker 2005).

Some writers (Siliotti 2001: 262–3, 331 n. 78; Usick 2002 implicitly by indexing together), perhaps following the suggestion of Louis Christophe (1967: 171, n. 5), have assumed that the Mr Fuller referred to by Irby and Mangles is to be identified with John Fuller, whose *Narrative of a Tour through Some Parts of the Turkish Empire* was published in 1829. But on opening Fuller's account it becomes immediately clear that he could not have been the companion of Straton, unless he made the same journey twice! In any case, Belzoni's claim that Straton, Fuller and Bennet avoided meeting him on their return to Thebes (detailed below) seems at variance with Belzoni's later comments on John Fuller (Dewachter 1970, 114, n. 6).

John Fuller is a somewhat elusive figure. His *Narrative* is one of the most entertaining accounts of travel in the region and betrays a facetious eye. Finati's memoir of 1830 (dictated to, and considerably supplemented by, William Bankes) states that John Fuller was a member of the Literary Fund Club (later the Royal Society of Literature). He was proposed for election to the Travellers Club by William Bankes and others in July 1823 (archive reference 0899/887) but, for some unspecified reason, not admitted as a member. He was later a member of the White Nile Association and the newly founded Royal Geographical Society.

John Fuller's travels took him from Naples through southern Italy (July 1818) and the Aegean to Smyrna, thence to Istanbul and from there to Cairo. Following the Egyptian tour he went through Palestine and Syria, eventually arriving in Athens in November 1820: he was one of the last of the British residents to leave in May 1821. It therefore seems highly unlikely that John Fuller would have travelled in Egypt in 1817, leaving at the end of the year, returned to Italy, begun the entire journey again in summer 1818 and made no reference at all to the first visit in his narrative. The Mr Fuller encountered by Irby and Mangles must be someone else, and is probably best identified with Fitzherbert Fuller.

While John Fuller's travels are well documented but his identity and life remain a little obscure, the contrary applies to the Rev. Fitzherbert Fuller, whose identity and career are well documented but whose travels do not seem to be. The Rev. Robert Fitzherbert Fuller was a member of the Fuller family of Brightling Park, Sussex (Salt 1966, 1968, 1969; Hodgkinson 2014). The family had made their fortune originally as gun-founders at Chiddingley and Heathfield, Sussex. They acquired sugar estates in Jamaica through marriage with the daughter of Fulke Rose (whose widow married Hans Sloane), and purchased the Brightling Park estate in 1705. A notable member of the family was 'Mad Jack' Fuller, MP (1757–1834), 'politician and eccentric' (Entract 2008), who was buried inside a pyramid, seated upright with a plate of mutton chops in front of him.

The Rev. Robert Fitzherbert Fuller was the youngest son of John Trayton Fuller (1743–1811) and the Hon. Anne Elliott (1754–1835). Anne Elliott was daughter of George Augustus Elliot, Lord Heathfield (1718–90), and Anne Pollexfen Drake (1726–72) (daughter of Francis Henry Drake, Fourth Baronet, and sister of Francis Drake, Fifth Baronet), whom he had married in 1748, and sister of Sir Francis Augustus Elliot, Second Lord Heathfield.

Fuller's father was the son of a younger son of the Brightling Park family, but a failure of male heirs in both his father's and his mother's families brought a sharp rise in the family's social position. The principal Fuller estates eventually passed to Robert Fitzherbert's eldest brother, General Sir Augustus Elliot Fuller, MP, of Rose Hill and Ashdown (1777–1857). Another brother, Thomas Trayton Fuller, was heir to his maternal uncle the Second Lord Heathfield, who was himself heir to the Drakes of Buckland Abbey. On the death of Lord Heathfield in 1813, unmarried, Thomas Trayton Fuller acquired the recently rebuilt Nutwell Court at Lympstone between Exeter and Exmouth: he was later to be created a baronet as Sir Thomas Trayton Fuller Elliot Drake. It must be this latter connection that brought Iusenhesumut to Exeter.

A number of earlier Fullers had attended Cambridge University, most at Trinity College, although Augustus, Robert Fitzherbert's eldest brother, attended St John's. Robert Fitzherbert broke with that tradition and went to Brasenose College, Oxford (as did his son and grandson). There are no papers of Robert Fitzherbert Fuller in public archives, and the graffiti that can be associated with this journey give no initial. Is there any evidence that confirms that Robert Fuller was Colonel Straton's travelling companion?

On Wednesday 1 September 1817, Charles Irby and James Mangles returned to Cairo from their journey and the 'opening' of the Great Temple of Ramesses II at Abu Simbel:

> On our arrival we found, at Mr Salt's house, Colonel Stratton (*sic*) of the Enniskillen dragoons, and Mr Fuller: these two travellers had come from making the tour of Palestine, having lastly arrived by land from Yaffa and Gaza. They embarked at Constantinople, having first made the tour of Greece. As they had not yet been to the pyramids, we were glad to have an opportunity of accompanying them. (Irby and Mangles 1823: 155)

They then noted that:

> Egypt begins to fill with English travellers: a few days ago Captain Bennett (dragoons) and Mr Jolliffe arrived from making the tour of Palestine. The former is gone up as high as Assuan with Colonel Stratton and Mr Fuller; the latter is obliged to return immediately to England. (Irby and Mangles 1823: 163)

Of this group of travellers, Joseph Straton is well known — and must have been well-known in his day — as a hero of Waterloo (Bierbrier 2012: 529). The spelling is usually Straton, but occasionally Stratton. He was aged about forty, having been born in 1778, the third son of Cololnel William Muter of Annefield, Fife, and his wife Janet Straton. As Joseph Muter he entered service in 1794, in the 2nd Dragoon Guards, later transferring to the 6th Regiment Inniskilling Dragoons and serving on the staff of the Duke of Gloucester and in the Peninsula campaign (1810). At Waterloo, after the death of Colonel Sir William Ponsonby, he was in command of the 'Union Brigade' (1st, 2nd and 6th Dragoons): he was wounded in action and his horse wounded twice. On inheriting the estate of his uncle, Joseph Straton of Kirkside, near Montrose, in 1816, he changed his name to Straton.[1]

---

1 Bierbrier 2012: 529 and earlier editions follow the contemporary obituaries in saying that he changed his name following the death of his aunt, Miss Straton, but see 'Stratons of Kirkside' in Straton 1939: 67–75 and *London Gazette*, November 1816.

Irby and Mangles state that Straton and Fuller had travelled through Greece and then sailed from Constantinople to Yaffa and thence overland to Gaza and Cairo. It is quite possible that they had already met Bennett and Jolliffe in Palestine. There is no obvious connection between Straton and Fuller, and they may have met while travelling, or possibly been introduced through the military connections of the families: Fuller's uncle, Lord Heathfield, had been a lieutenant colonel in the 6th Dragoons, among other possible contacts.

The Rev. Thomas Robert Jolliffe (1780–1872: Bierbrier 2012: 281) was educated at Trinity College, Cambridge, very shortly before William Bankes and Lord Byron. His own account — *Letters from Palestine descriptive of a tour through Galilee and Judaea, with some account of the Dead Sea, and the present state of Jerusalem* — was published in 1819; the second edition (1820) had *Letters from Egypt* added to it. The volume was dedicated to his father, Thomas Samuel Jolliffe (*c*.1747–1824), who had been MP for Petersfield, but most of the letters are addressed to 'Sir G*****T E**T, Bart.' (sometimes just 'G.E—'); he can be identified as Sir Gilbert East of Hall Place, Berkshire, who was married to Jolliffe's cousin Eleanor. One of Eleanor's brothers, George Jolliffe RN, had been killed at the Battle of the Nile (1 August 1798), and Thomas's own brother, Captain Charles Jolliffe, 23rd Foot (Royal Welsh Fusiliers), was killed at Waterloo (18 June 1815).

Jolliffe mentions his travelling companion, 'Captain B.', a couple of times, but the name Bennett appears only in the other sources. No other initial or name is given and he is more difficult to identify. He is probably the James Bennett (b. *c*.1786–87) who served in the 7th Dragoon Guards, and appears to have retired to Florence, where he died on 16 October 1865 aged seventy-eight and was buried in the Protestant cemetery with his wife Hannah (d. 1874). We learn from Jolliffe's letters that Bennett wanted to follow the route of the River Jordan from the Sea of Galilee to the Dead Sea.

Straton, Bennett and Fuller travelled south, visiting the excavations of Belzoni at Thebes. They arrived at Luxor on the evening of 9 October and went with Henry Beechey to the Valley of the Kings on 10 October. With Belzoni and Beechey they entered the newly opened tomb of Ramesses I, leaving a graffito dated 11 October 1817 (Christophe 1966; De Keersmaecker 2005). Later on the 11th they went to tombs at Gourna and to 'the little temple in the valley behind Memnonium' (Deir el-Medina). Belzoni tells us that:

> Next day, the 12th, the party could not proceed on their voyage, the wind being foul. On the 13th I caused some spots of ground to be dug at Gournou, and we succeeded in opening a mummy-pit on that day, so that the party had the satisfaction of seeing a pit just opened, and receiving clear ideas of the manner in which the mummies are found, though all tombs are not alike. This was a small one, and consisted of two rooms painted all over, but not in the best style. It appeared to me that the tomb belonged to some warrior, as there

were a great number of men enrolling themselves for soldiers, and another writing their names in a book. There are also several figures, & c. In the lower apartment we saw the mummies lying here and there one on another, without any regularity. To all appearance therefore this pit had been opened by the Greeks, or some other people to plunder it.

The same day we visited another mummy-pit, which I had opened six months before. The construction is somewhat similar to what I have just described, a portico and a subterraneous cavity where the mummies are. Here the paintings are beautiful, not only for their preservation, but for the novelty of their figures. There are two harps, one with nine strings, and the other with fourteen, and several other strange representations: in particular, six dancing girls with fifes, tambourins, pipes of reeds, guitars, & c. (Siliotti 2001: 200)

Belzoni suggests here that the tomb was opened in April 1817 or thereabouts. As Lise Manniche (1988: 158–69) has already shown, this is the 'Bankes tomb' that Irby and Mangles (1823: 143–7) visited (on Monday 18 August 1817), of which Straton (1820a) later wrote an account and from which Bankes acquired the sections of paintings now at Kingston Lacy House.

The departure of the group is not mentioned in Belzoni's account, and presumably took place on the 14th or 15th. Finati's own narrative states that they arrived at Luxor with a letter from Salt directing him to accompany them into Nubia. At Aswan, Finati had to procure a new boat for the journey into Nubia, and this took some time. He tells us that Bennett laid the blame upon him, and that it was only the kindness of Straton and Fuller that smoothed over the situation and persuaded Finati to continue (Finati 1830, II: 215–16). The party travelled south of the cataract almost as far as Wadi Halfa. They stopped at Abu Simbel only a few months after the opening of the Great Temple by Belzoni and his companions, and this party was only the second to enter it.

The journey south is further documented by a graffito at Philae (RDK 915 in De Keersmaecker 2005). This is to be found inside the first pylon of the temple of Isis, and names Straton, Bennett and Fuller. The graffito, undated, could have been written on either the outward or the return journey.

The return to Thebes is mentioned in passing in Belzoni's *Narrative*. He records the arrival of the Earl of Belmore's party along with Henry Salt (Siliotti 2001: 208–9). He notes that Belmore continued south, and then says that 'The three travellers were now come back from Nubia, but they passed on without stopping'.

This is contradicted by the other sources, and Belzoni clearly wrote in the light of the subsequent events at Luxor. Finati (1830, II: 218) notes the party's return to Luxor and that 'Lord Belmore's family arrived just about the same time, and also Mr Salt'. The Belmores continued south, leaving Salt in Luxor.

Belzoni's comment on the Straton party implies some sort of disagreement that had not been indicated earlier, but the evidence is to the contrary. The question also arises of the antiquities that Straton (and probably Fuller) had acquired. These would have been collected on the return journey or dispatched separately (assuming that they came directly from Belzoni and not from Salt). Nor is it likely that guests of Salt's would have passed without paying him the courtesy of a visit. Halls notes that after Belmore and his party had continued to Nubia, Salt and Belzoni had a major disagreement, and that one of those present was Straton (the others presumably being Fuller and Bennett).

> It was about this time that Mr Belzoni discovered his groundless jealousy towards Mr Salt in the presence of several English Travellers, one of whom I have been informed was Colonel, now Major-General Sir Joseph Stratton [sic], CB, FRS, and who appears to have been one of those gentlemen to whom Mr Salt alludes in his statement as having been present on the unpleasant occasion. (Halls 1834, II: 45)

Halls then continues with Stratton's statement on Salt's generous dealing with the situation. Finati certainly met Salt at Luxor during the return journey, as he was sent by him to go and join William Bankes at Acre: Belzoni wanted his wife and their 'servant', James Curtin (Morkot 2013), to travel with him, as she planned a visit to Jerusalem. Finati (1830, II: 219) tells us that he continued to Cairo (arriving probably some time in December) with 'the Colonel and his two companions, and where I parted from them but a few days after, they pursuing their way to Alexandria, having testified their satisfaction in my services, both in a written paper which they left with me, and by a liberal reward'. Finati eventually met Bankes in Jerusalem, where he also found 'my two fellow-labourers at Abousambul, Captains Irby and Mangles, all Lord Belmore's family and suite, Mrs Belzoni and her servant, and Mr Legh, an English traveller, whom I had never seen before'. Mr Legh was Thomas Legh of Lyme Park, Cheshire, who had already travelled in Egypt and into Nubia in 1813, publishing his account, with some of the earliest descriptions of the temples of Lower Nubia, in 1816 (Bierbrier 2012: 319–20; Legh 1816).

It seems that Straton, Fuller and Bennett left Alexandria in December 1817 or January 1818. Straton sent an account of the Abu Simbel temple to Dacier (Le Corsu 1966; Christophe 1967). In it he compared the statues with the work of Phidias, Praxiteles and Canova. Two letters from Straton to Dacier, one dated 9 September 1818, along with the account and other letters of Salt, are now in the Collège de France (Le Corsu 1966), and as Louis Christophe noted, challenge the idea of the 'war of the consuls'. Straton presented the same account as a lecture to the Royal Society in Edinburgh, and it was published in *The Edinburgh Philosophical Journal* (Straton 1820b). The main points of the lecture were printed in the *Monthly Magazine or British Register* on 1 August (Straton 1820c), and a week later this article was repeated in the *Weekly Entertainer and West of England Miscellany* published in Sherborne (Straton 1820d), demonstrating the wide spread of knowledge about and interest in important discoveries in Egypt at this time. Straton was elected to the Royal Society of Edinburgh on 8 January 1821.

The *Gentleman's Magazine* for July 1819 records:

> A few weeks ago, that accomplished and gallant officer, Col. Straton, of Enniskillen dragoons, presented to the Museum of the University of Edinburgh, through Professor Playfair, an Egyptian mummy, in a very high state of preservation. It was brought from Thebes by the Colonel himself, along with several other Egyptian remains, which he has also presented to the College. This mummy, to judge from its triple inclosure, rich and varied ornaments, and situation when in Thebes, must be the body of a person of the highest rank, and which was probably consigned to the catacombs 3000 years ago. (pp. 62–3)

Straton died in 1841 at Park Street, Grosvenor Square, having risen in rank to Lieutenant General and Companion of the Order of the Bath. There is a portrait of him by William Salter in the National Portrait Gallery (NPG 3758), which was the model for the figure in Salter's group of the Waterloo banquet of 1836 now at Apsley House. The published obituaries tell us that 'He was very economical, if not penurious, in his habits of life, considering the extent of his fortune, the residue of which, amounting it is supposed, to not less than, 70,000l, he has bequeathed to the University of Edinburgh' (*Gentleman's Magazine*, May 1841, 537). He was buried at Ecclesgreig, adjacent to his estate of Kirkside.

Robert Fitzherbert Fuller took his MA in 1819, and in the same year became Perpetual Curate of Lingfield and Crowhurst, Sussex. In 1836 he was presented by his brother to the living of Chalvington. He died on 22 August 1849 at Leamington Spa, and was buried in Lingfield church. He married Maria Ursula, daughter of Sir Robert Sheffield, and had several children (one of whom succeeded him as Rector of Chalvington).

Straton's mummy (A.UC.70C), coffin (A.UC.70 +A.UC.70A) and mummy board (A.UC.70B) are now in the National Museum of Scotland (Manley and Dodson 2010: 41–6, nos. 10–11; Niwinski 1988, 138, no. 182). The coffin is a typical late 21st Dynasty yellow-varnished type YV, but the lid is recarved from a New Kingdom coffin. The vignettes show the owner as female but the name is now unreadable. Manley and Dodson observe that while the coffin lid and mummy board are both of type YV, the coffin lid does not have the red braces (which are on the mummy board) of the latest, early 22nd Dynasty phase of this type and question whether the mummy, board and coffin all belonged together originally.

The lack of names makes a direct association between the Straton and Fuller mummies difficult to confirm, although they are of the same type and date. Bosse-Griffiths (1991) dated the Exeter–Swansea coffin to the 21st Dynasty on iconographical grounds. Niwinski (1988: 170, no. 368) places it early in the yellow type of the middle 21st Dynasty. There was originally an outer coffin associated with the inner coffin and mummy board. This outer coffin may have had identical decoration to the inner one, which would be typical for the 21st Dynasty, although no description survives; nor does the coffin.

Niwinski (1988: 22) notes two other coffins of similar date and type that were acquired by Belzoni: London, British Museum (BM) EA 6700 (Niwinski 1988: 150–1), an inner case of late 21st or early 22nd Dynasty date; and Brussels, Musée du Cinquantenaire E.5288 (Niwinski 1988: 112, no. 47), an outer coffin with name and titles of Butehamun, but apparently not used with the equipment now in Turin. One might suspect that the coffin later acquired by the British Museum (BM EA 6663: Niwinski 1988: 22, 150, no. 252) from the collection of the Earl of Belmore also has a Belzoni connection. This is an inner coffin type IIIa of mid- to late 21st Dynasty date.

The owner of the Exeter coffin and mummy board, Iusenhesumut, was a chantress of Amun and *nbt pr*. These titles indicate that she was a member of the elite, although her position within that is more difficult to determine: her parentage, husband and other relatives could have been holders of significant positions, but they are not named. A number of other funerary objects can be associated with her, indicating that she was well provided for (Quirke 1993: 313). Robert Ritner (2010: 176), in publishing a section of papyrus in Brooklyn Museum (37.1801E) which probably belongs to the same woman, noted that title *smȝy 'Imn* is 'relatively common and considered to be of the lower rank'. The Brooklyn papyrus (Ritner 2010: 172, pl. V) was originally in the collection of Edwin Smith (Bierbrier 2012: 515) and has a Theban provenance (Ritner 2010: 173). This papyrus provided the only reference to the name cited by Ranke (1935–52, II: 261, item 25; Ritner 2010: 179, n. 29) with the spellings *'Iw=s-n-ḥsw.(t)-Mw.t*, *'Is-ḥ-Mwt*, although he corrected it as *iw.s-m-ḥs.t-mw.t*. The Exeter mummy board spells the name with the *ns* hieroglyph (Gardiner's sign list F 20).

Ritner links the Brooklyn Papyrus with another Book of the Dead in Houston (31.72: Ritner 2010: 167–73). This document also has a Theban provenance, having been acquired by the donor, Annette B. Finnegan, from the dealer Mohareb Todrous (Bierbrier 2012: 542). The papyrus belongs to a *nb.t pr šm'yt n.(t) 'Imn-R' ny-sw.t ntr.w ḥs.(t) 'Mw.t* Nes-khonsu daughter of Ius-en-hesut-Mut. Once her mother is specified as *šm'yt n 'Imn*. Neither papyrus adds to our knowledge of the wider family connections.

Several shabtis in museum and private collections, all of typical 21st Dynasty type, carry the same name and titles. Janes (2002: 64–5, no. 32) published one example with the name *i(w).s-n-ḥs.(t)-Mw.t* and titles *nbt pr* and *šmꜥyt n 'Imn-Rꜥ nsw nṯrw*. He notes further examples that are probably attributable to the same owner that were sold in auctions between 1988 and 1997 (Janes 2002: 65 n. 8). The shabti in the British Museum (EA 33966; Janes 2002: 65 n. 7) was donated by the Rev. Greville Chester (Bierbrier 2012, 119–20). The acquisitions by Smith and Chester suggest that the cache was only partly exploited in the early 19th century and was perhaps reopened in its later years, or continued to be a source of artefacts over a long period.

A heart scarab of 'basalt?' was in the Hessisches Landmuseum, Darmstadt (Janes 2002: 65 n. 5; von Droste zu Hülshoff and Schlick-Nolte 1984, I: 25), but destroyed during an air raid in 1944. This carries the titles *nbt pr šmꜥyt n 'Imn-Rꜥ njswt nṯrw 'I<w>.s-n-ḥswt-mwt*. The presence of the heart scarab in the Darmstadt collection, allied with the reference to a shabti of Sety I being found in the wrappings, suggests that the mummy associated with the coffins had been tampered with, perhaps before their acquisition by Fitzherbert Fuller. Unfortunately, it is no longer possible to investigate the human remains from the coffin. If there really was a shabti of Sety I, as part of Fuller's collection, this would associate the material with Belzoni, who notes that the Earl of Belmore and his party were the first to be shown the tomb after its discovery, the discovery itself taking place in the period that Straton, Fuller and Bennett were in Nubia.

So far, it has not been possible to document the coffin's journey from Thebes to Exeter. Presumably it travelled back from Egypt either with, or about the same time as, Colonel Straton and Fitzherbert Fuller. One can only assume that the wider Fuller family were less than enthusiastic about having an ancient Egyptian lady take up residence in their house, fashionable as she may have been; so she, probably accompanied by her acquisitor, must have been put in a carriage (or ship?) and sent on the long journey from Sussex to Devon. Whether she went straight to the Cathedral Close and the recently formed Devon and Exeter Institution or spent a country house weekend at Nutwell Court is also in the realms of speculation: local newspapers may yet provide an answer. They may also answer the question as to whether the late 18th Dynasty royal head accompanied Iusenhesutmut on her travels.

Far from resting quietly in the Devon and Exeter Institution in Cathedral Close, Iusenhesumut's coffins and mummy have suffered a sorry history since their donation. Already in the middle of the nineteenth century enquiries were being made of the British Museum because the outer coffin was being eaten by maggots: it appears to have been destroyed before the transfer to the new RAMM in 1868. Anthony Adams (1990: 17) records that on 29 April 1971 the mummy was 'disposed of at Exeter Crematorium on the orders of the archae-ologist': no reason is given. This is a salutary lesson on changing attitudes to human remains in museum collections, and the Exeter mummy was not alone in being 'disposed of' at that time. Two years later the 'coffin itself was in the process of being hacked to pieces': this was actually the mummy board, which was restored and remains at Exeter. In his article Adams ascribes both of these destructions to the mummy and body of 'Amenhotpiy' although it is now clear that it was Iusenhesumut who suffered the fate. The inner coffin of Iusenhesumut is now in Swansea (W1982: Bosse-Griffiths 1991), having being given to the Wellcome Collection (now the Egypt Centre) on indefinite loan in 1982 by the RAMM (Bosse-Griffiths 1991: 6). Thanks to Gwyn and Kate Griffiths and their search for specific coffin scenes, Iusenhesumut's coffin has been conserved and restored (Watkinson and Brown 1995) and is on display, a positive end to a sorry tale.

Acknowledgements

My thanks to John Allan (former Curator, RAMM, Exeter) for encouraging this work in the late 1990s and to the current Curator, Tom Cadbury, for continued access to the collections. I am grateful also to Sally-Anne Coupar (Hunterian Museum, Glasgow), Carolyn Graves-Brown (Egypt Centre, Swansea), Bill Manley (National Museum Edinburgh), Deborah Manley, Peta Rée and John H. Taylor (British Museum), who have kindly answered questions and gen-erously provided information. My thanks to Sheila Markham and the Hon. Librarian and Library Committee of the Travellers Club for access to the club's records, and to John H. Taylor and Bill Manley for information on Straton's mummy, coffin and mummy board.

References

Adams, C. V. A. (1990), 'An investigation into the mummies presented to H.R.H. the Prince of Wales in 1869', *Discussions in Egyptology* 18, 5–19.

Belzoni, G. (1820), *Narrative of the Operations and Recent Discoveries within the Pyramids, Temples, Tombs and Excavations in Egypt and Nubia* (London: John Murray).

Bierbrier, M. L., (ed.) (2012), *Who Was Who in Egyptology*, 4th revised edn (London: Egypt Exploration Society).

Bosse-Griffiths, K. (1991), 'Remarks concerning a coffin of the 21st Dynasty', *Discussions in Egyptology* 19, 5–12.

Christophe, L. A. (1966), 'Qui, le premier, entra dans le grand temple d'Abou Simbel?', *Bulletin de l'Institut d'Égypte* 47, 37–45.

Christophe, L. A. (1967), 'Le voyage nubien du Colonel Straton', *Bulletin de l'Institut français d'archéologie orientale* 65, 169–75.

De Keersmaecker, R. (2005), 'Some graffiti at Philae', *The Association for the Study of Travel in Egypt and the Near East Bulletin* 23, 19–20.

Dewachter, M. (1970), 'Nubie — Notes diverses §5: quatre visiteurs d'Amada en mars 1819: le Révérend William Jowett, J. Fuller, H. Foskett et Nathaniel Pearce', *Bulletin de l'Institut français d'archéologie orientale* 70, 114–17.

Droste zu Hülshoff, V. von and Schlick-Nolte, B. (1984), *Aegyptiaca Diversa I: Museen der Rhein-Main-Region* (Mainz: Philipp von Zabern).

Entract, J. P. J. (2008), 'John Fuller [iv]' *Oxford Dictionary of National Biography* (Oxford: Oxford University Press), online edn, May 2008, www.oxforddnb.com/view/article/39364 (last accessed 24 August 2015).

Finati, G. (1830), *Narrative of the Life and Adventures of Giovanni Finati, Translated from the Italian as Dictated by Himself and Edited by William-John Bankes*, 2 vols. (London: John Murray).

Fuller, J. (1829), *Narrative of a Tour through Some Parts of the Turkish Empire* (London: John Murray).

Halls, J. J. (1834), *The Life and Correspondence of Henry Salt, Esq., F.R.S. & c. His Brittanic Majesty's Late Consul General in Egypt*, 2 vols. (London: Richard Bentley).

Hodgkinson, J. S. (2014), 'Fuller family (*per c.* 1650–1803)', *Oxford Dictionary of National Biography* (Oxford: Oxford University Press), online edn, September 2014, www.oxforddnb.com/view/article/47494 (last accessed 24 August 2015).

Irby, C. and Mangles J. (1823), *Travels in Egypt and Nubia, Syria and Asia Minor* (London: T. White).

Janes, G. (2002), *Shabtis: A Private View. Ancient Egyptian Funerary Statuettes in European Private Collections* (Paris: Cybèle).

Le Corsu, F. (1966), 'Une description inédite d'Abou Simbel: le manuscrit du colonel Straton', *Bulletin de la société française d'Égyptologie* 45, 19–32.

Legh, T. (1816), *Narrative of a Journey in Egypt and the Country beyond the Cataracts* (London: John Murray).

Luckhurst, R. (2012), *The Mummy's Curse: The True History of a Dark Fantasy* (Oxford: Oxford University Press).

Manley, B. and Dodson, A. (2010), *Life Everlasting: National Museums Scotland Collection of Ancient Egyptian Coffins* (Edinburgh: National Museums Scotland).

Manniche, L. (1988), *Lost Tombs: A Study of Certain Eighteenth Dynasty Monuments in the Theban Necropolis* (London and New York: Kegan Paul International).

Morkot, R. G. (2013), 'The 'Irish lad' James Curtin, 'servant' to the Belzonis', *Association for the Study of Egypt and the Near East Bulletin* 56, 16–19.

Niwinski, A. (1988), *21st Dynasty Coffins from Thebes* (Mainz: Philipp von Zabern).

Quirke, S. (1993), review of A. Niwinski, *Studies on the Illustrated Theban Funerary Papyri of the 11th and 10th Centuries BC*, in *Journal of Egyptian Archaeology* 79, 309–15.

Ranke, H. (1935–52), *Die ägyptischen Personennamen* (Glückstadt and Hamburg: J. J. Augustin).

Ritner, R. (2010), 'Two Third Intermediate Period Books of the Dead: P. Houston 31.72 and P. Brooklyn 37.1801E', in Z. Hawass and J. House Wegner (eds.), *Millions of Jubilees: Studies in Honor of David P. Silverman*, II (Cairo: Supreme Council of Antiquities), 167–83.

Salt, M. C. L. (1966), 'The Fullers of Brightling Park', *Sussex Archaeological Collections* 104, 63–87.

Salt, M. C. L. (1968), 'The Fullers of Brightling Park', *Sussex Archaeological Collections* 106, 73–88.

Salt, M. C. L. (1969), 'The Fullers of Brightling Park', *Sussex Archaeological Collections* 107, 14–24.

Siliotti, A. ed. (2001), *Belzoni's Travels: Narrative of the operations and recent Discoveries in Egypt and Nubia* (London: British Museum Press).

Straton, C. H. (1939), *The Stratons of Lauriston and their offshoots* (Exmouth).

Straton, J. (1820a), 'Account of the Sepulchral Caverns of Egypt', *Edinburgh Philosophical Journal* 3, 345–8.

Straton, J. (1820b), 'Account of the subterranean temple of Ipsambul', *Edinburgh Philosophical Journal* 3, 62–7.

Straton, J. (1820c), 'Account of the subterranean temple of Ipsambul, lately discovered in Egypt by Belzoni and Beechey, and described by Lieutenant-Colonel Stratton, in a paper read before the Royal Society of Edinburgh', *Monthly Magazine or British Register* (London), 1 August, 27–9.

Straton, J. (1820d), 'Account of the subterranean temple of Ipsambul', *Weekly Entertainer and West of England Miscellany* (Sherborne), 7 August 1820.

Usick, P. (2002), *Adventures in Egypt and Nubia: The Travels of William John Bankes (1786–1855)* (London: British Museum Press).

Watkinson, D. and Brown, J. (1995), 'The conservation of the polychrome wooden sarcophagus of Praise Mut', in C. E. Brown, F. Macalister and M. M. Wright (eds.), *Conservation in Ancient Egyptian Collections: Papers given at the Conference organised by the United Kingdom Institute for Conservation, Archaeology Section, and International Academic Projects, Held at London, 20–21 July 1995* (London: Archetype Publications), 37–46.

PART IV

Science and experimental approaches in Egyptology

29

Scientific studies of pharaonic remains: imaging

Judith E. Adams

In ancient Egypt the practice of desiccating human and animal remains by mummification in order to preserve them for the afterlife has resulted in a large number of specimens being available for analysis thousands of years later. The study of such artefacts can provide valuable insights into the way of life, the rituals practised and the health of the population during the period of life, and has excited public fascination through the ages. During the nineteenth and early twentieth centuries 'mummy unrollings' were popular, a pursuit in which mummies were unwrapped and dissected, with little documentation of the findings. This practice resulted in the destruction and loss of this valuable resource for scientific research, and is no longer considered ethical. The application of imaging to the study of mummified remains provides a method to 'peep inside' the wrapping and cartonnage of a mummy to reveal the contents and secrets without their destruction.

Wilhelm Roentgen's discovery of X-rays in December 1895 transformed medical diagnosis, and the application of X-rays to the study of mummies followed soon after this date (Boni, Ruhli and Chhlem 2004). Four months, later in 1896, Walter Koenig radiographed a mummified child and a cat from the Senckenberg Museum in Frankfurt, Germany. In the same year Thurston Holland obtained a radiograph of a mummified bird in Liverpool, UK (Holland 1937: 61). At this time the radiographic equipment would have been mobile and could be utilised on site but was quite simple, with limited tube rating (exposure factors were limited, so it may not have been possible for the X-ray beam to penetrate through the very thick and dense material of the coffin or cartonnage) and exposure times long at three minutes or more. W. M. Flinders Petrie, Professor of Egyptology at University College London and a major figure in the early archaeological sciences, applied X-rays to the examination of mummified human remains from Deshasheh, south of Cairo, in 1898 (Petrie 1898). In 1904 the anatomist and anthropologist Sir Grafton Elliot Smith, assisted by Howard Carter, applied X-ray examination to the mummy of Tuthmosis IV in Cairo, determining the age of the king at death (Smith 1912: Adams and Alsop 2008: 21). In 1931 R. L. Moodie surveyed the Egyptian and Peruvian mummies in the Chicago Field Museum in one of the earliest comprehensive radiographic studies of such collections (Moodie 1931). In 1960 P. H. K. Gray and collaborators documented the radiographic findings of some 193 ancient Egyptian mummies housed in various museums in the UK and Europe (Gray 1973), including the British Museum, the City of Liverpool Museum and the Rijksmuseum van Oudheden in Leiden, Netherlands. Since that time imaging has been increasingly applied in the study of human, and to a lesser extent to the study of animal, mummies (Adams and Alsop 2008: 22; McKnight 2010).

Computed tomography (CT) was introduced in 1972, initially to image the human brain, and it transformed the practice of neuroradiology (Hounsfield 1973). Subsequently whole body CT scanners with larger gantries were available from 1975. CT has significantly impacted on the clinical diagnosis and management in patients and is extensively used for these purposes; it is now the imaging technique most widely applied to the study of mummified remains. CT was first applied in 1979 to the study of mummies in Manchester (Isherwood, Jarvis and Fawcitt 1979) and in Canada (Harwood-Nash 1979). There has been a biomedical research programme in the study of Egyptian artefacts in the University of Manchester since the early 1970s, established and led by Professor Rosalie David and leading to the establishment in 2003 of the KNH Centre for Biomedical Egyptology in the University's Faculty of Life Sciences (David 1979; David 2008; McKnight, Atherton and David 2011). This programme of research has included imaging, initially in collaboration with Professor Ian Isherwood (Isherwood, Jarvis and Fawcitt 1979).

Technical aspects and developments of imaging methods

The principles of the interaction of X-rays with tissues and structures of different density (determined by atomic number and proton density) apply in both radiographs and CT in forming an image. In dense tissue such as bones, which contain calcium (which has a high atomic number of 20), and metal, most X-rays are absorbed and do not reach the medium (radiographic film, photosensitive cassettes or sensitive scintillation or electronic detectors) that records the X-ray photons passing through the item being imaged. These structures appear white in images. In areas of low-density material (air, fat) most X-ray photons pass through to reach the recording medium and will appear black. Structures of intermediate density will appear in varying shades of grey between these two extremes.

Radiographs

The early studies on mummies may have been performed with portable X-ray equipment on the sites of excavation or in museums; the image quality would have been limited. Image quality is superior if acquired on equipment based in hospital radiology departments, where such imaging is now generally performed. Images were initially captured on hard-copy silver-coated film, of which there would be only a single copy, and if under- or over-exposed the process had to be repeated. However, since the introduction of picture archiving and communication systems (PACS) in the early 2000s the image has been captured electronically to form a digital image. Initially this was done with computed radiography (CR), in which the imaging plate is housed in a cassette, as in traditional film or screen X-ray systems. More recently digital radiography (DR), in which the image is captured directly onto a sensitive flat panel detector without a cassette, has been increasingly used. DR therefore acquires the image more rapidly, utilises lower doses of ionizing radiation and has higher spatial resolution than CR. Digital images have the advantage of being able to be manipulated and viewed in multiple sites and on various devices with appropriate software,[1] but have lower spatial resolution, a measure of how well small objects can be visualised (0.25 mm in DR), than hard-copy film (0.1 mm).

Radiographs, however acquired, have the strengths of being widely available and inexpensive, but have the limitation of being 2D images of 3D objects, which result in superimposition of structures causing them to be less well seen (Figure 29.1). To overcome this to some extent, two views at right angles are generally performed, anterior posterior (AP) and lateral. Many groups who have applied imaging to the study of mummified remains have abandoned performing radiographs as they now take longer to perform than does the CT scan, which was not the case previously. However, radiographs have superior spatial resolution (0.25 mm) to CT (0.6 mm), so we continue to acquire them as we find that they provide useful information.

Computed tomography (CT)

When this technology was first introduced in 1972 a pencil beam of X-rays rotated around a patient and the emerging beam was measured by a detector. Later a fan beam of X-rays and an arc of detectors were used, and by rotating these around the patient many hundreds of transmitted radiation readings were obtained; with powerful computing these were displayed as a transverse axial slice through the body. Initially these were individual single 2D sections 5–10

---

1   e.g. Apple Dicom viewer, www.osirix-viewer.com/ (last accessed 3 January 2015).

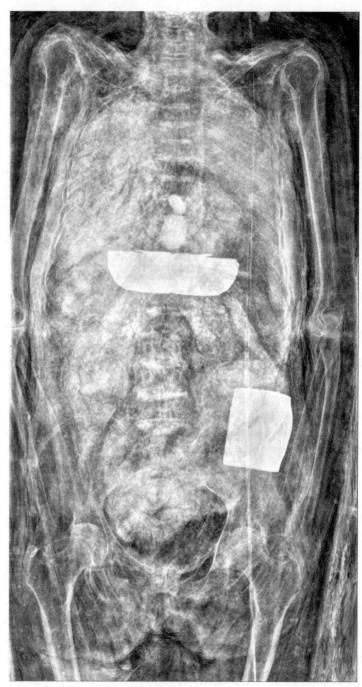

29.1 Radiograph (antero-posterior) of a mummy (no. 5053a) showing high-density amulets or artefacts. (Courtesy of Manchester Museum, University of Manchester.)

mm in thickness. Each slice is made up of individual picture elements (voxels) which are given a value depending on the X-ray attenuation of the contents (in Hounsfield Units, or HU) which makes possible the quantitative measurement of the voxel contents.

Great technological developments have occurred in CT over the past two decades which have resulted in faster scanning, thinner slice acquisition and 3D volumetric reformations. These advantages have been acquired by a rotating X-ray tube and rings of detectors (initially 4, then 16, 32, 64, 128 and a maximum of 256). This process, known as multi-detector spiral CT (MDCT), permits rapid acquisition of images; in original scanners each 2D section took twenty seconds to acquire, and now the entire torso is acquired in this time; it gives improved spatial resolution (0.6 mm generally) and the ability to manipulate the data to reconstruct images in the coronal or sagittal planes and to acquire 3D volumetric images with surface rendering depending on what structures are to be depicted. From the latter the mummy bundle can be 'unwrapped' to display its contents (Figures 29.2a–c).

More recently, dual-energy CT has been introduced. In this there are two X-ray tubes positioned at 90° to each other in the scanner gantry. These can be operated at the same energy (kV), permitting even more rapid image acquisition, or at two different energies, enhancing visualisation and quantitation of high-density structures such as calcium and bone. This results in superior quantitation (measurement of density and size) to determine the composition of structures which might aid differentiating, such as amulets made of stone, wax or metal, and improved spatial resolution (0.3 mm). Also, with sophisticated and often time-consuming manipulation of the data using special software packages, spectacular images can be obtained which enhance public perception and appreciation of the contents of mummies, for instance in the exhibition 'Ancient Lives, New Discoveries' at the British Museum (Taylor and Antoine 2014).

The strengths of CT are rapid acquisition of images, quantitation and 3D manipulation of data. The limitations of the technique involve expense, access to clinical CT scanners and the large amount of data acquired, which takes up considerable storage space in PACS. For an adult human mummy approximately 3,500 transverse axial slices are acquired, and with reformations there may be in excess of 7,000 images.

Fluoroscopy

In this method the X-ray photons transmitted reach a phosphor screen and are intensified by electronic or geometric means. The image can be recorded photographically by a 'spot' camera for static images, or on a television monitor, which allows real time imaging. This may be relevant in imaging mummies

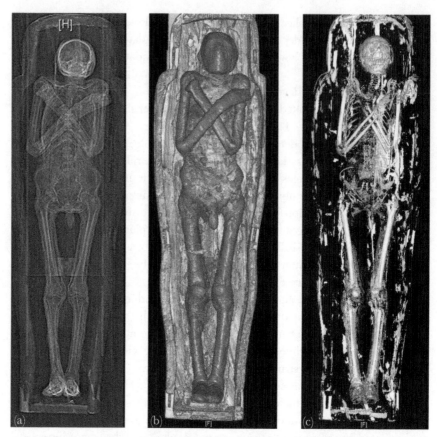

29.2 CT scans of a mummy (no. 9354) (all images courtesy of Manchester Museum, University of Manchester):
(a) antero-posterior scan projection (scout) image. (b) 3D volumetric surface rendered image to show mummy in wrappings. (c) 3D image with higher attenuation surface rendering demonstrating skeleton within the coffin and wrappings.

when endoscopy is being performed and it is important for identifying the anatomical position of the end of the endoscope, for instance when a biopsy is being taken (Notman *et al.* 1986).

Other clinical imaging techniques
Ultrasound scanning (US) and magnetic resonance imaging (MRI) are important imaging techniques that are widely used in clinical medicine. However, both depend on body water and so are not applicable to dessicated mummified tissues unless they are rehydrated, which leads to putrefaction and tissue damage; consequently these techniques are rarely performed.

Practical aspects

So that all the images of an individual mummy or specimen can be found easily in PACS and the radiographs and CT images stored in the same digital 'package' it is essential that mummies are 'booked in' to be scanned, as are patients, before the imaging session starts. Patients have to be booked in with a surname and forename. It has been found to be useful if the surname for the relevant specimen is always recorded as 'Mummy' and the first name is the museum accession number and some description of the item (e.g. MM for Manchester Museum, followed by the museum accession number, e.g. 11630, and description or name, e.g. Demetria; this would give the forename MM 11630 Demetria). A valuable asset is also a team of a few, experienced radiographers who are enthusiastic and willing to work outside normal working hours, as it is essential that such imaging of ancient artefacts never interferes with clinical imaging of patients. After the imaging session the images obtained must be sent promptly to PACS so as to avoid inadvertent loss, as there will be limited storage on the local CT scanner or radiographic equipment hard drive.

In Manchester we perform both radiographs (CR and DR) and MDCT with reformations in all the mummies and artefacts we have studied. Over the past three decades we have imaged over 100 human mummies or remains and about 250 animal mummies. For some mummies which were imaged in the 1970s we have repeated the imaging over the past decade to take advantage of the technical improvements that have occurred and the scientific advances in knowledge that they offer. There are issues of insurance and transportation of the valuable items from museums and their safe keeping and careful handling during imaging, which have to be addressed. This is ensured by having appropriate personnel present during the session who are experienced in handling the artefacts, so that radiologists and radiographers can concentrate on optimising the image quality.

All the imaging of mummies has taken place out of hours in the various radiology departments in the Central Manchester University Hospital NHS Foundation Trusts, and we ensure that the sessions never interfere with clinical imaging of patients. Initially the imaging took place in the adult department of the Manchester Royal Infirmary, where there are two CT scanners. However, with the increasing clinical demand for CT in adults, which required an extension of routine CT working hours from 8.00 a.m. to 8.00 p.m. and additional heavy emergency use outside these hours, access for imaging of mummies became problematic. Consequently such imaging has moved to the children's radiology department, where use of CT is much less than in an adult department because of the 'ALARA' (As Low As Reasonably Achievable) principle that is applied to ionising radiation exposure to patients; because CT involves significant radiation doses it is used much less frequently in children than in adults, making access more feasible.

Application of imaging to the study of human mummies

The main attribute of imaging in the study of mummies is that it provides a non-invasive method of examination. The images can provide information about mummification practices used and important aspects of the person whose mummified remains are being studied (Adams and Alsop 2008; Chhem and Brothwell 2008; Jackowski, Bollilger and Thali 2008).

State of body in cartonnage and wrappings
Imaging can give information on the disposition of the body within the cartonnage and wrappings and the condition of the mummy. If the mummy has not been kept in ideal conditions, ligaments and tendons across joints (e.g. sacroiliac joints) tend to break under shear forces and become dislocated, resulting in disruption of the skeleton.

Wrapping and amulets
The material wrappings are better demonstrated on CT than on radiographs, but the latter can indicate the site of metallic amulets within the wrappings and other decorations of high atomic number material (e.g. gold paint, glass or ornamental stones; see Figure 29.1). The positions of such decorations and artefacts can indicate re-wrapping of a mummy.

Mummification process
As most of the organs were removed before mummification, the cranium, thorax and abdomen of mummies will be largely filled with air, packages, resin, the skeletal remains and desiccated soft tissue. The latter will attenuate X-rays to a greater extent than they do in the living human. The radiographic contrast difference between this desiccated soft tissue and air will be greater than under normal clinical conditions, and it is important that the appearances are not misinterpreted as disease (e.g. ankylosing spondylitis; Chhem, Schmit and Faure 2004; Rhuli, Chhem and Boni 2004). Resin residue can be identified in the dependent parts of the body (posterior of skull vault, spinal canal, abdomen, thorax), confirming that the body was in a supine position when the mummification process was undertaken

Packages and artificial appendages
Organs such as the intestines, liver, heart, lungs and spleen were often removed before mummification and were either placed in canopic jars or replaced in

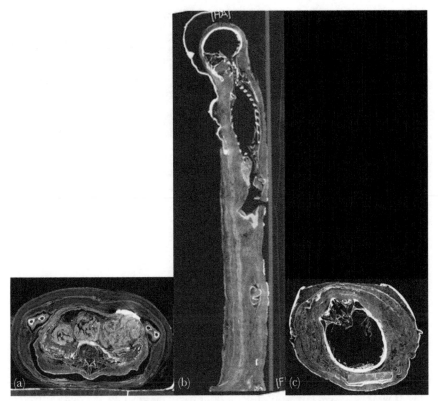

29.3 CT scans of mummification processes (all images courtesy of Manchester Museum, University of Manchester):
(a) axial section through abdomen with high density (white) metal over left anterior abdomen. (b) sagittal reformation of body showing packing in mouth and neck.
(c) axial section through head showing high density false eyes.

packages into the cavities of the body or between the limbs, which can be visualised on imaging (Figure 29.3a). As the mummified body had to closely resemble a lifelike individual, packing was used in the cheeks (infra-temporal fossa), oropharynx, neck and elsewhere in the soft tissues, which is evident on images (Figure 29.3b). The soft tissues of the eyes and other structures would shrink in size on desiccation, and false eyes were placed within the orbits (Figure 29.3c); an artificial phallus may have been fashioned and rods and other items may be evident which provided support (Figure 29.3c). Some mummies have been found to have artificial limbs; these were usually restoration limbs, added after mummification in persons who had lost a limb before death, in order to make the body whole in the afterlife, rather than prostheses for use during life (Finch 2013).

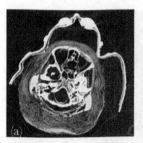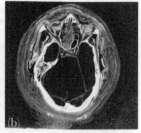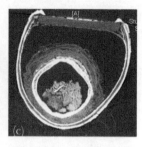

29.4 CT scans of ex-cerebration (all images courtesy of Manchester Museum,
University of Manchester):
(a) axial section through skull base showing bone destruction through left ethmoid
air cells. (b) in a different mummy there is packing in the bone defect in the right
ethmoid air cells, both proof that the brain was removed though the nose.
(c) material within the skull vault has an undulating surface of brain tissue proving
the ex-cerebration did not occur.

Organ removal

The intestinal organs were generally removed through an incision in the left
side of the abdomen, the position of which may be evident from a metal cover
(Figure 29.4), or though the perineum, which can be demonstrated to be defi-
cient on CT.

The brain was removed before mummification, via an anterior approach,
with instruments through the ethmoid air cells and cribriform plate on either
side (Figure 29.3a). The consequent bone destruction can be demonstrated
on both radiographs and CT (Figure 29.4a). The brain was also sometimes
removed through the foramen magnum, at the junction between the posterior
skull and the cervical spine, but there will be no radiological evidence of this
on imaging. Mostly the skulls of mummies are filled with air; sometimes there
is resin layered posteriorly within the skull vault, and only occasionally can
the gyri of remnants of brain be identified on imaging (Isherwood, Jarvis and
Fawcitt 1979; Figure 29.4b). From the CT scans of the head of the mummy
facial reconstruction can be carried out (Wilkinson 2010; Figure 29.5).

Imaging of forensic anthropology

Images of the skeletal remains can provide information about the age of the
mummified person (in children unerupted teeth and open growth plates;
Figure 29.6) and the gender (oval pelvic shape in females, pear shape in males),
and perhaps give insight into diet through teeth cusps eroded by sand in food,
and dental caries and related abscesses (Leek 1986), lifestyle and disease during
life and the cause of death (Ruhli, Chhem and Boni 2004).

However, there is often sparse information on the latter as life expectancy
was lower than it is in modern times and acute systemic infections would

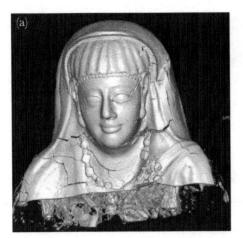 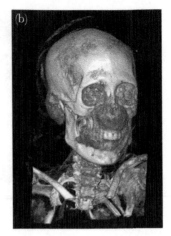

29.5 CT scans of head (all images courtesy of Manchester Museum, University of Manchester):
(a) with surface rendering for cartonnage. (b) for bone surfaces, from which data facial reconstruction can be performed.

commonly have accounted for death, events which leave no skeletal signatures. Degenerative changes in the spine and joints or skeletal diseases that are more common in the elderly (e.g. osteoporosis), if present, may suggest that the person was of more advanced age. Harris growth arrest lines (thin horizontal sclerotic lines in the ends of long bones) indicate that some episode of illness or malnutrition at that stage of skeletal development caused cessation of enchondral ossification; the provisional zone of cartilage calcified is not resorbed as is normal, and remains as an indicator of disease. Pre-mortem fractures in long bones have evidence of healing (callus formation). Osteomyelitis causes periosteal reaction, cloacae and sequestra. Septic arthritis will cause joint narrowing and juxta-articular bone destruction or later healing by bone ankylosis (Isherwood, Jarvis and Fawcitt 1979). In the elderly there may be features of osteoporosis (thinned cortices, reduced trabecular number, prominent vertical striation in the vertebrae of the spine as the horizontal trabeculae are lost preferentially, and fractures in sites of the skeleton rich in trabecular bone such as the spine) or degenerative joint disease (osteophytes, subchondral sclerosis, cyst formation, joint space narrowing). However, degenerative changes may also indicate that the person had undertaken heavy manual labour rather than having a sedentary lifestyle.

Tramline high density in soft tissues indicates calcification in arteries, which may reflect arthero-sclerosis or diabetes (Sandison 1962; Abdelfattah *et al.* 2013). Calcification in the bladder wall is most likely to indicate bilharzia infection; other infestations may cause soft tissue calcification.

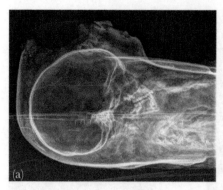 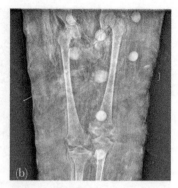

29.6 Radiographs of a child mummy (all images courtesy of Manchester Museum, University of Manchester):
(a) lateral radiograph of head showing un-erupted teeth. (b) antero-posterior radiograph of knees showing open growth plates in distal femora and proximal tibia.

Artefacts

Mummification can cause changes on images which may mimic disease processes. The cartilage in joints and intervertebral discs may appear more radiodense, through dessication, than in living humans and may be adjacent to air in mummies, resulting in greater contrast difference. Joints may appear narrowed as a consequence; the absence of associated arthritic changes, whether erosive (juxta-articular erosions) or degenerative (osteophytes, subchondral cyst and sclerosis), helps to distinguish the narrowed joint as being due to mummification rather than pre-morbid arthritis. Intervertebral discs may also be calcified. This was initially considered to be due to onchronosis (alkaptonuria), an inborn error of tyrosine metabolism, but has now been confirmed to be artefactual and due to mummification (Wells and Maxwell 1962), with the deposition of natron in the disc. The dessicated paravertebral ligaments may appear denser and more prominent because of increased contrast difference between ligaments and adjacent air in body cavities. These features must not be misinterpreted as the paravertebral ossification of ankylosing spondylitis; a normal sacro-iliac joint excludes this pathological diagnosis. Forestier's (senile) hyperostosis (diffuse idiopathic skeletal hyperostosis, or DISH) also causes paravertebral ossification, and has been misinterpreted as ankylosing spondylitis in the mummy of Ramesses II (Chhem, Schmit and Faure 2004), although there are distinct radiographic appearances that distinguish these two conditions.

Application of imaging to animal mummies

A wide variety of animal mummies have been examined (McKnight 2010), including cats, dogs, birds of prey (kestrels, sparrowhawks), other birds (ibis), insectivores, Nile crocodiles and fish or parts thereof. Imaging can non-invasively confirm whether the mummy contains an animal skeleton or does not (this is known as a pseudo-mummy; Figure 29.7) and from the skeletal characteristics can confirm the type of animal. Unlike in human mummification there is little evidence on imaging that evisceration and removal of the brain were undertaken in the mummification of animals. There is often little evidence of disease or clue as to how the animal was killed before being mummified. As with human mummies, if a pathological feature is present, such as a fracture,

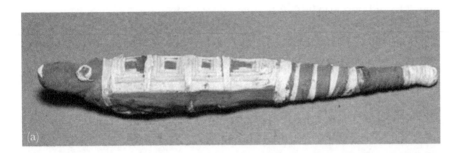

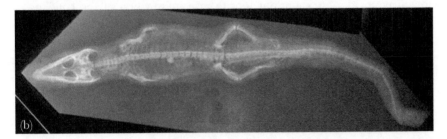

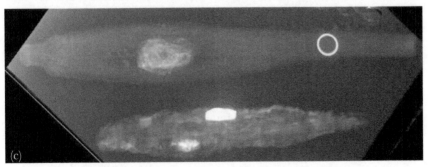

29.7 Animal mummies (courtesy of Manchester Museum, University of Manchester, images provided by Lidija M. McKnight):
(a) Nile crocodile mummy bundle. (b) crocodile skeleton confirmed on radiograph.
(c) radiographs of two animal bundles which appear externally to be crocodiles but contain no crocodile skeleton (pseudo-mummies).

it is important to define whether this is a pre-mortem feature (with evidence of callus around the fracture site; Atherton *et al.* 2012) or an artefact related to mummification or a post-mortem event. There are some challenges in imaging animal mummy bundles. They are often small in size, meaning that optimising spatial resolution is paramount. Clinical general-purpose CT scanners have limited spatial resolution as there are restrictions to acceptable maximum doses of ionising radiation to humans, and the gantry (ring) size is large so as to accommodate the human torso, so may not be ideal for imaging small animal bundles. High-resolution CT (HRpCT) has been developed to image trabecular and cortical bone structure in peripheral skeletal sites in humans, with spatial resolution of 130 μm. Micro-CT scanners are available to scan small objects *in vivo* or *in vitro* with much higher spatial resolutions of between 10 and 60 μm. These could offer advantages in the imaging of small animal mummies: exposure times in such scanners are often long, but movement is not a problem in these cases (Adams 2015).

Conclusion

Imaging provides an important tool to give information of the contents of a mummy, both human and animal, without damage to the mummy or its wrappings, and offers insight into the life and traditions of ancient civilisations from which they are drawn (Chhem and Rhuli 2004). Radiographs were widely applied in the past, but now MDCT is the one most widely utilsed, and in some studies is the only one. For all such imaging, high-quality equipment and skilled technical radiographic staff are important, as is having radiological in addition to Egyptological expertise for the interpretation of imaging features and for differentiating between pre-mortem disease, post-mortem changes and artefacts (technical changes and those due to the mummification process).

Acknowledgements

Thanks to the Clinical Directors of Radiology in the Central Manchester University Hospitals NHS Foundation Trust (CMFT) for permitting use of the imaging equipment out of hours, to radiographers who performed the imaging and to the CMFT Research Endowment for funding provided.

References

Abdelfattah, A., Allam, A. H., Wann, S., Thompson, R. C., Abdel-Maksoud, G., Badr, I., Amer, H. A. R., Nur el-Din, A. el-Halim, Finch, C. E., Miyamoto, M. I., Sutherland, L., Sutherland, J. and Thomas, G. S. (2013), 'Atherosclerotic cardiovascular disease in Egyptian women: 1570 BCE–2011 CE', *International Journal of Cardiology* 167 (2), 570–4.

Adams, J. E. (2015), 'Imaging of animal mummies', in L. M. McKnight and S. D. Atherton-Woolham (eds.), *Gifts for the Gods: Ancient Egyptian Animal Mummies and the British* (Liverpool University Press), 68–71.

Adams, J. E. and Alsop, C. W. (2008), 'Imaging in Egyptian mummies', in R. David (ed.), *Egyptian Mummies and Modern Science* (Cambridge and New York: Cambridge University Press), 21–42.

Atherton, S., Brothwell, D., David, R. and McKnight, L. (2012), 'A healed femoral fracture of *Threskiornis aethiopicus* (sacred ibis) from the Animal Cemetery at Abydos, Egypt', *International Journal of Palaeopathology* 2, 45–7.

Boni, T., Ruhli, F. J. and Chhem, R. K. (2004) 'History of paleopathology: early published literature, 1896–1921', *Journal of the Canadian Association of Radiology* 55 (4), 203–10.

Chhem, R. K., and Brothwell, D. R. (2008) *PaleoRadiology: Imaging of Mummies and Fossils* (Berlin and Heidelberg: Springer-Verlag).

Chhem, R. K., and Ruhli, F. J. (2004), 'Paleoradiology: current status and future challenges', *Journal of the Canadian Association of Radiology* 55 (4), 198–9.

Chhem, R. K., Schmit, P. and Faure, C. (2004), 'Did Ramesses II really have ankylosing spondylitis? A reappraisal', *Journal of the Canadian Association of Radiology* 55 (4), 211–17.

David, A. R. (ed.) (1979), *The Manchester Museum Mummy Project: Multidisciplinary Research on Ancient Egyptian Mummified Remains* (Manchester: Manchester University Press).

David, R. (2008), 'The background of the Manchester Mummy Project', in R. David (ed.), *Egyptian Mummies and Modern Science* (Cambridge and New York: Cambridge University Press), 3–9.

Finch, J. (2013), 'The Durham Mummy: deformity and the concept of perfection in the Ancient World', in R. David (ed.), *Ancient Medical and Healing Systems: Their Legacy to Western Medicine*, supplement to *Bulletin of the John Rylands University Library of Manchester* 89 (Manchester: Manchester University Press), 111–32.

Gray, P. H. K. (1973), 'The radiography of mummies of ancient Egyptians', *Journal of Human Evolution* 2, 51–3.

Harwood-Nash, D. C. F. (1979), 'Computed tomography of ancient Egyptian mummies', *Journal of Computer Assisted Tomography* 3, 768–73.

Holland, T. (1937), 'X-rays in 1896', *Liverpool Medico-Chirurgica Journal* 45, 61.

Hounsfield, G. N. (1973), 'Computerized transverse axial scanning (tomography), 1: Description of system', *British Journal of Radiology* 46 (552), 1016–22.

Isherwood, I., Jarvis, H., and Fawcitt, R. A. (1979), 'Radiology of the Manchester mummies', in A. R. David (ed.), *The Manchester Museum Mummy Project: Multidisciplinary Research on Ancient Egyptian Mummified Remains* (Manchester: Manchester University Press), 25–64.

Jackowski, C., Bolliger, S. and Thali, M. J. (2008), 'Common and unexpected findings in mummies from ancient Egypt and South America as revealed by CT', *Radiographics* 28 (5), 1477–92.

Leek, F. F. (1986), 'Dental health and disease in ancient Egypt with reference to the Manchester mummies', in A. R. David (ed.), *Science in Egyptology: Proceedings of the 'Science in Egyptology' Symposia* (Manchester: Manchester University Press), 35–48.

McKnight, L. M. (2010), *Imaging Applied to Animal Mummification in Ancient Egypt* (Oxford: Archaeopress).

McKnight, L. M., Atherton, S. D. and David, A.R. (2011), 'Introducing the ancient Egyptian Animal Bio Bank at the KNH Centre for Biomedical Egyptology, University of Manchester', *Antiquity* 85, 329.

Moodie, R. L. (1931), *Roentgenological Studies of Egyptian Peruvian Mummies* (Chicago: Field Museum of Natural History).

Notman, D. N. H., Tashjian, J., Aufderheide, A. C., Cass, O. W., Shane, O. C., Berquist, T. H., Gray, J. E. and Gedgaudas, E. (1986), 'Modern imaging and endoscopic techniques in Egyptian mummies', *American Journal of Roentgenology* 146, 93–6.

Petrie, W. M. F. (1898), *Deshasheh 1897* (London: Egypt Exploration Fund).

Ruhli, F. J., Chhem, R. K. and Boni, T. (2004), 'Diagnostic paleoradiology of mummified tissue: interpretation and pitfalls', *Journal of the Canadian Association of Radiology* 55 (4), 218–27.

Sandison, A. T. (1962), 'Degenerative vascular disease in the Egyptian mummy', *Medical History* 6, 77–81.

Smith, G. E. (1912), *The Royal Mummies* (Paris: Imprimerie de l'Institut Français d'Archéologie Orientale).

Taylor, J. H. and Antoine, D. (2014), *Ancient Lives, New Discoveries: Eight Mummies, Eight Stories* (London: British Museum Press).

Wells, C. and Maxwell, B. M. (1962), 'Alkaptonuria in an Egyptian mummy', *British Journal of Radiology* 35, 679–82.

Wilkinson, C. (2010), 'Facial reconstruction-anatomical art or artistic anatomy?', *Journal of Anatomy* 216 (2), 235–50.

30

Education, innovation and preservation: the lasting legacy of Sir Grafton Elliot Smith

Jenefer Cockitt

Sir Grafton Elliot Smith (1871–1937) is known to many in Egyptology and palaeopathology as an early pioneer in these fields. His work on ancient Egyptian mummification and the Archaeological Survey of Nubia (ASN) during the early twentieth century is extensively referenced and quoted. While it is recognised that his methods were not always perfect by modern standards, there are few who would deny that Elliot Smith played a pivotal role in the development of the scientific study of human remains. Despite this recognition, studies of Elliot Smith's career in archaeology and anthropology tend to focus more on his controversial views on cultural diffusionism. The two biographies produced by his colleagues after his death (Dawson 1938b; Elkin and Mackintosh 1974) provide relatively brief descriptions of his work in these areas, which is understandable given that his greatest achievements came from his main area of research, anatomy. As a consequence, a comprehensive assessment of his legacy to both palaeopathology and Egyptology is long overdue.

The man and the reputation

The work and ideas of Grafton Elliot Smith were extremely polarising both to his contemporaries and to those who succeeded him. His theory of cultural diffusionism was based on 'the view that evolutionary development had occurred only once, on the banks of the Nile, and that civilisation had subsequently diffused from this single point' (Burley 2008: 46). Although others, including W. H. R. Rivers (1911: 389), had previously raised the notion that cultural ideas and practices were transmitted through the migration of people, it was Elliot Smith who identified the origin of these ideas as Egypt. This both challenged the established theory of Darwinian socio-cultural evolution, which was considered to be heretical by some anthropologists even many years after his death (Pretty 1969: 27), and argued against the role of any other ancient culture in the development of civilisation. The theory created strong feelings in supporters and opponents alike who fiercely defended their views.

Despite growing opposition to these diffusionist theories from the 1920s onwards (Elkin 1974), there were few, if any, who questioned Elliot Smith's credentials in the subjects of ethnology and social anthropology. His tenacity and ability to carry out a phenomenal amount of research across a diverse range of subjects appear to have allowed the anatomist and physical anthropologist to expand his expertise into other areas. However, in the years since his death, Elliot Smith's reputation has suffered, probably in large part because of his diffusionist theories. It has even been suggested that he was responsible for the Piltdown hoax (Millar 1972: 236), although there is no evidence to support this. Despite this, his work on ancient Egyptian mummification remains widely quoted and his involvement in the origins of palaeopathology appears well established (Aufderheide 2003: 13; Baker and Judd 2012: 213).

There is little doubt that his reputation as an anatomist was considerable and well earned. It was due largely to this reputation, and the convenience of his having just taken the chair of anatomy in Cairo, that Elliot Smith was first asked to examine the ancient Egyptian skeletons found in the Predynastic cemetery at Naga ed Deir in 1901 (Smith 1923: 112). From this point onwards, he was invited to study a wide variety of skeletal and mummified remains, quickly becoming regarded as 'the' expert in this area. His involvement extended beyond Egypt and Nubia and into areas with similar collections of human remains, such as the mummies from Torres Strait and skeletal material from the Levant.

Elliot Smith was well known for his unorthodox approach to research; he enjoyed debate with both colleagues and students and the results of proposing new or radical theories that challenged the status quo. There is a tendency for people today to regard his work, and therefore the man himself, as rather solemn and serious, though this may not be a completely accurate picture. Many of his colleagues described him as having an excellent, if slightly mischievous, sense of humour. As well as a dedicated scientist he was also an excellent artist, producing many line drawings for his own research (Wingate Todd 1937: 523). Although his workload was often phenomenal, he took this in his stride side with his only real breaks being periods of inactivity when he 'mused' (Jones 1938: 146). These periods would often be followed by intense research or writing (Harris 1938: 181). His capacity for focused research and dedication to a subject, once his interest was piqued, has led to recent suggestions that he may have been autistic (Crook 2012: 11–12).

Egypt and the beginning of a career in anthropology

It is tempting to see Elliot Smith's move to Cairo as an event that drastically altered the path of his research career; this was, however, not the case. Elliot Smith's early neurological studies focused on the brain, specifically the part that controlled personality and social integration. His interests in the social aspects of anthropology and their relationship to anatomy were therefore already formed when he started studying ancient Egyptian remains (Wingate Todd 1937: 523). Although Elliot Smith's initial involvement with archaeologists was formed largely from a desire to support their work and to further his anatomical research (Smith 1908a: 25) this soon gave way to the exploration of his own anthropological interests – expressly, human cultural development and evolution.

Elliot Smith's work on ancient human remains can be seen as innovative from the beginning, though not necessarily because his study techniques were different from those of any other anatomist at the time. Rather, he obliged those who requested his support, took the time to study skeletal remains in detail and, unlike many contemporaries, was prepared to work in the field. He saw considerable potential in ancient human remains to help answer modern anatomical questions and provide evidence for the evolution of anatomical features (Smith 1908a: 25). As his primary research area was neuroanatomy it is not surprising that much of his research focused on the skull and the brain. He found mummified brains still in situ in the skeletal remains he first encountered at Naga ed Deir and compared these ancient examples with those of the modern population. He highlighted the research potential of mummified brains (Smith 1902) and went on to secure a large collection of them from the ASN.

A request from Gaston Maspero at the Egyptian Museum, Cairo, to study the mummy of Tuthmosis IV in 1903 led to a new line of enquiry for Elliot Smith (Smith 1903b) and the beginning of a study of considerable importance to the future of anthropology and Egyptology. Although others had unrolled and studied ancient Egyptian mummies before, there were few who had approached this as a scientific study. The use of radiology to study Tuthmosis IV was not the first time a mummy had been X-rayed (William Flinders Petrie X-rayed a mummy in 1897: Petrie 1898), but it was the first time this had been done as part of a thorough scientific investigation, providing an early echo of modern mummy studies. Much was learned by Elliot Smith about the process of mummification from his studies of the mummies of Tuthmosis IV and a number of 21st Dynasty priests that he was also permitted to study (Smith 1903a). However, his examinations were restricted largely to observations following the unwrapping of the body; this changed when later in the same year Maspero gave him permission to dissect the mummy of a priestess (Smith 1906a). The ability to use

anatomical study methods had a significant impact upon Elliot Smith's knowledge of mummification and began the studies for which he is remembered.

Although today there is considerable criticism of the dissection of mummies,
Elliot Smith did not take this decision frivolously. Dawson (1938a: 39) notes
that Elliot Smith did not want to begin his studies on the 'precious' bodies
of the pharaohs and that dissections were initially partial and private. The
numbers of dissections may have increased over time but regard was still paid
to the opinions of the curators or excavators of mummies. For example, during
the ASN only mummies that were not well preserved and/or were not suitable
for museum display were studied by Elliot Smith and his colleagues (Smith
1910: 66). By modern standards the technique of anatomical dissection is not
an acceptable study method but it was used very successfully for many years,
with other researchers following in Elliot Smith's footsteps. As an anatomist,
he made dissection the basis of both his teaching and his research. There were
few, if any, other options open to him at this time for investigating the process
of mummification; it would be many decades before computed tomography
(CT) scanning was developed. It is apparent that without his work in this area
understanding of the process of mummification in a number of different regions
would be significantly less advanced.

Elliot Smith's reputation as an anatomist can be seen clearly in the work he
did relating to ancient Egyptian mummification. He was already experienced
in the study of the dead and in working with both hard and soft tissues. His
previous research had trained him to look for anomalies in the tissues he studied, which he found in abundance in the mummies of Egypt. As was typical
for Elliot Smith, he familiarised himself with the work of those who had gone
before him (such as Pettigrew and Fonquet) and with the surviving historical
sources (Herodotus and Diodorus Siculus) and set about assessing their evidence through his own research (Smith 1906b). Although he verified many of
the details provided by the historical accounts using the bodies he studied, he
went well beyond this tentative beginning. Already predisposed towards looking for differences between mummies from different historical periods from his
studies in Egyptology and his work with George Reisner, Elliot Smith went on
to clearly identify stages in the development of artificial mummification from
the earliest periods of Egypt's history through to the Coptic Period (Smith and
Dawson 1924).

The considerable volume that Elliot Smith published about the process of
mummification shows very clearly the developments being made in the area at
that time, despite the scant evidence often available to him. His theories about
the origins of mummification were amended as time went on, with artificial
mummification initially thought to be unlikely during the Old Kingdom (Smith
1906b: 4). This theory was later amended in light of the discoveries made by

Petrie and Reisner of well-dated Old Kingdom mummies. Elliot Smith appears to have often sought patterns from very small numbers of available bodies, and in some instances evidence was provided by a single example (i.e. Smith and Dawson 1924). The later periods of Egyptian history in particular proved difficult for Elliot Smith: 'Our information from Egypt itself is so meagre, that for later periods we have to rely very largely upon the data afforded by the examination of a very large series of mummies from Nubia' (Smith and Dawson 1924: 121). Many of Elliot Smith's theories about mummification from the Ptolemaic to Coptic Periods in particular came from what was discovered during the ASN, work that was actually carried out by Wood Jones (Jones 1910). Despite all of this, Elliot Smith's conclusions for these periods are still considered accurate, despite the growing number of mummies that have been studied from these later periods.

Arguably Elliot Smith's greatest contribution to the study of mummification and the area in which he remains unsurpassed is his study of the subcutaneous packing that had been carried out mainly during the 21st Dynasty. Before Elliot Smith's work, the leading scholar in this area was Fonquet; Elliot Smith disagreed with him almost immediately (Smith 1906b: 13) and set about reanalysing the mummies studied by Fonquet and providing enhanced descriptions against which Fonquet's work could be compared. These descriptions are, anatomically, exceptionally detailed, and to date no scholar has provided anything to rival them. Later, when asked to study mummies from other cultures, Elliot Smith sought other signs of packing or moulding of the body shape. In his eyes this method was like a fingerprint identifying ancient Egyptian influence; as such mummification became one of the identifying features of his cultural diffusionism theory (Smith 1915).

Innovation in the field: the Archaeological Survey of Nubia

Elliot Smith's osteological studies began almost as soon as he reached Cairo in 1901, but his most significant work in this area was undoubtedly carried out during the ASN (1907–11). The measurements he made on skeletal remains were standard for the time, with his ideas in this area possibly being influenced by the work of Alexander Macallister while in Cambridge. It is, however, in the recording methods he used that the innovative nature of Elliot Smith becomes apparent. From the time he worked at Naga ed Deir, Elliot Smith made use of pre-printed cards for the detailed recording of a body (Smith and Jones 1910: 10). These cards, when used during the ASN, included boxes for noting a number of skeletal measurements, places to record the age, sex, location, condition of the teeth and degrees of suture closure and space for comments. His decision to develop these cards is likely to have been encouraged or at least influenced by

George Reisner, who used similar cards for recording graves and grave goods and is well known to have kept meticulous excavation records.

The skeletons found in Nubia were studied in situ during the excavations and again back in the laboratory. Measurements were made, checked, and revised as required, with as many measurements and observations as possible being made on bodies that were too fragile to retain (Smith 1910a: 8). Focus was not restricted to intact adult human skeletons as in many similar surveys at the time, and partial skeletons, children and animals were also studied. Although Elliot Smith worked alongside two colleagues – Frederick Wood Jones and Douglas Derry, both future professors of anatomy in their own right – there is no doubt that the driving force behind the work was Elliot Smith. Even when he left Cairo for Manchester and became involved in other plans Elliot Smith continued working on the ASN material which he had shipped to him (Smith 1910). He tried to maintain the same meticulous attention to detail with this work as he had when working on the small number of bodies found at Naga ed Deir, despite the fact that the Nubian survey produced more than 7,000 bodies.

Much has been made of Elliot Smith's role in the foundation of palaeopathology, which is not surprising as he was responsible for some of the earliest published work in this area. Despite this, the anatomists involved had no intention of turning their hands to pathology. Frederick Wood Jones recalls that 'the anatomist was forced to turn pathologist' during the ASN (Jones 1938: 145). Elliot Smith's own contribution was restricted largely to case studies of unusual pathologies or those identified for the first time in ancient remains (such as a case of gout and the discovery of a mummy with an old appendicitis). The main focus of his research was anatomical, involving the identification of racial origin and familial relationships. The majority of the pathological reports for the ASN were produced by Wood Jones and Derry, whose roles in the survey are often largely eclipsed by their famous colleague. Although the pathological research conducted during the ASN has drawn criticism (Waldron 2000: 387) there was a determined effort on the part of Elliot Smith to bring in expert help. A number of pathologists are recorded as having been consulted to confirm specific diagnoses, including Marc Armand Ruffer, and where diagnosis was uncertain Elliot Smith ensured that detailed anatomical descriptions of pathologies were recorded to support future studies (e.g. Derry 1909: 42). Input from experts was not restricted to bodies recently excavated, and the surviving recording cards from the ASN testify that experts such as Thomas Strangeways, an eminent pathologist, continued to be consulted once specimens were taken back to the UK.

During the course of his studies into ancient Egyptian and Nubian human remains Elliot Smith identified some of the first examples of medical treatment carried out in this region. Although providence may have provided these

examples, Elliot Smith's fascination with the development of culture and ethnology meant that he read much into them. His studies of the splints found at
Naga ed Deir in Egypt and Hesa in Nubia are an excellent example of this; he
provided detailed descriptions of each one, compared and contrasted them and
assessed their usefulness by modern standards. He took his assessment further
by comparing the splints with examples found in modern-day Egypt (Smith
1908c: 734). This is typical of the approach he took to ancient medicine: drawing comparisons with modern, traditional forms of medicine and looking for
evidence of evolving ideas. The introduction he wrote to Bryan's book on the
Ebers Papyrus (1930) could almost have been written today. It succinctly summarises the few positive examples of medical treatment found among ancient
remains and the problems in linking written evidence provided by the medical
papyri to the physical evidence.

The Archaeological Survey of Nubia collections

It was perhaps a result of his training in anatomy that Elliot Smith left his most
lasting legacy: the ASN collections. As an anatomist he was used to searching for
suitable specimens that demonstrated particular anatomical features or unique
or unusual variations. It is therefore not surprising that he recognised the potential in ancient material and in the ASN material in particular for research and
education. He was already familiar with the Royal College of Surgeons (RCS)
collections, having produced between 1899 and 1901 a descriptive and illustrated
catalogue of the mammalian and reptilian brains curated there (Dawson 1938b:
221–2). This made it a logical repository for the major portion of the osteological
and pathological material excavated from the ASN. A number of other institutions were interested in the material according to Elliot Smith (Smith 1908b),
and in all probability he enjoyed the kudos of bringing a major collection to
London. This became known as the Nubian Pathological Collection (Molleson
1993) and was by far the most important of the ASN collections, although other
significant collections were also put together at Manchester and University
College London by Elliot Smith and Derry.

Elliot Smith recognised very early on in his anthropological career that
provenance was extremely important. This led to the production of a card index
system for the Nubian Pathological Collection in which each specimen had its
own card with a description of the important features and information about
age, sex, date and location of the body. Specimens that showed similar features
were cross-referenced on each card. It is apt to use the word 'specimen': Elliot
Smith prepared his ancient specimens much as he would his modern ones. If
a feature of interest was identified (e.g. a healed appendicitis discovered in the
abdomen of young female mummy; Smith 1908a: 32, pl. XXIV) then the body

was dissected and this area of interest was kept as an anatomical specimen. In
the majority of cases, the location of the rest of the body is unknown. In the
case of fractured bones, both the left and right bones were kept to show both
the broken and unbroken examples. The Nubian Pathological Collection also
had a predominance of mummified heads and skulls, in line with Elliot Smith's
own interests. Much as he considered the different types of archaeological
information useful to anatomists and archaeologists, the interests of anatomists,
anthropologists and ethnologists were considered when putting together the
ASN collections. The majority of examples of pathology and trauma were
retained in the RCS collection, along with what were at the time termed curios
(mummified body parts including brains, hair, etc.). The Manchester collection
(Elliot Smith's personal collection while he occupied the chair of anatomy) had
an abundance of complete skeletons used for studies into racial origin.

Sadly, time has not been kind to these collections. The RCS was bombed
during the Second World War, which resulted in the destruction of a considerable proportion of the collection, including most of the index (Molleson 1993:
136). The Manchester and UCL collections (now at the Duckworth Laboratory,
University of Cambridge) have also suffered significant losses over the years,
primarily through the removal of skeletons from the specially designed boxes
that Elliot Smith had built. These had a special compartment for the head and
a longer section for the postcranial skeleton; the skull and the box were marked
with the provenance of the body but it was not thought necessary to mark
individual bones. Unfortunately, over time all of these boxes have been lost
or replaced, leaving large parts of the collection now unprovenanced. A lack
of surviving written sources related to the ASN material has made it difficult
to determine what was in these collections originally. However, careful study
of the bulletins and anatomical report for the 1907–08 season makes this possible. Elliot Smith recorded the number of bodies retained from each cemetery
and whether they had been studied in the field or not. He also noted whether
samples such as intestinal contents were retained and highlighted the finds
of pathological and anatomical interest. This was not, however, maintained
for the subsequent seasons when Elliot Smith was not present in Egypt, and
although far fewer bodies were found during the last three seasons, there is a
notable absence of information about bodies from these excavations.

Despite the loss of a significant number of the ASN human remains and
the problems in verifying the provenance of many bodies or skeletal elements,
the surviving part of the collection remains extremely important, representing
a significant study collection for palaeopathologists and osteologists today. The
material comes from an important region at the cusp of two ancient civilisations, which makes it politically significant for the study of both countries.
The nature of the excavation as a rescue project adds a further dimension, as

the area now sits below the waters of Lake Nasser. The collections contain a significant number of rare, if not unique, examples of pathology and trauma, and provide a partial demographic representation of the population of Lower Nubia from the A-Group to the Coptic period. The ASN also stands as a testament to the achievements of Elliot Smith and his colleagues Wood Jones and Derry. Few anatomists at that time would have had the dedication, patience and foresight to have assisted with excavations and studied and collected such a vast number of human and animal remains. What survives both in terms of the human remains and the written sources represents a significant and still largely untapped resource.

An educational legacy

The importance Elliot Smith attached to education and the enjoyment he found in it has been well documented by his colleagues (Stopford 1938). This was not restricted to anatomy; especially in later years Elliot Smith also taught widely on anthropology, with the links between the subjects being explored and used as a teaching tool. The Anatomical Museum at the University of Manchester was considerably enhanced by him, with archaeological material from the ASN, Egypt and possibly other areas being added to the collection. At this time Elliot Smith's teaching focus was entirely anatomical, but he still made considerable use of ancient human remains in his teaching as well as his research. His move to University College London (UCL) in 1919 prompted a change in this approach, and he began to devise ideas for a new multidisciplinary department focused on the study of 'Human Biology' (Harris 1938: 175).

The concept of human biology that Elliot Smith developed at UCL with his colleagues (particularly W. H. R. Rivers before his death in 1922) was intended to revolutionise the way anatomy was studied by combining for the first time anatomy, histology, anthropology, psychology and the arts. This new institute of anatomy was to re-establish the importance of anatomy and instigate further research into human evolution. Elliot Smith sought funding from the Rockefeller Foundation for his project; however, he ultimately lost out to Bronislaw Malinowski, a social anthropologist at the London School of Economics. Malinowski's proposal favoured a social science methodology in the study of human life and culture, which the Rockefeller Foundation felt was 'more scientific' than Elliot Smith's anatomically focused proposal (Fisher 1986: 6). In fact, the decision has also been seen as a judgement of the theories advocated by each scholar; in the end, cultural diffusionism was considered too extreme by the Rockefeller Foundation (Fisher 1986: 6), and the department Elliot Smith had envisaged was never funded.

Harris (1938: 178–9) has described the way in which Elliot Smith ran his department at UCL as 'bedlam'; the eclectic mix of research areas may have suited Elliot Smith but it was beyond the comprehension of many of his colleagues and students. Despite this, the ideas of Elliot Smith do have some parallels with modern-day bioarchaeology departments, where multidisciplinary studies are the norm and scientists, medics, anthropologists, archaeologists and historians often work together. Elliot Smith's concept for the teaching of anatomy could not be separated from his theory, however, and as a result both were rejected.

Aufderheide (2003: 13) has highlighted the fact the Elliot Smith did not record the methodology he used to study Egyptian mummies. Several options present themselves as to why he failed to do this: the descriptions may have been in notes which are now lost, he may have intended to write these up but failed to do so (there are numerous papers where this was the case; see Dawson 1938a: 43), or it may simply be that he saw no reason to do so. Elliot Smith's attention to detail was meticulous, so it is possible that if he did not write this down it was because he felt the method of anatomical dissection was well established and did not require repetition. Although he did not provide a precise methodology, Elliot Smith did provide detailed descriptions of his findings, especially in his study of a number of 21st Dynasty priests. The level of anatomical detail used to describe, particularly, the methods of subcutaneous packing used on these mummies is sufficient to guide the reader step by step through his investigations and could potentially serve to help someone else carry out the same procedures. Elliot Smith did train a number of colleagues in his study methods, notably Wood Jones (during the ASN) and Douglas Derry (whose studies included the mummy of Tutankhamun). As the invasive study of mummies has given way to non-invasive methods such as CT scanning it is unlikely that anyone would now try to replicate his work. By contrast, the detailed descriptions of osteological measurements made by Elliot Smith and colleagues during the ASN (Smith 1908a; Smith and Jones 1910), allowed others such as Batrawi (1945) to follow the same methodology.

Although there are few surviving archival sources relating to Elliot Smith's work, the number of published books and papers written by him is considerable. During his lifetime his work was actively sought and print runs often sold out, even towards the end of his career when his diffusionist theory began to lose significant ground. Many of his papers were written versions of presentations he gave, providing a lasting record of them. Although his theories of cultural diffusionism may be of little value to those studying human evolution today, the liberal 'scattering' of case studies within his publications in this area remain useful to those interested in his work on ancient remains, as they often fill in some of the gaps found in his osteological reports. More conventional value however is found in his work on mummification, and the books produced (in particular *The Royal Mummies* of 1912 and *Egyptian Mummies* of 1924, which he co-authored with Warren Dawson) still provide a basis for those studying ancient Egyptian mummies.

Conclusion

It has in the past been easy for the achievements of Sir Grafton Elliot Smith in the study of ancient human remains to become obscured by the controversy of his diffusionist theories and the renowned brilliance of his anatomical career. The extent of his impact can however been seen in the lasting legacies he left: in short an innovative approach to the study of skeletal and mummified remains, a vast and unique collection of human remains from Egypt and Nubia and the foundation of a research area that continues to educate and fascinate many today. In the decades that have passed since his death there have been many discoveries and developments in this area but the work of Sir Grafton Elliot Smith remains among the first of these achievements.

References

Aufderheide, A. C. (2003), *The Scientific Study of Mummies* (Cambridge: Cambridge University Press).

Baker, B. J. and Judd, M. A. (2012), 'Development of paleopathology in the Nile valley', in J. E. Buikstra and C. A. Roberts (eds.), *The Global History of Paleopathology* (Oxford: Oxford University Press), 209–34.

Batrawi, A. (1945), 'The racial history of Egypt and Nubia', *Journal of the Royal Anthropological Institute of Great Britain and Ireland* 75 (1–2), 81–101.

Bryan, C. P. (1930), *Ancient Egyptian Medicine: The Papyrus Ebers* (London: Ares Publishers Inc.).

Burley, A. (2008), 'A note on the publication of James Leslie Mitchell's "Grafton Elliot Smith: a student of mankind"', *Notes and Queries* 55 (1), 46–8.

Crook, P. (2012), *Grafton Elliot Smith, Egyptology and the Diffusion of Culture: A Biographical Perspective* (Eastbourne: Sussex Academic Press).

Dawson, W. (1938a), 'A general biography', in W. Dawson (ed.), *Sir Grafton Elliot Smith: A Biographical Record by his Colleagues* (London: Jonathan Cape), 17–112.

Dawson, W. (ed.) (1938b), *Sir Grafton Elliot Smith: A Biographical Record by his Colleagues* (London: Jonathan Cape).

Derry, D. E. (1909), 'Anatomical Report (B)', *The Archaeological Survey of Nubia Bulletin* 3 (Cairo: National Printing Department), 29–36.

Elkin, A. P. (1974), 'Elliot Smith and diffusion of culture', in A. P. Elkin and N. W. G. Mackintosh (eds.), *Grafton Elliot Smith: The Man and his Work* (Sydney: Sydney University Press), 8–15.

Elkin, A. P. and Mackintosh, N. W. G. (eds.) (1974), *Grafton Elliot Smith: The Man and his Work* (Sydney: Sydney University Press).

Fisher, D. (1986), 'Rockefeller philanthropy and the rise of social anthropology', *Anthropology Today* 2 (1), 5–8.

Harris, H. A. (1938), 'At University College, London', in W. Dawson (ed.), *Sir Grafton Elliot Smith: A Biographical Record by his Colleagues* (London: Jonathan Cape), 169–84.

Jones, F. W. (1910), 'Mode of burial and treatment of the body', in G. E. Smith and F. W. Jones (eds.), *The Archaeological Survey of Nubia Report for 1907–1908*. II: *Report on the Human Remains* (Cairo: National Printing Department), 181–220.

Jones, F. W. (1938), 'In Egypt and Nubia', in W. Dawson (ed.), *Sir Grafton Elliot Smith: A Biographical Record by his Colleagues* (London: Jonathan Cape), 139–50.

Millar, R. (1972), *The Piltdown Men* (London: Gollancz).

Molleson, T. (1993), 'The Nubian Pathological Collection in the Natural History Museum, London', in W. V. Davies and R. Walker (eds.), *Biological Anthropology and the Study of Ancient Egypt* (London: British Museum Press), 136–43.

Petrie, W. F. (1898), *Deshasheh 1897* (London: Egypt Exploration Fund).

Pretty, G. L. (1969), 'The Macleay Museum mummy from Torres Straits: a postscript to Elliot Smith and the diffusion controversy', *Man* 4 (1), 24–43.

Rivers, W. H. R. (1911), 'The ethnological analysis of culture', *Science* 34 (875), 385–97.

Smith, G. E. (1902), 'On the natural preservation of the brain in the ancient Egyptians', *Journal of Anatomical Physiology* 36 (4), 375–80.

Smith, G. E. (1903a), 'Report on the four mummies of the XXIst Dynasty', *Annales du Service des antiquités de l'Égypte* 4, 158–61.

Smith, G. E. (1903b), 'Report on the physical characters of the mummy of the pharaoh Thothmosis IV', *Annales du Service des antiquités de l'Égypte* 4, 112–15.

Smith, G. E. (1906a), 'An account of the mummy of a priestess of Amen, supposed to be Ta-Usert-Em-Suten-Pa', *Annales du Service des antiquités de l'Égypte* 7, 155–82.

Smith, G. E. (1906b), 'A contribution to the study of mummification', *Mémoires de l'Institut égyptien* 5, 1–53.

Smith, G. E. (1908a), 'Anatomical report (A)', *The Archaeological Survey of Nubia Bulletin* 1 (Cairo: National Printing Department), 25–36.

Smith, G. E. (1908b), Letter to Sir Arthur Keith, School of Medicine, Cairo, 26 May 1908, London, Royal College of Surgeons Archive, MS0018/1/15/16.

Smith, G. E. (1908c), 'The most ancient splints', *British Medical Journal* 1 (2465), 732–4.

Smith, G. E. (1910), Letter to Sir Arthur Keith, Victoria University of Manchester, Manchester, 30 June 1910, London, Royal College of Surgeons Archive, MS0018/1/15/16.

Smith, G. E. (1912), *The Royal Mummies* (Paris: Imprimerie de l'Institut Français d'Archéologie Orientale).

Smith, G. E. (1915), *The Migrations of Early Culture: A Study of the Geographical Distribution of Mummification* (Manchester: Manchester University Press).

Smith, G. E. (1923), *The Ancient Egyptians*, 2nd edn (London: Harper and Brothers).

Smith, G. E. and Jones, F. W. (1910) (eds.), *The Archaeological Survey of Nubia Report for 1907–1908*, II: *Report on the Human Remains* (Cairo: National Printing Department).

Smith, G. Elliot and Dawson, W. R. (1924), *Egyptian Mummies*, reprinted 1991 (London: Kegan Paul).

Stopford, J. S. (1938), 'The Manchester period', in W. Dawson (ed.), *Sir Grafton Elliot Smith: A Biographical Record by his Colleagues* (London: Jonathan Cape), 151–68.

Waldron, H. A. (2000), 'The study of the human remains from Nubia: the contribution of Grafton Elliot Smith and his colleagues to palaeopathology', *Medical History* 44 (3), 363–88.

Wingate Todd, T. (1937), 'The scientific influence of Sir Grafton Elliot Smith', *American Anthropologist* 39, 523–6.

31

Making an ancient Egyptian contraceptive: learning from experiment and experience

Rosalind Janssen

It is a great pleasure to dedicate this chapter to Professor Rosalie David as an educator who has been at the forefront of university adult education. Having single-handedly set up her innovative Certificate in Egyptology at the University of Manchester, she then ran a consistently oversubscribed course for some twenty-five years, enabling successive cohorts of locally based adult learners to study Egyptology seriously for the first time. I was privileged to be involved as the programme's external examiner for several years during the 1990s, and witnessed several completers subsequently publish their dissertations; I was particularly delighted to be asked to append the foreword to that by Peter Phillips (2002). It is a testament to her inspirational teaching that several of Rosalie's students subsequently went on to make a considerable mark on our discipline; I think particularly of the late Bob Partridge in this regard. Others are still actively involved in adult education with the editing of publications such as *Ancient Egypt* magazine, in the running of their own, now long-standing, Egyptology societies and as sought-after lecturers at conferences both at home and abroad. It is those firm foundations laid by Professor David as an educator and the resultant reputation of the University of Manchester as a provider of Egyptology for adult learners that has enabled the current Egyptology Online distance learning courses, run by Joyce Tyldesley and Glenn Godenho from the Faculty of Life Sciences, to prove equally popular to a now global audience. This is particularly significant when we have in recent years witnessed the sad demise of adult learning provision in the UK with the amalgamation or, in most cases, the complete closure of several long-established university departments of continuing education.

The aim of this chapter is to describe and discuss one recent experimental learning session of my own which involved the recreation of an ancient Egyptian contraceptive. Links to a similar prescription in the Kahun Gynaecological Papyrus mean that it stands as a further acknowledgement both of Professor David's outstanding contribution to both the study of Egyptian medicine and of her seminal inception of the Kahun Project with its in-depth analysis by experts of the pottery, metals and textile evidence from the site (David 1986). In my current role as a lecturer in education, I finally come full circle from those early days when Rosalie and I worked together on her Certificate in Egyptology to explore what recent educational theory has to tell us about the value of learning from experiment and experience.

The context

The session in question formed part of a ten-week course conducted for the University of Oxford's Department for Continuing Education (OUDCE) during the Michaelmas Term of 2013 under the title 'A day in the life of an ancient Egyptian village'. Six female learners signed up for the course, all of whom were in the retired age category. The aim was to draw on archaeological and textual information from the surviving workmen's villages at Giza, Lahun, Amarna, and Deir el-Medina to critically assess various work activities and daily life pursuits by tangibly recreating them within a classroom setting. Work activities such as farming and gardening, furniture making, stone working, writing and painting, and food and beer preparation were set alongside various leisure pursuits: personal hygiene, music and musical instruments and the world of play.

The practical craft making drew its inspiration from the University of Swansea's 'Experiment and Experience: Ancient Egypt in the Present' conference (10–12 May 2010) (Graves-Brown 2015), which was made available to a wider audience by streaming the proceedings online.[1] Participants were encouraged to include physical demonstrations to support their papers, and further reference will be made below to my own textile demonstration at this conference.

Meanwhile, the learning objectives of the OUDCE course were firstly to enable students to learn how to recreate and critically experience the reality of work activities and leisure pursuits and, secondly, to assess the similarities and differences between daily life in ancient and modern Egyptian villages. Thus, as shown in Figure 31.1, students worked in pairs attempting to recreate figured ostraca by drawing on broken flower pots from a garden shed using reed brushes sourced from a neglected ornamental grass growing in the university car park.

1 Podcasts from the conference can be found online at www.egypt.swan.ac.uk/index. php/conferences/397-technology-podcasts (last accessed 12 August 2015).

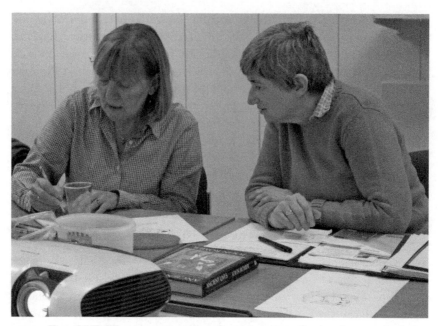

31.1 Two OUDCE students recreate a figured ostracon by drawing on a broken flower pot. (Photograph by the author.)

The pigments comprised brick dust laboriously ground down by the son of one of the students, made soluble in egg white. Plate 12 shows an attempt to replicate the fine ostracon showing a monkey scratching a girl's nose housed in the Petrie Museum of Egyptian Archaeology, University College London (UC 15946), as illustrated on the front cover of Page's book on the Petrie ostraca (1983). Even more fundamental was the in-depth discussion that took place immediately after each experiment, as evidenced by the conclusions drawn from the ostraca activity which I wrote up on the whiteboard as an aide-memoire (Figure 31.2).

The experiment

Making the contraceptive was the activity that took place during week 5 as the practical element of the personal hygiene topic. We followed the prescription from Papyrus Ebers 783:

> Beginning of the prescriptions prepared for women/wives (*hemut*) to allow a woman (*set*) to cease conceiving (*iur*) for one year, two years or three years; *qaa* part of acacia, carob (*djaret*), dates; grind with one *henu* (450 ml) of honey, lint is moistened with it and placed in her belly (*iuf*). (Translated in Nunn 1996: 196)

The week before, the six students had been instructed to liaise with their partners to source between them a pestle and mortar, a measure, dates, honey and lint as

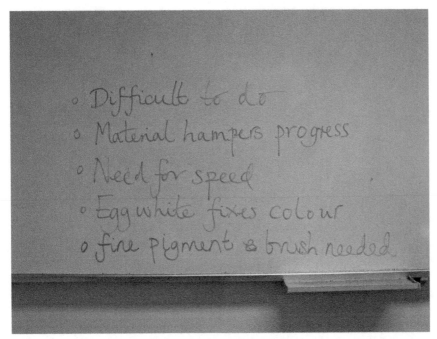

31.2 Discussion points from the ostraca activity as written up on the whiteboard. (Photograph by the author.)

their contribution to the experiment. In turn, I sourced acacia gum capsules as the cheapest form of this product available through the internet, together with natural carob drops, the more readily available powder not fulfilling the 'grind' of the prescription and the more realistic chips being prohibitively expensive.

On the day itself the students worked in their pairs to grind the roughly measured and proportioned acacia, carob and dates with the carefully measured honey. Following some vigorous grinding, carried out over a ten-minute period, the end results were examined. The experiment was later re-run with a group of students at London's City Literacy Institute (popularly known as City Lit; see Figure 31.3).

It was quickly discovered that the consistency of the products in the three mortars varied considerably, depending on whether the pairs had used runny or set honey. Since the former produced a liquid gooey mess when placed on the lint, it was quickly determined that the honey used by the ancient Egyptians must have been of the considerably more practical firmly set variety. It is noteworthy that honey similarly features in prescription Kahun 22, which specifies: 'a *hin* (450 ml) of honey, sprinkle over her vagina [*kat*], this to be done on a natron bed' (as quoted in Szpakowska 2007: 213), leading Nunn (1996: 196) to comment that this 'might be spermicidal by means of its osmotic effect'.

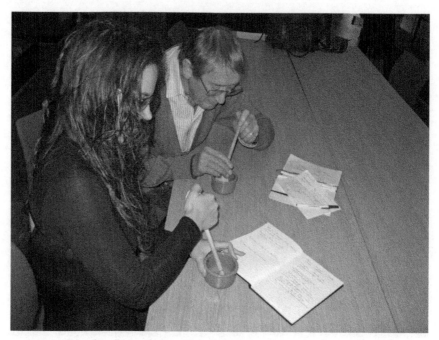

31.3 Two City Lit students grinding the ingredients for the contraceptive.
(Photograph by David Taylor.)

During the ensuing discussion considerable doubts were not surprisingly
expressed as to the optimistic 'up to three years' shelf-life of the product
(Figure 31.4). The students were all of the opinion that the only possible explanation could be that putting this concoction anywhere near the vagina would,
to quote Szpakowska (2007: 213) in reference to the use of crocodile dung in the
contraceptive prescription Kahun 21, 'quickly quench any amorous advances'.

Educational analysis

The literature on learning is understandably vast, but within the plethora it
is possible to identify three major models of learning. These have been aptly
summarised by three of my colleagues at University College London's Institute
of Education (UCL-IOE) as comprising the reception, construction and co-construction models (Watkins, Carnell and Lodge 2007). The reception model, most
dominant during the twentieth century, can be defined as learning equating to
being teacher-led: 'she taught me'. The construction model is one where learning
comprises individual sense-making as a result of discussion: 'I made sense of'. By
contrast, the co-construction model develops higher-order skills in that learning
involves building knowledge with others through dialogue: 'we worked out that'.

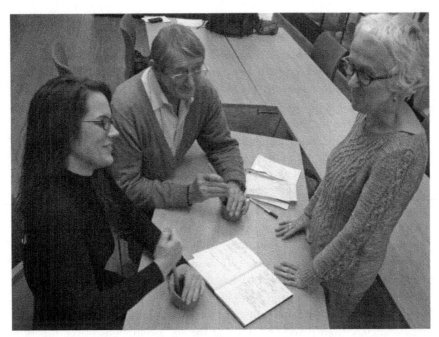

31.4 The author discussing the experiment with two City Lit students. (Photograph by David Taylor.)

It can thus be seen as a collaborative learning product, which is very much what my interactive OUDCE course was all about. The students benefited in the manner described by eleven-year-old Annie: 'You learn more because if you explain to people what you do, you say things that you wouldn't say to yourself, really. So you learn things that you wouldn't know if you were just doing it by yourself' (Watkins *et al.* 2002: 5). Similarly, the OUDCE students worked together in a process of mutual problem-solving, such as when discussing the constituency of the honey, to create a joint product and understanding. Such collaborative work is rated by school pupils as being twice as effective as individual activities for promoting their learning (Watkins, Carnell and Lodge 2007).

Drawing on earlier seminal work headed by the Institute of Education's then Reader in Education Chris Watkins (2001, 2002), he and his colleagues (Watkins, Carnell and Lodge 2007: 19) further discuss the concept of effective learning, which they define as 'an activity of *making* meaning – construction – not simply of receiving. The social dimension is always present, and in social contexts collaboration supports learning.' Once again, this conforms to the organisation of the OUDCE course with its integral collaboration in the prior sourcing of materials. The social context was always strong, taking us on a visit to the Petrie Museum and culminating in an end-of-term Deir el-Medina feast or Christmas party around a theme of food and beer preparation.

As to the educational significance of this learning experience, a useful model is the adaptation by Chris Watkins and his colleagues (2002) of the classic experiential learning theory (ELT) of David Kolb (1984). Kolb's learning model comprises a four-stage cycle: Do, Review, Learn, Apply. As such it demands that time is taken for reflection on a learning activity, for, according to Kolb (1984: 38), *'Learning is the process whereby knowledge is created through the transformation of experience'* (author's italics). What has been learned then feeds into future action (is applied), and then subsequent action is reviewed. Watkins *et al.* (2002) have incorporated an extra cycle in the reflection model which promotes learning about learning and thereby addresses the potential complexity of the process. Learning thus becomes the larger focus of their revised Do, Review, Learn, Apply cycle. The learner in this model becomes in fact a meta-learner, who is more versatile and is able to apply new learning across a wider range of contexts.

Finally, it is useful to consider Malcolm Knowles (1973, 1980, 1989; Knowles, in Knowles and Associates 1984) and his theory of andragogy, which states that adults learn in fundamentally different ways from children (thus distinguishing andragogy from pedagogy). One of the six assumptions of the theory is that adults learn by experience; this is based on the premise that, as a person matures, he or she accumulates a growing reservoir of experience that can become an increasing resource for learning. Then we have the somewhat disputed geragogy as first propounded by Lebel (1978). Focusing exclusively on the learning of older people, this envisages a search for meaning as a key educational activity. Thus Cusack (1991: 10) has emphasised lifelong education as 'a process of making meaning from experience, from life experience and from the learning experiences provided'.

Two experiential learning situations illustrate the fundamental differences between andragogy and geragogy. The online stream from my textile demonstration at the Swansea 'Experiment and Experience' conference mentioned above shows a team of volunteers – in the guise of Swansea Egyptology students – attempting to create pleats using four replica boards. Working in pairs and urged on by their 'overseer of the laundry' Jane, these young students attempt to push Second World War linen into the grooves of so-called pleating boards housed in the Egyptian Museums of both Turin and Florence and the British Museum. The end results are largely disappointing to the eye, to the extent that the plenary focuses on some fascinating alternative explanations for these ancient artefacts. Yet when the experiment was subsequently recreated in 2013 with my OUDCE students, using exactly the same boards and pieces of linen, perfect pleats were obtained. These Oxford students, all of whom it will be remembered were in the retired age group, provided their own explanation for their success: 'We were taught dressmaking by our mothers and grandmothers, unlike young people today.'

There is no doubt that the making of the contraceptive was responsible for achieving one of the three learning outcomes of the course: 'to explore the practical reconstruction of daily life activities through a critical contemporary lens'. It was also great fun at the time, a never-to-be-forgotten experience in which, looking back with hindsight and reflexivity, we realise that we all became meta-learners. Notwithstanding, at the time we all expressed considerable relief that we could not complete the Kolb experiential learning cycle in which the learner makes meaning out of the experience. None of us were of an age to test the final product.

References

Cusack, S. A. (1991), 'Making meaning from experience: toward an integrative theory of lifelong education', *Journal of Educational Gerontology* 6 (1), 7–15.

David, A. R. (1986), *The Pyramid Builders of Ancient Egypt: A Modern Investigation of Pharaoh's Workforce* (London: Routledge and Kegan Paul).

Graves-Brown, C. (2015), *Egyptology in the Present. Experiential and Experimental Methods in Archaeology* (Swansea: Classical Press of Wales).

Knowles, M. S. (1973), *The Adult Learner; A Neglected Species* (Houston: Gulf Publishing).

Knowles, M. (1980), *The Modern Practice of Adult Education* (Chicago: The Association Press).

Knowles, M. S. (1989), *The Making of an Adult Educator* (San Francisco: Jossey-Bass).

Knowles, M. S. and Associates (1984), *Andragogy in Action: Applying Modern Principles of Adult Learning* (San Francisco: Jossey-Bass).

Kolb, D. A. (1984), *Experiential Learning: Experience as a Source of Learning and Development* (Englewood Cliffs, NJ: Prentice Hall).

Lebel, J. (1978), 'Beyond andragogy to geragogy', *Lifelong Learning: The Adult Years* 1 (9), 16–28.

Nunn, J. F. (1996), *Ancient Egyptian Medicine* (London: British Museum Press).

Page, A. (1983), *Ancient Egyptian Figured Ostraca in the Petrie Collection* (Warminster: Aris and Phillips).

Phillips, J. P. (2002), *The Columns of Egypt* (Manchester: Peartree).

Szpakowska, K. (2007), *Daily Life in Ancient Egypt: Recreating Lahun* (Oxford: Wiley-Blackwell).

University of Swansea (2010), 'Experiment and Experience: Ancient Egypt in the Present', conference, 10–12 May, programme at www.egypt.swansea.ac.uk (last accessed 3 January 2015).

Watkins, C. with Carnell, E., Lodge, C., Wagner, P. and Whalley, C. (2001), 'Learning about learning enhances performance', *NSIN Research Matters* 13 (Spring), 1–9.

Watkins, C., Carnell, E., Lodge, C., Wagner, P. and Whalley, C. (2002), 'Effective learning', *NSIN Research Matters* 17 (Summer), 1–8.

Watkins, C., Carnell, E. and Lodge, C. (2007), *Effective Learning in Classrooms* (London: Paul Chapman).

32

Iron from the sky: the role of meteorite iron in the development of iron-working techniques in ancient Egypt

Diane Johnson and Joyce Tyldesley

The earliest evidence for the large scale smelting of iron ores in Egypt dates to the sixth century BC (Petrie 1886: 39); this strongly suggests that iron production technologies developed much later in Egypt than in neighbouring territories. However, archaeology has shown that some elite Egyptians were buried with iron grave goods long before iron production became common within their land (Carter 1927: 122, 135–6; Carter 1933: 89–92). The origin of the iron used in the manufacture of these artefacts, and the methods by which this iron was worked, have been much debated (Wainwright 1944: 177–8; El-Gayer 1995: 11–12). This chapter discusses an experimental approach designed to assess the role of meteorite iron in the development of Egyptian iron-working techniques. The authors, who first met as student and tutor on the University of Manchester Certificate in Egyptology programme, are delighted to have the opportunity of dedicating it to Professor Rosalie David.

Pre-'Iron Age' iron artefacts in Egypt

Although the ancient Egyptians had access to iron ores (Lucas 1948: 268–75; El-Hinnawi 1965: 1497–1509), there is no evidence that these ores were exploited as a source of metal before the First Persian Period (Ogden 2000: 166; Garland and Bannister 1927: 85). In spite of this, a small number of iron artefacts have been recovered from archaeological contexts predating 600 BC. All known metallic iron artefacts reportedly dating from the Predynastic Period to the 18th Dynasty are listed in Table 32.1. From the 19th to the early 22nd Dynasty there is very little information about the use of metallic iron in Egypt (Waldbaum 1978: 15–16). Iron then starts to become increasingly conspicuous in the archaeological record.

Table 32.1 Reported Predynastic to 18th Dynasty iron artefacts

Artefact	Find location:	Date	Notes, reference
Iron beads[a]	Gerzeh cemetery: tomb 67 (7 beads), tomb 133 (2 beads)	3300 BC	Wainwright 1912; Petrie and Wainwright 1912
Ring	Armant (tomb 1494)	Predynastic/Early Dynastic	Probably of later date[b]
Plate of iron	Great Pyramid, Giza	4th Dynasty[c]	Recovered outer stonework joint; Petrie 1883; Craddock and Lang 1989
Iron oxide residue on *pesesh-kef* design wand	Khufu's mortuary temple, Giza	4th Dynasty	Reisner 1931; Dunham and Young 1942
Pickaxe	Abusir	6th Dynasty[c]	Maspero 1883
Mass of iron rust	Abydos temple	6th Dynasty	Petrie 1903; Petrie 1910: 104
Pesesh-kef amulet blade[a]	Tomb of queen Ashait, Deir el-Bahri, Thebes	11th Dynasty	Brunton 1935
Spear head	Buhen, Nubia	12th Dynasty[d]	Randall-Maclver and Woolley 1911
Part of a chisel and hoe	Unknown	17th Dynasty[c]	Maspero 1883
2 corroded iron lumps	House in Amarna	18th Dynasty	Griffith 1924; analysis proved it to be a rich smelting product
1 dagger blade,[a] 1 model headrest,[a] 1 eye of Horus amulet, 16 miniature blades[a]	KV 62, Thebes	18th Dynasty	All found wrapped with the mummy except for the set of miniature blades, which were located in a box in the Treasury (Carter 1927; Carter 1933)
Arrowhead	Malkata palace, Amenhotep III, Thebes	18th Dynasty	Hayes 1959
Iron pin	Abydos	18th Dynasty	Garstang 1901; part of box.

a   Confirmed nickel-rich.
b   Noted at excavation as being possibly intrusive and therefore maybe of a later date, before it could be analysed it was lost during transfer in post (Mond and Myers 1937).
c   Date authenticity in doubt because of lack of archaeological evidence.
d   Style inconsistent with this frequently suggested date.

Unfortunately, several of the artefacts included in Table 32.1 do not come from sealed or well-documented archaeological contexts; this raises the possibility of contamination by the accidental inclusion of later-dating artefacts, and this in turn creates significant uncertainty in the interpretation of these artefacts. Some, such as the 'iron plate' recovered from the Great Pyramid, are likely to have little antiquity (Craddock and Lang 1989: 57–9). Our work therefore concentrates on the iron artefacts – predominantly high-status funerary objects – recovered from the three sound and well-documented archaeological contexts.

The Predynastic Gerzeh Cemetery

Nine iron beads were discovered in the late Predynastic cemetery at Gerzeh: seven in grave 67 (SD 53–63) and two in grave 133 (SD 60–3) (Wainwright 1912: 255–9). Not only are these beads the earliest known examples of iron-working in Egypt, but they are also probably the earliest example of worked iron in the Near East. Analysis has shown that the beads are composed of iron with a chemistry and microstructure consistent with meteorite iron (Wainwright 1912: 255–9; Desch 1928: 440–1; Johnson *et al.* 2013: 997–1006).

The 11th Dynasty Deir el-Bahri tomb of Ashait

A *Pesesh-kef* amulet – a ritual implement used in the 'Opening of the Mouth' ceremony performed on the mummy at the entrance to the tomb, transforming it into a latent being with potential for life – with a damaged iron blade and silver head was found in the robbed tomb of queen Ashait, a secondary wife of Montuhotep II (Brunton 1935: 213–17). It was confirmed that the iron is significantly nickel-rich at approximately 11 per cent by weight (Desch 1928: 440–1). This is consistent with it being meteorite iron.

The 18th Dynasty tomb of Tutankhamun in the Valley of the Kings

Tutankhamun's tomb yielded various iron artefacts. A set of sixteen model blades of six different designs with wooden handles was found in the Treasury. Each appears to have been beaten into flat sheets of sub-millimetre thickness and shaped (Carter 1933: 89–92). All other iron in this tomb was found with the mummy.

A miniature iron headrest, which had been relatively crudely constructed by welding together pieces of iron (probably at too low a temperature), was found directly behind the mummy's head on the inside of the gold mask (Carter 1927: 109). Uniquely, this was completely non-rusted. Similar headrest models were typically made from haematite (Waldbaum 1978: 22).

Wrapped with the mummy, on the right side of the thorax, was a thin, flat piece of iron which had been shaped into an 'eye of Horus' amulet and attached to a golden bracelet (Carter 1927: 122). Also wrapped with the mummy, along the right thigh, was a dagger with an iron blade, rock crystal pommel and sheet gold scabbard. This iron dagger is, as noted by its excavator, extremely sharp; unlike the other iron artefacts discovered in the tomb, it had been expertly produced (Carter 1927: 135–6).

The 'eye of Horus' amulet has no published chemistry. The other artefacts have iron chemistry recorded as nickel-rich, and this convinced the Egyptian Museum in Cairo that they were produced from meteorites (Bjorkman 1973: 124). However, more recent analysis of the dagger blade gave 3 per cent nickel content by weight: this is more suggestive of a smelted origin, and possibly production by the use of nickel-rich laterites (Helmi and Barakat 1995: 287–9; Photos 1989: 403–21). It seems probable that this dagger was imported into Egypt.

Natural sources of iron in antiquity

Worldwide, only two natural forms of metallic iron are known to occur, and both of these are rare. The first is telluric iron, of which the only confirmed exploited source is on Disko Island, Greenland (Buchwald 1992: 139–76). The second naturally is meteorite iron: iron which falls from the sky in the form of a meteorite. This may be found across the world, and has been used as a source of metal by many cultures at various points in time (Prufer 1961: 341–52; Burke 1986: 229–36; Buchwald 1992: 139–76; McCoy et al. 2008). Meteorite iron is, by its nature, in limited supply, although occasionally very large masses do occur. The South African Hoba meteorite, for example, has a 61 tonne mass (Spencer 1932: 1–19; Spargo 2008: 85–94).

Meteoric iron has been exploited worldwide in the manufacture of practical tools and weapons. A good example of this type of use is provided by the Cape York fragmented meteorite from Greenland (Buchwald 1992: 139–76). Cape York's 'Woman' meteorite was discovered surrounded by over 10,000 basalt hammer-stones, each with a mass between 1 and 10 kg. Some of these basalt stones had been sourced up to 50 km away and transported to the site as tools hard enough to break and fragment iron (Buchwald and Mosdal 1985: 1–49; Craddock 1995: 107). But not all meteorite iron has been restricted to the utilitarian sphere. To take just one example, Native American Indians recognised meteorites and considered them important in the context of burial and the afterlife (Nininger 1938: 39–40). Many examples of both worked meteorites (Grogan 1948: 302–5) and non-worked ones (Brady 1929: 477–86) have been found in their burial grounds.

Meteorite iron has a very distinctive chemistry and structure, but with processes and oxidation it can become difficult to distinguish meteorite iron from other sources of iron. In particular, the naturally nickel-rich meteorite iron frequently starts to become depleted of nickel during severe oxidation. Meanwhile, the occasional use of nickel-rich iron ores in antiquity has been known to produce nickel-enriched iron. It can therefore be dangerous to assume that all nickel-rich iron is meteorite iron. Ultimately, this can be determined only by the detailed structural and chemical analysis of individual artefacts.

In Egypt, at the beginning of the 19th Dynasty a new hieroglyphic word appeared, *bꜣ3-n-pt*, which literally translates as 'iron from the sky' (Harris 1961: 50–62). Why this new word appeared in this exact form and at this time we do not know, but we do know that the word was applied to all metallic iron. Although there had been occasional textual links between iron and the sky (Reiter 1997), no such clear link had previously been made. An obvious explanation for the creation of the new word is that a major impact event or large shower of meteorites had occurred, causing the Egyptians to realise that iron might quite literally fall from the sky. An ancient crater caused by the massive impact of an iron meteorite is known from southern Egypt. Although its exact age remains unknown, nearby archaeology suggests that the crater formed within the last 5,000 years (Folco *et al.* 2010: 804).

Evidence of ancient iron-working techniques

Structural examination of the Gerzeh beads has revealed that they were manufactured from small fragments of iron bent into a tube shape (Wainwright 1912: 255–9; Johnson *et al.* 2013: 997–1006). It seems likely that small boulders were used as hammer-stones; tube formation may have required some heating. No Egyptian records describe this processing technique, but this method was applied both by the prehistoric Inuit (who had a similar technology to the Predynastic Egyptians) working small fragments from the Cape York meteorite (Buchwald 1992: 139–76) and by the American Indians of the Hopewell Mounds, Ohio (McCoy *et al.* 2008).

We can derive some evidence for metal bead production by examining the copper beads which are relatively plentiful in Predynastic Egypt. These appear to have been manufactured from thin sheets of copper (less than 0.5 mm thick) curved around a small rod. Specific metal-working tools are unknown from this time, but more generalised tools such as small hammer-stones would have been ideal for use in bead production. Old Kingdom metal-working scenes, such as that in the 6th Dynasty Saqqara tomb of Mereruka (Duell 1938: pl. 30), show the hammering of copper, the use of blowpipes to achieve high temperatures for copper smelting and the use of insulating small blocks of stone or wads of clay to allow handling of hot crucibles. In a scene from the 5th Dynasty tomb of Wepemnefert at Giza (Hassan 1936: pl. 74) we can read the metal-workers'

discussion; this shows a working knowledge of the importance of heat annealing to avoid the embrittlement of the copper through work hardening. It is
possible that the heating methods which developed in early Egypt for successful
hammering and shaping of copper were simply applied to iron.

Experimental methods and results

Source materials: meteorite iron

Numerous types of meteorite exist. Their exact composition and structure is
dependent on their formation mechanisms, with the majority dating to formation some four and a half billion years ago. Three types of meteorite are
identified as containing sufficient metallic iron to be a practical source of iron
(McSween 2000):

1. Octahedrites are iron meteorites formed within the core of differentiated
   bodies (such as small planets or large asteroids), which were subsequently
   broken up by an impact event. The structures seen are large inter-grown
   crystals of iron nickel alloys: taenite, which is nickel-rich (approximately
   30 per cent by weight) and kamacite, which has a lower nickel content
   (approximately 6–8 per cent by weight).
2. Ataxites are iron meteorites formed by melting and recrystallisation to an
   extent where they are almost devoid of observable texture; this results in a
   significant overall nickel enrichment.
3. Pallasites are stony iron meteorites composed of metal similar to the
   octahedrites, intermixed mainly with large olivine crystals.

Experimental production of thin iron sheets

A granite stone and anvil were used to beat small pieces of meteorite iron at
room temperature in an attempt to compress them. The first attempt was made
using pallasite iron. The thickness at the start was 2–3 mm. The first blow of the
hammer smashed a small accessory mineral inclusion, the fragments of which
were collected and analysed by scanning electron microscopy with energy-
dispersive X-ray spectroscopy; this showed it to be the iron-nickel phosphide
mineral Schreibersite $(FeNi)_3P$. With continued beating over approximately five
minutes, fractures formed across the iron which ultimately caused the sample
to fragment with very limited compression (Figures 32.1 and 32.2). Similar
attempts were made with octahedrite iron and these yielded the same result;
fragmentation along the internal interfaces. In contrast, ataxite iron compressed
well using the stone tools, which worked with similar ease to modern steel. Very
little splitting or cracking developed in this process.

Samples of the same meteorites were then heated to progressively higher
temperatures from 200 to 800°C. Further attempts were made to compress the
samples using the same stone tools, but again all samples significantly fractured

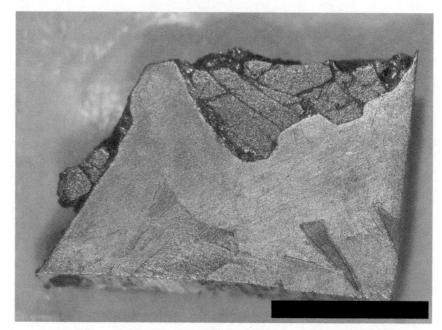

32.1 Pallasite meteorite iron, Seymchan, at the start of the experiment as a thick slice. Scale bar = 1cm. (Photograph by Diane Johnson.)

with the exception of the ataxite samples (see Figures 32.3 and 32.4 for octahedrite before and after attempts to compress at 800°C). The only meteorite iron successfully compressed at both room and high temperature was the ataxite meteorite iron, which has mechanical properties similar to modern steel.

Another method of producing a thin sheet of meteorite iron from octahedrites and possibly pallasites is to use the plate-like crystal structure of the meteorite iron itself. When these meteorites alter and rust, the surface will often expose layers or leaves of iron. These are separated from the main mass, where interfaces of the layers act as defect weakness points; they form thin sheets, with little or no compression needed to bend into tube shapes.

Further experiments were performed using a modern circular saw that partially cut through a thick piece of octahedrite meteorite iron. The remaining intact section was pulled by hand to separate the two pieces, producing thin slices generally along the boundaries. Other methods of producing thin sheets of meteorite iron are also possible: for example the use of abrasive grinding of either oxidised or fresh metal to create a sufficiently thin fragment.

Forming tube-shaped beads

An abrasive block of granite was used to smooth and flatten all sides of the meteorite iron obtained using the processes described above. Additional

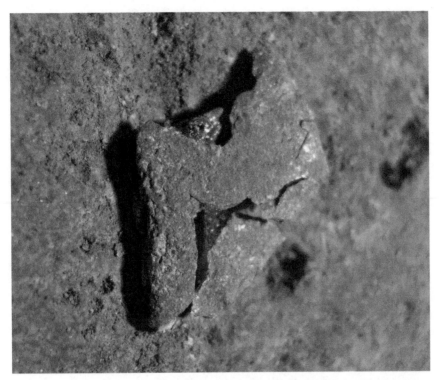

32.2 Pallasite meteorite, Seymchan, after attempts to compress by hitting with a granite hammer-stone and anvil at room temperature. (Photograph by Diane Johnson.)

samples were cut from octahedrite and pallasites iron using a modern circular saw; it was noted that cutting meteorite iron with a modern circular saw was very time-consuming, but using modern grinding technology was comparatively rapid.

A small granite block with a thin groove (approximately 0.5 cm wide) was used to form bends within the small sheet of meteorite iron. After placing the iron across the top of this groove and then placing a copper rod on top of the iron, a granite hammer-stone was used to hit the rod onto the iron, bending the sheet into the underlying groove. An iron rod and a small rod-shaped hard twig were also used with the same result. By slightly repositioning the iron and repeating the process, an open tube was produced. This could be closed into a complete tube with further light hammering, using a smaller rod to hold the bead in place.

Because of the problems encountered in the early experiments while working at room temperature, all tube-making attempts were conducted after heating the iron to 800°C, and the iron was bent into shape while still glowing

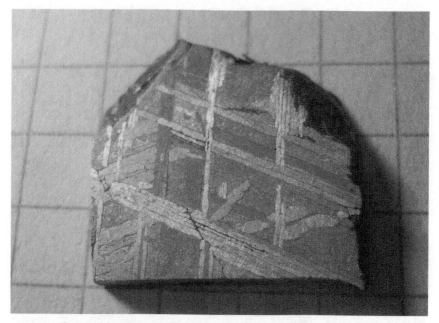

32.3 Octahedrite meteorite iron, Muonionalusta, Sweden, at the start of the
experiment as a thick slice. (Photograph by Diane Johnson.)

hot. The results were remarkably similar in bead cross-section structures to
those of one of the original Gerzeh iron beads; a comparison optical image of
an experimentally produced bead can be seen in Figure 32.5; a virtual X-ray
slice through the end of the Gerzeh iron bead in the collections of Manchester
Museum (acc. no. 5303) can be seen for comparison in Figure 32.6.

Scanning electron microscope analysis of iron micro-structure with mechanical working

The octahedrite iron meteorite known as Muonionalusta (found in
Muonionalusta, Sweden) was chosen for experiment, partly because of its type
and also because it is a large meteorite fall with no known associated ethical
issues that might constrain destructive analysis. A thin slice of this meteorite
was made using a circular saw and the surface of the sample was polished. It
was then analysed using a scanning electron microscope imaged with a back-
scatter electron detector. The slice was then beaten lightly for approximately
three minutes with a small granite hammer-stone, and was then re-polished
and imaged again in the scanning electron microscope. Comparisons of the
two show differences in the iron microstructure, as after beating the meteorite
iron the bright linear bands of nickel-rich taenite have undergone distortion to
appear in as non-linear thin bands.

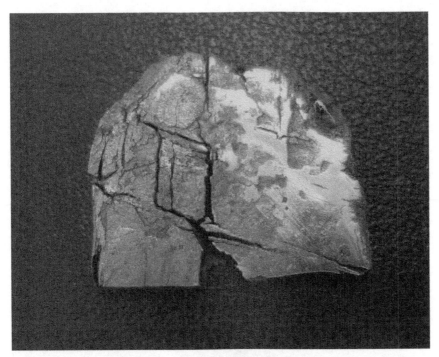

32.4 Octahedrite meteorite iron, Muonionalusta, Sweden, after attempts to compress by hitting with use of a granite hammer-stone and anvil heated in a furnace up to 800°C. (Photograph by Diane Johnson.)

Polishing and treatment of the iron bead

When the tube-shaped bead was formed it could be easily polished using abrasives, the ancient and modern techniques being almost identical. The cleaning of the bead starts with a coarse gain abrasive – either loose grains which the iron is pushed against or a small rough flat block of stone which the bead is rubbed against – which removes any thick oxides formed during the heating process. Progressively finer grain abrasives are then used until a bright and smooth surface is achieved.

It was observed that during the heating process a colour change occurs on the surface of the iron as a consequence of a thin oxide layer forming. This layer is sufficiently thin to create a bright iridescent pattern caused by light diffraction. If desired, this thin oxide layer may be replaced on the fully formed cleaned bead by reheating it until a colour change is observed. On the basis of the evidence of Predynastic grave contents, bright colours and shiny materials are likely to have been highly valued, so this colour change would probably have appealed to Predynastic metal-workers. Two experimental replica beads with thin colour oxide layers can be seen in Plate 13.

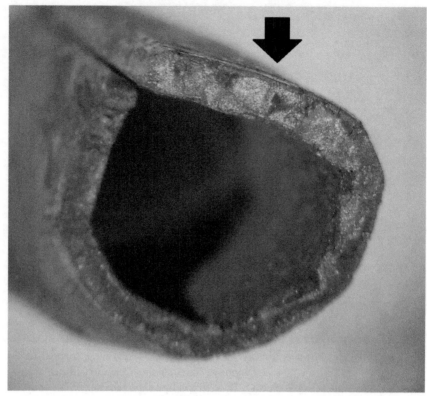

32.5 Replica bead produced by bending meteorite iron around a rod and over a groove cut into granite. (Photograph by Diane Johnson.)

Discussion

The Gerzeh beads suggest that meteorite iron was worked by the Predynastic Egyptians, despite the difficulties of working with this generally brittle material. Three main stages are involved in iron bead production, as follows.

1. Sourcing the meteorite iron

The iron could simply have come from a small, local meteorite fall, which would be unlikely to have formed an impact crater. The high density of the fresh or weathered iron meteorite would allow it to be identified as an unusual material; it may, or may not, have been recognised as being of celestial origin. As a rare material the iron is likely to have had significant value, and its ownership probably indicated a high social or religious status. Alternatively, the iron could have been imported into Egypt as a high-value trade item. This suggestion is supported by other non-local materials recovered from the Gerzeh

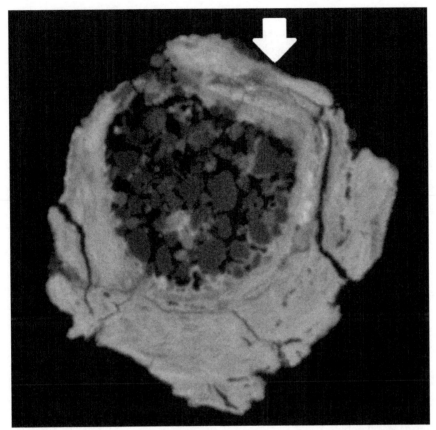

32.6 X-ray computed tomography data showing one end of a Gerzeh iron bead, Manchester Museum 5303. (Courtesy of Manchester Museum, University of Manchester.)

graves, including shells, obsidian and lapis lazuli (Stevenson 2006: 47). In addition, there are a limited number of large ancient meteorite falls in the region (Grady 2000: 680) which require further investigation to assess them as possible iron sources.

2. Making the thin flat iron sheet

Our experimental work has shown that the thin iron sheets needed to produce the beads could have been made by a number of methods, but it is highly unlikely that they were made by compressive hammer blows alone. The only meteorite iron that is readily compressive into thin sheets comes from ataxite meteorites; however, the microstructures observed in our previous study indicate that the Gerzeh beads were formed from an octahedral meteorite (Johnson *et al.* 2013).

The use of high temperatures while attempting compression with a hammer-stone is also insufficient to make a thin meteorite iron sheet. The method used in antiquity is likely to have involved a cleaving or fracturing through the octahedrite structure along edges of its crystal planes. This would have required limited amounts of striking with a hammer-stone. Further thinning could be achieved by use of abrasive techniques which were clearly achievable at this time.

3. Bending the iron sheet into a tube

The bending process employed to produce the tube shape was generally successful at high temperature, although any small defect present on the edge of the iron sample had a strong tendency to extend as a tear propagating along any intersecting crystal plane. Temperatures of 800°C would probably be uncommon in Predynastic Egypt, but could have been achieved by certain methods, including a well-built fire positioned to achieve maximum wind flow, the use of bellows, the use of charcoal and the use of closed up-draught kilns. Marl ware, which requires high temperatures for successful firing, was likewise being produced at this time (Wilkinson 1999: 33–6).

Summary

In early Egypt iron was a rare, exotic material, apparently sourced from meteorites. The iron artefacts known to predate the traditional Egyptian 'Iron Age' are predominantly high-status funerary objects. The exact origin of these artefacts and the processes by which they were worked into important symbolic forms is still debated.

The Predynastic Gerzeh iron beads are currently the earliest known example of the purposeful working of metallic iron in the Near East. Their production method can be inferred by studying their macroscopic and microscopic structures; these suggest at least a basic knowledge of high-temperature methods, combined with hammer bending and grinding. Further experimental archaeology is ongoing to determine whether it is possible to achieve the production of tube-shaped beads at lower temperatures.

Egyptologists have long wondered why the 'Iron Age' developed so late in Egypt (e.g. Ogden 2003: 262–3). It has been suggested that this may have been due to an inability or reluctance to develop the necessary technologies to work iron. However, the evidence of iron-working in Predynastic times suggests that this may not have been the case. A shortage of fuel may have been a consideration. Alternatively, it may be that the lack of interest in producing practical worked iron artefacts was a deliberate choice, inspired by the knowledge that iron fell from the sky. Was iron too closely related to the gods to play a part in daily life?

Acknowledgements

The authors would like to acknowledge the Manchester X-ray Imaging Facility, University of Manchester, for expertise and X-ray CT scanning; Manchester Museum, University of Manchester for the loan of a Gerzeh iron bead; the Petrie Museum of Egyptian Archaeology, University College London, for access to its collection; Dr Tim McCoy (Smithsonian Institute, Washington DC); Mr Denys Stocks and Professor Paul T. Nicholson (Cardiff University) for advice on ancient technical aspects of bead production; and Professor Monica Grady (Open University) for discussions on meteorite iron. We would also like to acknowledge the practical assistance provided during iron-working experiments as well as the engineering advice of Mr Chris Hall (Open University).

References

Bjorkman, J. K. (1973), 'Meteors and meteorites in the ancient Near East', *Meteoritics and Planetary Science* 8, 91–132.

Brady, L. F. (1929), 'The Winona meteorite', *American Journal of Science* 18, 477–86.

Brunton, G. (1935), '*Pesesh kef* amulets', *Annales du Service des antiquités de l'Égypte* 35, 213–17.

Buchwald, V. F. (1992), 'On the use of iron by Eskimos in Greenland', *Materials Characterisation* 29 (2), 139–76.

Buchwald, V. F. and Mosdal, G. (1985), 'Meteoritic iron, telluric iron and wrought iron in Greenland, Meddelelser om Grønland', *Man and Society* 9, 1–49.

Burke, J. G. (1986), *Cosmic Debris: Meteorites in History* (Oakland, CA, and London: University of California Press).

Carter, H. (1927), *The Tomb of Tut.ankh.Amen*, II: *The Burial Chamber* (London: Cassell), reprinted 2001 (London: Duckworth and Co.).

Carter, H. (1933), *The Tomb of Tut.ankh.Amen*, II: *The Annex and Treasury* (London: Cassell), reprinted 2000 (London: Duckworth and Co.).

Craddock, P. T. (1995), *Early Metal Mining and Production* (Edinburgh: Edinburgh University Press).

Craddock, P. T. and Lang J. (1989), 'Gizeh iron revisited', *Historical Metallurgy* 27 (2), 57–9.

Desch, C. H. (1928), *Reports on the Metallurgical Examination of Specimens for the Sumerian Committee of the British Association* (London: British Association).

Duell, P. (1938), *The Mastaba of Mereruka*, I (Chicago: Oriental Institute Publishing).

Dunham, D. and Young, W. J. (1942), 'An occurrence of iron in the Fourth Dynasty', *Journal of Egyptian Archaeology* 28, 57–8.

El-Gayer, E. S. (1995), 'Predynastic iron beads from Gerzeh', *Institute for Archaeo-Metallurgical Studies* 19, 11–12.

El-Hinnawi, E. E. (1965), 'Contributions to the study of Egyptian (UAR) iron ores', *Economic Geology* 60 (7), 1497–1509.

Folco, L., Di Martino, M., El Barkooky, A., D'Orazio, M., Lethy, A., Urbini, S., Nicolosi, I., Hafez, M., Cordier, C., van Ginneken, M., Zeoli, A, Radwan, A.

M., El Khrepy, S., El Gabry, M., Gomaa, M., Barakat, A. A., Serra, R. and El Sharkawi, M. (2010), 'The Kamil Crater in Egypt', *Science* 329 (5993), 804.

Garland, H. and Bannister C. O. (1927), *Ancient Egyptian Metallurgy* (London: Griffin).

Garstang, J. (1901), *El Arabah: A Cemetery of the Middle Kingdom* (London: Bernard Quaritch).

Grady, M. M. (2000), *Catalogue of Meteorites* (Cambridge: Cambridge University Press).

Griffith, F. Ll. (1924), 'Excavations at el-'Amarnah, 1923–24', *Journal of Egyptian Archaeology* 10, 299–305.

Grogan, R. M. (1948), 'Beads of metal iron from an Indian mound near Havana, Illinois', *American Antiquity* 13 (4), 302–5.

Harris, J. R. (1961), *Lexicographical Studies in Ancient Egyptian Minerals* (Berlin: Akademie Verlag).

Hassan, S. (1936), *Excavations at Giza 1930–1931*, II (Cairo: Government Press).

Hayes, W. C. (1959), *The Scepter of Egypt II* (Wellfleet, MA: Harper and Brothers).

Helmi, F. and Barakat, K. (1995), 'Micro analysis of Tutankhamun's dagger', in F. A. Esmael (ed.), *Proceedings of the First International Conference on Ancient Egyptian Mining & Metallurgy and Conservation of Metallic Artifacts* (Cairo: Egyptian Antiquities Organization), 287–9.

Johnson, D., Tyldesley, J., Lowe, T., Withers, P. J. and Grady, M. M. (2013), 'Analysis of a prehistoric Egyptian iron bead with implications for the use and perception of meteorite iron in ancient Egypt', *Meteoritics and Planetary Science* 48 (6), 997–1006.

Lucas, A. (1948), *Ancient Egyptian Materials and Industries* (London: Edward Arnold and Co.).

Maspero, G. (1883), *Guide du visiteur au Musée de Boulaq* (Cairo: Boulaq Museum).

McCoy, T. J., Marquardt, A. E., Vicenzi, E. P., Ash, R. D. and Wasson, J. T. (2008), 'Meteoritic metal from the Havana, Illinois Hopewell Mounds', *Lunar and Planetary Science Conference* 39, 1984, abstract 1391.

McSween, H. Y. Jr. (2000) *Meteorites and their Parent Planets*, 2nd edn (Cambridge: Cambridge University Press).

Mond, R. and Meyers, O. H. (1937), *Cemeteries of Armant*, I (London: Egypt Exploration Society).

Nininger, H. H. (1938), 'Meteorite collecting among ancient Americans', *American Antiquity* 4, 39–40.

Ogden, J. (2000), 'Metals', in P. T. Nicholson and I. Shaw (eds.), *Ancient Egyptian Materials and Technology* (Cambridge: Cambridge University Press), 166.

Ogden, J. (2003), 'Why was there no Egyptian iron-age?', in B. Manley (ed.), *The Seventy Great Mysteries of Ancient Egypt* (London: Thames and Hudson), 262–3.

Petrie, W. M. F. (1883), *The Pyramids and Temples of Gizeh* (London: Field and Tuer).

Petrie, W. M. F. (1886), *Naucratis*, I: *1884–5* (London: Egypt Exploration Fund).

Petrie, W. M. F. (1903), *Abydos*, II (London: Egypt Exploration Fund).

Petrie, W. M. F. (1910), *Arts and Crafts of Ancient Egypt* (Edinburgh: T. N. Foulis).

Petrie, W. M. F. and Wainwright, G. A. (1912), *The Labyrinth, Gerzeh and Mazghuneh* (London: British School of Archaeology in Egypt).

Photos, E. (1989), 'The question of meteorite versus smelted nickel-rich iron: archaeological evidence and experimental results', *World Archaeology* 20 (3), 403–21.

Prufer, O. H. (1961), 'Prehistoric Hopewell meteorite collecting: context and implications', *Ohio Journal of Science* 61 (6), 341–52.

Randall-MacIver, D. and Woolley, C. L. (1911), *Buhen* (Philadelphia: University Museum Philadelphia).

Reisner, G. A. (1931), *Mycerinus* (London: Humphrey Milford).

Reiter, K. (1997), *Die Metalle im Alten Orient unter besonderer Berücksichtigung altbabylonischer Quellen* (Munster: Ugarit-Verlag).

Spargo, P. E. (2008), 'The history of the Hoba meteorite part 1; nature and discovery' *Monthly Notes of the Astronomical Society of Southern Africa* 67 (5–6), 85–94.

Spencer, L. J. (1932), 'Hoba (South West Africa), the largest known meteorite', *Mineralogical Magazine and Journal of the Mineralogical Society* 23 (136), 1–19.

Stevenson, A. (2006), *Gerzeh: A Cemetery Shortly before History* (London: Golden House Publications).

Wainwright, G. A. (1911), 'Pre-dynastic iron beads in Egypt', *Man* 11, 177–8.

Wainwright, G. A. (1912), 'Pre-dynastic iron beads in Egypt', *Revue Aachéologique* 19, 255–9.

Wainwright, G. A. (1944), 'Rekhmire's metal-workers', *Man* 44, 94–8.

Waldbaum, J. C. (1978), *From Bronze to Iron: The Transition from the Bronze Age to the Iron Age in the Eastern Mediterranean* (Göteborg: Paul Åstroms Förlag).

Wilkinson, T. A. H. (1999), *Early Dynastic Egypt* (London: Routledge).

33

A bag-style tunic found on the Manchester Museum mummy 1770

Susan Martin

1770 is the accession number given to a mummy once held in the Manchester Museum Egyptology collection. There has been much debate over the date and gender of this mummy and whether it has been re-wrapped at some point in its history. 1770 is now, however, strongly believed to be the mummy of a female adolescent (David 1984: 41), and both the textiles and the human remains are considered to be contemporary and of Ptolemaic date (Cockitt, Martin and David 2014: 95–102; Martin 2008).

In June 1975 a multidisciplinary team lead by Rosalie David undertook an unwrapping and dissection of 1770: the team included specialists in dentistry, facial reconstruction, conservation, diagnostic radiology, histopathology, entomology and organic chemistry (David 1978: 85–6; Tapp 1979). The poorly preserved condition of both the body and the wrappings meant that a literal unwrapping of 1770 was not a viable option. The textiles were generally too fragmentary to enable the routes that they took around the body to be easily followed for any great distance, and the human remains were not well enough preserved to withstand the handling involved in an unwrapping. Instead it was decided that a dissection that worked along the mummy in sections in an organised and systematic manner was the most practical course of action. This strategy reflected the largely biomedical interests and strengths of the research team and resulted in a method that ultimately favoured the salvage of human material. At the time of the dissection the study of the textiles from 1770 did not feature prominently in the interests of the research team, and the wrappings received only minimal attention. The wrappings were, however, divided into numbered units as they were removed from the mummy and were then carefully retained and stored in the collections of the Manchester Museum; recently these wrappings have been revisited and studied in detail (Martin 2008).

This chapter explores one particular textile from the wrappings of 1770, which forms a largely complete simple bag-style tunic. Evidence of previous use was apparent in a number of the 190 units of textile removed from 1770; however, this bag tunic was by far the most outstanding example. The position of this garment among the mummy wrappings, the garment's condition and its overall construction are described; issues surrounding the manner in which the tunic might have been worn are discussed; and in particular, the notably large neck opening that the garment was found to have is evaluated.

Description of the extant 1770 tunic

The tunic was removed from below the centre back section of 1770; it had been roughly folded to form a pad measuring approximately 20 × 20 cm, and would have constituted part of the first layer of wrappings encountered by modern investigators directly below the thin strips of textile that made up the latticed decoration present on the outer surface of the mummy (Figure 33.1).

When the tunic was first examined for this study, one arm opening and a shoulder seam were clearly visible on the outer surface of the folded pad, as were extensive portions of a bottom hem. By lifting some of the folds, where the cloth was well preserved and flexible, a side seam could also be located. While it was clear from these features that the textile formed some type of garment, treatment by a specialist textile conservator was required to relax and unfold the tunic before it could be fully understood.

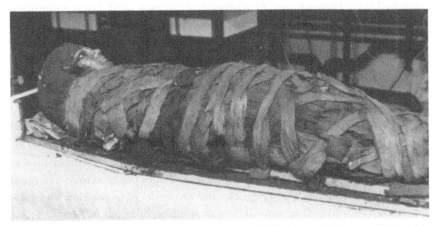

33.1 Mummy 1770 before dissection. (Courtesy of Manchester Museum, University of Manchester.)

As the tunic was relaxed it became apparent that some sections had suffered considerable damage. However, the surviving areas of the tunic can be described as follows. On one side of the tunic the shoulder seam, arm opening and side seam are virtually complete. The neckline continues from the shoulder seam for one face of the tunic; the bottom hem of the tunic is also complete for this same face. Much, but not all, of the bottom hem of the second face of the tunic has also survived. On the other side of the garment the lower portion of the second side seam is also present but the upper part of the tunic on this side is missing, resulting in the absence of the second arm opening and shoulder seam. Also the second face of the neckline is not present. The central section of the tunic has suffered a great deal of damage, and only a few narrow areas of remaining cloth still join the upper and lower portions of the tunic in this region. It is apparent from the surviving shoulder seam that the tunic is inside out, and must have been like this when folded and placed on the mummy by the embalmers.

The probable form of the 1770 tunic when complete

The majority of the extremities of the 1770 tunic survive (Plate 14), making it possible for a largely complete picture of the likely original form of the garment to be pieced together (Figure 33.2). From the sections of the tunic that survive it is possible to construct the following description of the garment when complete.

The tunic was formed from two separate rectangles of cloth of a well-woven but not particularly fine fabric. It is likely that the two pieces of cloth used to construct the tunic are from the same original web, as their overall appearance and their technical specifications are so similar. Both are a warp-faced medium plain weave, with an average yarn count per centimetre of 19 × 9. The warp threads are slightly packed at the selvedge edges but other than this the selvedges are plain. All of the yarns are s-spun with a medium to loose twist. Small variations in yarn diameter (0.5 mm to 0.8 mm) and colour give a slight longitudinal striped effect to the cloth.

One rectangle of fabric formed the front face of the tunic, and the second rectangle formed the back face of the tunic. This method of construction would seem to be unparalleled among extant Pharaonic bag tunics. It is more usual for a bag tunic to be formed from a single length of cloth which has been folded in half at the shoulders, with an opening then being cut for the head to pass through (Vogelsang-Eastwood 1993: 134–5). The two rectangles of fabric from which the 1770 tunic was formed measure 80 cm in width and 83 cm in length. These dimensions fall somewhere between those commonly recorded for garments intended for adults and garments intended for children (Vogelsang-Eastwood

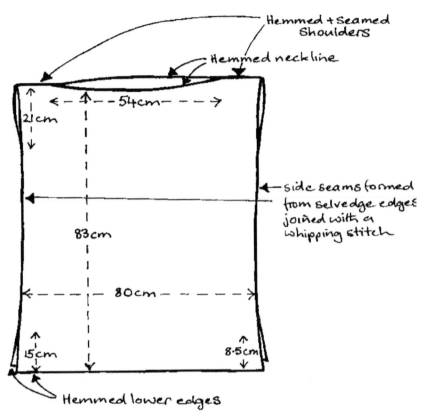

Hemmed + Seamed Shoulders

Hemmed neckline

54cm

21cm

side seams formed from selvedge edges joined with a whipping stitch

83cm

80cm

5cm

8·5cm

Hemmed lower edges

33.2 The likely form of the 1770 bag-tunic when complete. (Created by the author.)

1993: 139–41). Therefore, the 1770 tunic can be considered to be a relatively small garment perhaps intended for an adolescent.

The two pieces of fabric that make up the 1770 tunic were cut from full widths of cloth with both selvedge edges present. The edges of the selvedge were positioned along the sides of the tunic. The cut edges that formed the top and the bottom of the tunic were finished with hems. The bottom hems and the surviving shoulder hem (the hemming of the shoulders does not continue over the neckline) are both stitched in a very neat and regular fashion. The stitching is carried out in the manner shown in Figure 33.3a. There are two stitches per centimetre, and the stitching is obvious on the outer surface of the tunic. The shoulder seam was then formed by joining the hemmed top edges at the outer side of the rectangles of fabric in the manner shown in Figure 33.3b; again there are two stitches per centimetre, and the surviving shoulder seam extends 13 cm in from the outer edge of the garment.

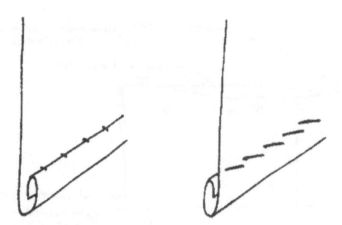

33.3a Diagram of folded and stitched hem. (Created by the author.)

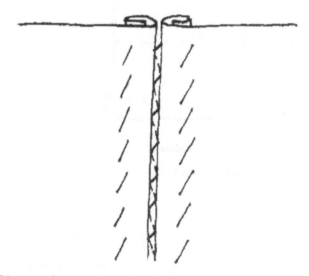

33.3b Diagram of a seam where the edges of the fabric are hemmed before the seam is made. (Created by the author.)

The single face of the neckline that survives continues straight across from the surviving shoulder seam, making it clear that the 1770 tunic did not have the cut out 'keyhole' neckline typical of bag tunics (Vogelsang-Eastwood 1993: 134–5). There is no way of knowing whether the straight section of neckline that survives would have been intended as the neckline for the front face or the back face of the tunic. It is also impossible to determine whether the missing face would have taken the same form as this or would have been cut and styled differently. It is possible that the half of the neckline no longer in existence may have been worn to the front and that a vertical slit may have existed creating a T-shaped neck opening. In either case, if the surviving shoulder seam is complete, and the opposite shoulder seam would have matched it in length, then the neck opening on this garment would have measured about 54 cm across from one shoulder to the other. This measurement is notably large: a similarly styled neck opening in a comparable tunic of otherwise similar dimensions measures a much smaller 32 cm from shoulder to shoulder (Crowfoot 1989).

The neckline of the 1770 tunic is hemmed in a similar manner to the seams that run across the top of the shoulders but has been sewn separately. The rolled edge of the neckline is completed in a continuous round, and has been sewn using a single ply thread as opposed to the two-ply thread used for the shoulder hems and seam. The stitching of the neckline is less even than the stitching of the shoulder hems and the bottom hem. In some places there are two stitches per centimetre while in other places there is only one.

The front and back face of the tunic are joined with stitching at each side. The side seam that survives intact on the left of the garment has been stitched for a distance of 53 cm. A gap of about 21 cm has been left at the top of the side seam to create an opening for the arm to pass through. This arm opening has not been finished in any further manner and is edged simply by the selvedge edges of the cloth. There is no evidence that sleeves had ever been attached to the tunic: no marks indicating previous stitching are present around the arm openings. The size of the arm opening, at 21 cm, is relatively small (Vogelsang-Eastwood 1993: 134–5), again indicating that the garment was probably not intended for a fully grown adult.

The side seams also do not continue all the way down to the bottom of the garment: the left one ends 8.5 cm from the bottom hem while the right one ends 15 cm from it. This appears to be a deliberate styling device, the motivations for which may have been either practical or aesthetic. The latter of these two options is perhaps the more convincing: arguably these slits would have allowed the wearer greater ease of movement, but the garment is already loosely cut and would not have reached to the lower legs where such a feature would have been more likely to serve a practical purpose.

The stitching of the two side seams is not alike and even within one seam the stitching varies, indicating that the seams have probably been repaired over time. This strongly suggests that the garment had been worn before it became part of the wrappings for 1770. Although irregular, and in places messy, the side seams are generally stitched in a manner similar to that shown in Figure 33.3c. The bottom edges of both the front and the back face of the tunic are hemmed in a similar manner to the shoulder and neck edges (Figure 33.3a).

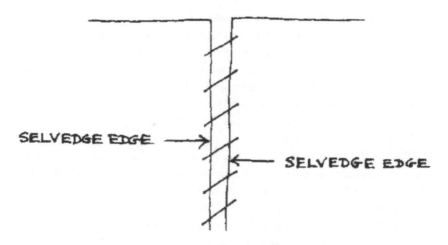

33.3c Diagram of a seam where two selvedge edges are joined with a whipping stitch. (Created by the author.)

Who wore the 1770 tunic and how would it have been worn?

Evidence would point to the fact that the 1770 tunic had been used before it was incorporated into the mummy bundle. There are clear signs of wear on the fabric, and some of the seams and hems appear to have been repaired. Whether the tunic would have been worn by 1770, a female adolescent of high status, is less clear.

The relatively modest length and width of the 1770 tunic (Vogelsang-Eastwood 1993: 139–41) and its small arm opening indicate a tunic that is likely to have been intended for use by an adolescent. Even on a younger person the tunic would not have been a long garment: at most the hemline would have reached to the level of the knee. Artistic depictions showing tunics in use provide some evidence to suggest that while full-length tunics would have been worn by both men and women in ancient Egypt the shorter version would have been worn only by men (Vogelsang-Eastwood 1993: 144–54). Arguably, therefore, the 1770 tunic would seem to have been intended for use by a male adolescent, while 1770 is thought likely to be the mummy of a female (David 1984: 41).

If the interpretation of the neckline previously made is correct and the neck opening did in fact measure 54 cm across from one shoulder seam to the other, the shoulders of an adolescent of average build would have easily passed through the neck opening if the garment was worn loose. If the garment was indeed intended for an adolescent, the tunic would, at the very least, have had to be carefully gathered and pleated to avoid it falling off the shoulders of the wearer. To achieve this effect the tunic would have to have been belted in some manner: with either a sash, a kilt, or a wrap-around skirt of some kind. In support of this theory it is common for artistic representations to show the full-length bag tunic worn alone, while shorter versions are often depicted in combination with a kilt and/or a sash (Riefstahl 1970). Even bearing in mind these various approaches, the neck opening of the 1770 tunic would still seem to be unusually large: this leads us to consider two other possible solutions for wear.

Firstly, the neck of the tunic could have been narrowed by some form of pinning. It has been argued that Roman military tunics may have been fastened at the shoulder in this manner (Fuentes 1987). However, a careful examination of the top edge of the 1770 tunic produced no evidence of the use of pins with this garment.

Secondly, the idea that the tunic was actively designed as a garment intended to be worn falling off one shoulder should also be explored. If one looks beyond Egypt to the wider Roman world, artistic representations of tunics intentionally worn fully off one shoulder can be found (Croom 2000: 38, fig. 3; Strong 1923: pl. XLIII): these are usually depictions of farm-workers and labourers wearing short tunics with their right arm and the right side of their chest exposed. An empty right arm opening is often clearly visible hanging at waist level in the folds of the tunic, showing that the wearer had chosen to extract his right arm from a two-armed garment (Figure 33.4a) and was not wearing a tunic that been designed with only one arm opening on the left-hand side. To enable a tunic to be worn in this manner the neck opening would have had to be large, as in the 1770 tunic. Other images can be found that depict short-sleeved tunics worn with both arm openings in use but with a knot tied at the nape of the neck (Figure 33.4b), presumably to reduce the size of the neck opening in a tunic that was designed with the option of being worn off one shoulder (Bandinelli 1971: pl. 175; Croom 2000: 38–9; Fuentes 1987; Houston 1965: 97). 1770 would almost certainly have been an individual of high status, and therefore this interpretation of the tunic would further support the theory that it was a garment that was worn by someone other than 1770.

Conclusion

The dissection of 1770 in the mid-1970s was a rare event, but as non-invasive research techniques have improved and attitudes towards the use of human remains for purposes of research have, in general, changed it is now regarded as an event that is unlikely to occur again. The access that the dissection of 1770 gave to the mummy's wrappings should therefore be recognised as a very rare and a very important textile research opportunity.

The dissection of 1770 made possible the study of a dated collection of

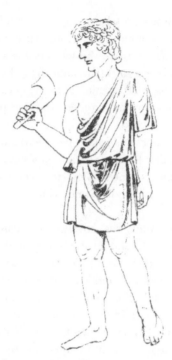

33.4a Bag-tunic with two arm openings with one shoulder exposed, depicted on a vine dresser in the Torre del Padiglione relief. (Created by the author after Fuentes 1987, Fig. 1, citing Strong 1923, Tav. XLIII.)

textiles that, as re-used items, presents an important opportunity to comment on the everyday use of textiles in Ptolemaic Egypt. The 1770 tunic in particular provides a rare chance to study an everyday garment of Ptolemaic date: to comment on its construction, and to consider how it might have been worn and by whom.

The 1770 tunic is of a simple bag style and of relatively small dimensions. It conforms closely in overall appearance to the standard definition of a bag tunic; however, in several details of its construction it is unusual. Firstly, it is constructed from two separate pieces of cloth as opposed to one longer piece that has been folded in half. Secondly, its neck opening has been formed from the top edges of these two separate pieces of cloth and has not been cut out in the keyhole shape more commonly seen. Finally, this straight horizontal neck opening is notably large.

While there is strong evidence to suggest that the tunic would have seen use before it became part of the 1770 wrappings, who would have actually owned and worn this garment is less clear. In terms of its dimensions the tunic would have been a suitable size for use by 1770 in life. However, short bag

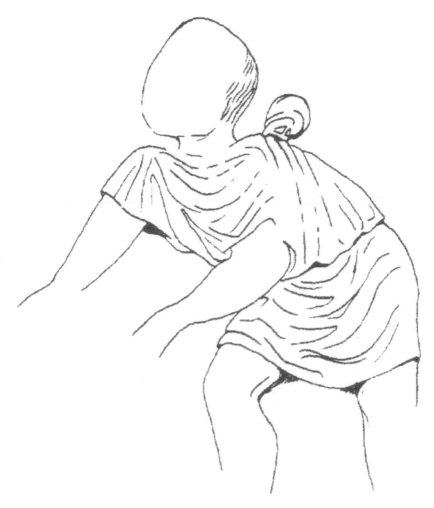

33.4b Knotted tunic worn by an olive harvester, adapted from a depiction of a second-century AD bas relief in the Museo Arqueológico Provincial, Cordova. (Created by the author after Fuentes 1987, Fig. 2, citing Bandinelli 1971: pl. 175.)

tunics have been more commonly associated with male wearers while 1770 is believed to be the mummy of an adolescent female. Added to this the styling of the neckline could, arguably, suggest a garment used by someone engaged in physical work. This interpretation is at odds with the obvious high status of 1770. Thus, while from the evidence available it would seem likely that the tunic had indeed been used, it seems less likely that it had been a part of 1770's wardrobe in life.

References

Bandinelli, R. B. (1971), *Rome, the Late Empire: Roman Art AD 200–400* (London: Thames and Hudson).

Cockitt, J. A., Martin, S. O. and David, A. R. (2014), 'A new assessment of the radio-carbon age of the mummy no. 1770', *Yearbook of Mummy Studies* 2 (Munich: Verlag Dr Friedrich Pfeil), 95–102.

Croom, A. T. (2000), *Roman Clothing and Fashion* (Stroud: Tempus Publishing).

Crowfoot, E. (1989), 'A Romano-Egyptian dress of the first century BC?', *Textile History* 20 (2), 123–8.

David, A. R. (ed.) (1978). *Mysteries of the Mummies: The Story of the Manchester University Investigation* (London: Book Club Associates).

David, A. R. (1984). 'Introduction', in A. R. David and E. Tapp (eds.), *Evidence Embalmed: Modern Medicine and the Mummies of Ancient Egypt* (Manchester: Manchester University Press), 3–42.

Fuentes, N. (1987), 'The Roman military tunic', in M. Dawson (ed.), *Roman Military Equipment: The Accoutrements of War. Proceedings of the Third Roman Military Equipment Research Seminar* (Oxford: Archaeopress), 41–76.

Houston, M. G. (1965), *Ancient Greek, Roman and Byzantine Costume and Decoration* (London: Barnes and Noble).

Martin, S. O. (2008), 'Ancient Egyptian Mummy Wrappings from the Mummy 1770: A Technological and Social Study' (PhD dissertation, University of Manchester).

Reifstahl, E. (1970), 'A note on ancient fashions: four early Egyptian dresses in the Museum of Fine Arts, Boston', *Bulletin of the Museum of Fine Arts Boston* 68, 244–9.

Strong, E. (1923), *La scultura romana da Augusto a Constantino*, II (Florence: Fratelli Alinari).

Tapp, E. (1979), 'The unwrapping of a mummy', in A. R. David (ed.), *The Manchester Museum Mummy Project: Multidisciplinary Research on Ancient Egyptian Mummified Remains* (Manchester: Manchester University Press), 83–93.

Vogelsang-Eastwood, G. M. (1993), *Pharaonic Egyptian Clothing* (Leiden: Brill).

34

'Palmiform' columns: an alternative design source

J. Peter Phillips

The proposition advanced in this chapter was first suggested to the author by the late Robert B. Partridge (1951–2011) (see Bierbrier 2012: 417), and was first mentioned briefly in my book *The Columns of Egypt* (Phillips 2002: 16–18). Bob Partridge studied for the Certificate in Egyptology at the University of Manchester under Dr (now Professor) David. In his later life he became a prominent member of the Egyptology community both in the UK and worldwide, and was a strong supporter of Rosalie's work.

Column types

From the 4th Dynasty onwards, the ancient Egyptians used a limited number of column types in the construction of their monumental buildings. These types held particular significances and followed strict design and location criteria. It is likely that designs used in domestic architecture, which were made of perishable materials that have not survived, were more freely interpreted than the monumental forms they inspired. The stone columns employed in temple construction fall into two broad categories: those whose design is based upon plant forms of some variety and those, such as octagonal and sixteen-sided columns, which are ultimately derived from simple pillars with a square cross-section by progressive removal of the corners.

Although the types of temple column remained basically unchanged for thousands of years, they did evolve very gradually. The papyrus cluster columns erected in Amenhotep III's reign in Luxor temple evolved, via the elaborate type of columns raised during Akhenaten's reign at Akhetaten, into the papyrus bud columns of Ramesside temples. The campaniform ('bell-shaped') papyrus columns of Luxor temple, each of which represents, on a massive scale, a single stem of papyrus with an open flower, appear in stone there for the first time since they were utilised in Djoser's Step Pyramid complex as symbolic of northern Egypt. These columns evolved in the Late Period into the elaborate floral capitals of the composite columns seen in Ptolemaic and Roman temples.

The most common type of 'plant' column surviving from the Old and New Kingdoms is the papyrus cluster (or papyrus bundle) column. The design of this column is clearly based upon a bundle of stems of the papyrus plant, with unopened flowers, bound together. The individual elements of the shaft are triangular in cross-section, like stems of papyrus; the overall bulging profile of the column represents the shape of the papyrus plant, and even the leaves at the base of the papyrus stems are copied in stone.[1]

The palmiform column

There is one type of column, however, first seen in the Old Kingdom, which was virtually unchanged throughout the remainder of pharaonic history and was still being erected alongside composite columns in the Ptolemaic Period. It is the type customarily known as 'palmiform' because of its resemblance to the date palm trees that grow everywhere in Egypt.

Ludwig Borchardt was the first to classify 'plant' columns in a formal way in his slim volume *Die aegyptische Pflanzensäule* (1897). In the early chapters of this work, Borchardt defines lotus, lily and papyrus columns and then goes on to describe *Palmensäulen* (palm columns). Borchardt says of the palmiform design:

> Bei dieser Art von Säulen können wir auf die Beschreibung der ihr zu Grunde liegenden Pflanze und der ägyptischen Darstellungen derselben verzichten, da seit dem Bekanntwerden der ersten Säulen dieser Art es nie zweifelhaft war, welche Pflanze in dem architektionisch ausgebildeten Säulentypus gemeint war, und da auch gar keine Möglichkeit vorliegt, diese Pflanzensäule mit irgend einer anderen zu verwechseln, was bei den bisher abgehandelten eher möglich und auch leider reichlich der Fall war. Es mag daher die hier gegebene Abbildung ... und der Hinweis auf die Beschreibung der Dattelpalme 'Phoenix dactylifera L.' genügen, welche sich sehr ausführlich in der Description de l'Egypte, Teil 19, S. 436 ff. und Tat. 62 findet. (Borchardt 1897: 44)
>
> With this type of column we can dispense with the description of the plant it is based on and the Egyptian representations of the same, since there has never been any doubt about the plant represented by this column type since it has become known, and as there is no possibility of confusing this plant column with any other, as might have been the case, and unfortunately

---

1   For a full discussion of the classification and evolution of column types, the reader is referred to Phillips 2002, within which are many relevant illustrations which cannot be included in this chapter because of space constraints.

occurred frequently, with the previously discussed [column types]. Therefore the image reproduced here ... and the reference to the very detailed description of the date palm *Phoenix dactylifera L.* suffices, which can be found from page 436, and on Plate 62, in Part 19 of *Description de L'Egypte.*[2]

While I cannot disagree with Borchardt's statement regarding other plant column types (papyrus cluster columns are very frequently referred to as lotus columns, for example, even in academic journals), I must take issue with his opening statement. I am of the opinion that there is considerable doubt as to the 'plant it is based on'.

It is clear that by the time of the Roman occupation of Egypt, this type of column was indeed thought by its builders to represent the date palm. Beneath the capitals, the upper part of the shaft is sometimes carved to represent the characteristic triangular-shaped pattern seen on the trunks of date palm trees (caused by the removal of old dead fronds as the tree grows). In some cases, such as in the outer courtyard of the temple of Isis at Philae, bunches of dates are carved at the base of the fronds of the capitals and above the horizontal bands at the top of the shafts (Phillips 2002: 17, figures 34a, b). Herodotus in his *Histories* (II, 169) describes the temple of Neith at Sais, which he visited early in the 27th Dynasty, as 'a great cloistered building of stone, decorated with pillars carved in imitation of palm trees' (De Sélincourt and Marincola 2003: 165). This identification had already become established by the time of Nectanebo I, since there exist the remains of palmiform capitals with carved bunches of dates from the Mammisi that was erected by him at Dendera (Phillips 2002: 159).

However, the earliest extant columns of this type to be erected in stone were found in the Valley Temple and Memorial Temple of Sahura (*c*.2487–2475 BC) at Abusir, as described by Borchardt in his excavation report (1910) and illustrated in Figure 34.1. It is easy to see that the significance and origin of this column type could have been forgotten in the intervening two millennia, and they may not in fact have been inspired by the date palm tree.

Description

The Sahura columns of this type are monolithic and carved from granite. They have shafts with a circular cross-section that taper gradually without any of the bulge characteristic of papyrus columns. Apart from a simple inscription identifying the pharaoh, the shafts are undecorated. The capitals represent fronds of some type which are bound around the top of the shaft. The binding 'rope' is depicted wound around the shaft five times, and below this there is a U-shaped

---

2   Translation by Birgit Schoer.

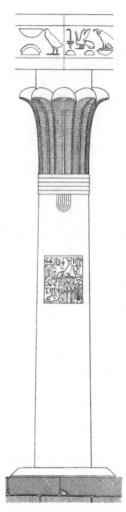

34.1 A typical 'palm' column from the Sahura mortuary complex at Abusir.
(Created by the author after Borchardt 1910: Blatt 9.)

carving. This U shape is always arranged to be as visible as possible, for instance facing outwards to an open courtyard. Monolithic granite columns of this type bearing the cartouche of Ramesses II and other pharaohs are to be seen at several locations in Egypt, such as Tanis, but it is likely that they originated in the Old Kingdom and had been re-used several times. The fact that they are carved from single blocks of granite transported hundreds of miles from Aswan would have made them very valuable.

Six monolithic granite palmiform columns were excavated by Naville in 1891 from the pronaos of Herakleopolis Magna and sent to museums: the British

Museum (EA 1123), the Manchester Museum (1780), Bolton Museum and Art
Gallery (1891.14.1/1891.14.2), the South Australian Museum at Adelaide (inventory number not known), the Museum of Fine Arts, Boston (91.259), and the
University Museum, University of Pennsylvania, Philadelphia (E636). Detailed
analysis by Yoshifumi Yasuoka (2011: 31–60) of the inscriptions on these columns
confirmed that they were indeed usurped by Ramesses II from originals almost
certainly of Old Kingdom date. Yasuoka also speculated that the re-use of these
columns at the Herakleopolis Magna pronaos may have been supervised by
Khaemwaset, fourth son of Ramesses II.

Antecedents

The design of all stone 'plant' columns is probably based on prototypes made in
wood, which themselves copy the original plants. In the case of the 'palmiform'
column this is certainly true, as earlier wooden examples on a small scale have
survived in the 'cabin' of Khufu's solar boat reconstructed beside his pyramid
at Giza. The finial of the carrying chair found in the tomb of Khufu's mother,
Hetepheres, also has exactly the same design as this type of column capital
(Phillips 2002: 18, fig. 38). There seems little doubt that wooden columns of this
design were used in Khufu's palaces.

Palm fronds or feathers

The identification of these columns as originally representing the date palm has
a number of problems, and it is my contention that they could also represent
large ostrich feathers bound around a pole as in Figure 34.2. If the intention
had been to represent a date palm tree, in the same way as the papyrus columns
represent the papyrus plant, the ancient Egyptians would have had no difficulty
in carving the column shaft in the characteristic pattern of the trunk of a date
palm tree. When they wished to identify a column as a bundle of papyrus stems,
they carved these in a realistic manner. Instead, apart from any inscriptions, the
shafts of 'palm' columns are completely smooth, indicating that the Sahura ones
represent substantial poles made of some other type of wood. Strong wooden
poles of large dimensions were not available to the ancient Egyptians from their
native trees; this perhaps implies that the shafts represent cedar poles imported
from Lebanon similar to the flagpoles placed in front of temple pylons. In
its turn, this implies that the poles being represented were prestigious items,
something that could not be said of palm tree trunks.

The capital represents fronds of some type bound to the shaft with a rope.
If the intention was to represent a date palm tree, there would be no point
in attaching cut fronds to a pole: it would be much more effective to carve a

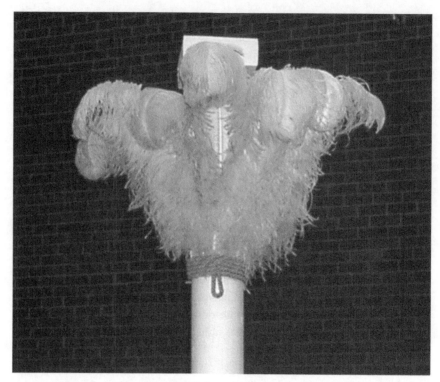

34.2 Ostrich feathers bound round a pole. (Photograph by R. B. Partridge.)

complete tree. The carving of the fronds does show similarities to the fronds of a date palm, but also to large ostrich feathers.

If real palm fronds had been bound round a pole in this fashion they would have needed to be replaced at very frequent intervals; otherwise they would have shrivelled and turned brown and brittle, or drooped untidily as they do on an unmanaged date palm tree. Viewed from above, the capital does not have the sharp jagged appearance of palm fronds, but rather the soft curl of feathers. A surviving capital in the Mit Rahina site museum illustrates this point well (Figure 34.3).

Ostrich feathers

Ostriches were well known to the ancient Egyptians. Depictions of them appear on Predynastic pots and, in the scene from the south wall of the forecourt of the temple of Beit el-Wali, both live ostriches and ostrich feathers are shown being presented as tribute to Ramesses II (Roeder 1938: 31–42, pls. 32–4). Ostrich-feather fans were also used: the handle of one in the form of a head

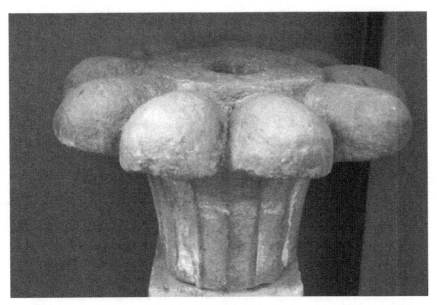

34.3 A 'palm' column capital in the Mit Rahina site museum. (Photograph by R. B. Partridge.)

of Hathor is on display in the Nebamun Gallery of the British Museum with modern feathers attached (EA 20767). The fan originated in Thebes, dates to the New Kingdom and was purchased by Wallis Budge in 1888. Because of the difficulty of capturing the birds, we might expect that ostrich feathers were a luxury and would have been displayed in royal palaces as symbols of the wealth of the pharaoh. Ostrich feathers tied in this way round a cedar pole would have been permanent and much more attractive and decorative than palm fronds. According to W. M. Flinders Petrie, a column capital found by him at the site of an Amarna palace and depicted in his volume *Tell el-Amarna* was decorated with coloured inlays in a pattern that resembles the cloisonné work used in jewellery to depict feathers (Petrie 1894: 10, pl. VI; Phillips 2002: 246–7, fig. 502).

The feather of Maat

In many depictions of the Book of the Dead on papyri and elsewhere, the heart of the deceased is shown being weighed on scales against the feather of Maat, representing justice and order. The goddess Maat was depicted with a feather on her head, and human figures wearing feather headdresses are depicted on Predynastic pottery and inscriptions. The feather, therefore, had a religious significance. Used on column-capitals in palaces and temples, they would have emphasised the stability of the kingdom and the maintenance of Maat. The palm frond has no such obvious connotations.

Binding

At the top of the shaft below the capital are carved five horizontal rings around the shaft's circumference. It seems entirely reasonable to assume that these represent successive turns of a rope used to bind the fronds of the capital to the shaft. The same five rings also appear below the capital of the papyrus cluster columns that make their first appearance in stone in the 5th Dynasty at Abusir (Phillips 2002: 52–3), where they can be taken to represent rope binding together a number of separate papyrus plants. When they are similarly used in Luxor temple on the campaniform papyrus columns that appear to represent single papyrus plants with open flowers, their use can be explained only as an artistic convention analogous to their use on the papyrus cluster columns. The Amenhotep III columns were created over a thousand years after the Sahura ones. There is no trace of this 'binding' on the attached campaniform papyrus columns in Djoser's Step Pyramid complex (Phillips 2002: 40, fig. 71).

However, on the Sahura 'palm' columns, and only on this type of column, a further device is shown below the binding: a U shape. At first glance, this seems to represent three nested U-shaped narrow ropes, but could as easily be intended to show two nested U's with a space between the ropes. How can this device be explained?

The carving of the binding may represent the kind of 'whipping' that is still used today to fasten objects tightly to a pole. The problem encountered by anyone attempting this task is that of securing the ends of the rope so that it does not unravel. This is accomplished by the method shown in Figure 34.4.

The rope is firstly laid along the length of the pole and subsequently doubled back on itself to the original start point (1). It is then wound several times round the pole and the doubled end of the rope (2). The remainder of the rope is then passed through the loop at the bottom of the binding (3), and by pulling on the loop of rope from the top end of the binding (4) the loose end of the rope can be pulled under the binding, and thus hidden from sight and tightly secured (5). This may be the situation depicted in the binding of the papyrus cluster columns. When complete, this kind of binding is not only effective but also permanent, in that it is unable to be undone except by cutting the binding rope.

In a speculative alternative to the method of 'whipping' just described, the starting doubled length of rope can again be doubled (6), then wound as before and passed through the double loop at the bottom of the binding (7). If the resulting U is tightened by pulling first on the right-hand side of the loop at the top of the binding (8) and then on the left-hand side of the same loop (9),

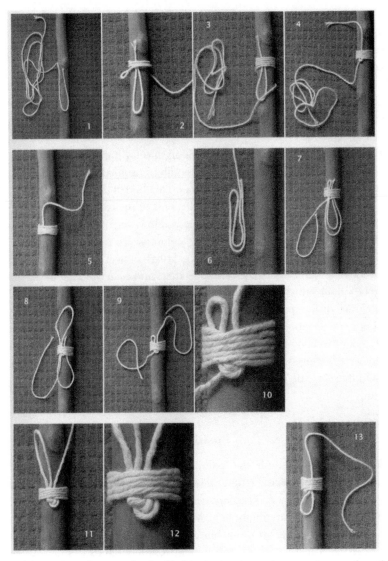

34·4 Illustration of two methods of 'whipping', using string round a wooden stick.
(Photographs by the author.)

without actually pulling the open end of the rope under the binding (10), and
the end of the rope is passed through the hole in the U and tucked under the
binding (11), the end is again secured. The final result resembles the double U
of the carving (12), although the narrowness of the rope in the Sahura carving is
not replicated. This discrepancy could perhaps be explained as artistic licence,
since ancient Egyptian art rarely respects true proportions.

The binding itself, being more important, is carved full size, while the method of securing the end of the rope is relatively insignificant and therefore carved on a lesser scale. Interestingly, the ropes in the U carved in the reign of Hakor of the 29th Dynasty, at the temple of Amun at Hibis in Kharga Oasis, are of the same width as the binding rope above, and show two nested U's (Phillips 2002: 157, figs. 304–5). A similarly large double U is shown on the previously mentioned surviving column in Nectanebo I's Mammisi at Dendera (Phillips 2002: 159, fig. 309).

However, this second method of binding has an important advantage over the first. If the outside U is pulled, the binding is immediately released without the need to cut the rope (13). Thus the second method of binding, with the double loop, provides a method by which the elements of the capital could be changed frequently if they were in fact palm fronds. However, it is also relevant if the fronds were ostrich feathers. The stone columns are copies of wooden ones, which would have stood in mud-brick buildings subject to frequent alteration. The wooden column shafts, the ostrich feathers and even the rope of the binding would be valuable materials that could be re-used in later constructions.

A clump of live papyrus plants, bound together at the top of their stems, could not conceivably have been used to support a roof, so the stone papyrus cluster columns copy either earlier wooden models of the plants, or the plants themselves growing symbolically on the 'mound of creation' within the temple. It would therefore be irrelevant to represent removable binding on this type of column.

Positioning

In Sahura's Valley Temple the 'palmiform' columns form the entrance portico and in his Memorial Temple they surround the outer courtyard (Phillips 2002: 52, fig. 99; Plate 15). They are used in small palaces attached to both the Ramesseum and the large temple at Medinet Habu (Phillips 2002: 254–5, fig. 522), and their presence in the cabin of Khufu's boat suggests that they may have been used in prominent positions in Khufu's palaces. They were used in Akhenaten's palaces at Amarna and in the palace of Apries at Memphis (Phillips 2002: 258, figs. 530–1). If the objective of their positioning was to impress the visitor, ostrich feathers would have been much more successful than date palm fronds.

Conclusion

Although the 'palmiform' columns may have imitated date palm fronds tied round a pole, and by the Late Period they were undoubtedly thought to be stone versions of date palm trees, it is quite conceivable that their origins in the Old Kingdom had been forgotten. There is a very real possibility that early palaces and temples were adorned with valuable imported ostrich feathers bound around imported cedar poles, and that these were copied firstly in miniature in carved wood, and later on a grand scale in granite (transported with huge effort from Aswan), making a statement of enormous wealth and power.

References

Bierbrier, M. L. (ed.) (2012), *Who Was Who in Egyptology*, 4th edn (London: Egypt Exploration Society).

Borchardt, L. (1897), *Die aegyptische Pflanzensäule: Ein Kapitel zur Geschichte des Pflanzenornaments* (Berlin: E. Wasmuth).

Borchardt, L. (1910), *Das Grabdenkmal des Königs S'ahu-re I: Der Bau* (Leipzig: J. C. Hinrichs).

De Sélincourt, A. (trans.) and Marincola, J. M. (ed.) (2003), Herodotus, *The Histories*, revised edn (London: Penguin).

Petrie, W. M. F. (1894), *Tell el-Amarna* (London: Methuen).

Phillips, J. P. (2002), *The Columns of Egypt* (Manchester: Peartree).

Roeder, G. (1938), *Der Felsentemplel von Bet el-Wali* (Cairo: Institut français d'archéologie orientale).

Yasuoka, Y. (2011), 'Some remarks on the palm columns from the pronaos of Herakleopolis Magna', *Journal of Egyptian Archaeology* 97, 31–60.

35

Scientific evaluation of experiments in Egyptian archaeology

Denys A. Stocks

I first met Professor Rosalie David in 1979 as an enrolled member of her introductory course in Egyptology. The meeting with Rosalie changed the direction of my life, for in 1980 I enrolled for her Certificate in Egyptology course, which later led to a research degree, a teaching qualification and a position as a teacher of design and technology, and of history.

About ten years earlier I had commenced an ancient Egyptian technology research project incorporating craftworking techniques, which involved the manufacture of replica and reconstructed tools made from wood, stone, copper, bronze and other materials for test and evaluation. I constructed a home workshop containing a furnace for casting the copper and bronze tools, the first ones cast being replicas of anciently designed flat and crosscut tapered chisels.

During an interview with Rosalie, mainly to discuss the subject area for the Certificate in Egyptology dissertation, I showed to her some of my cast copper chisels, and she mentioned that they were similar to copper chisels in the basement store and in the display cases of the Manchester Museum. I also pointed out six indentations on each replica chisel's edged taper, created by a hardness testing machine. We discussed the use of scientific methods to assist with the evaluation of a chisel's hardness and its associated capability for cutting types of wood and stone. Rosalie expressed a commitment to scientific methods for supporting future evaluations of experiments completed as part of my ancient Egyptian technology research project. In 1986, she kindly made contacts within the University of Manchester on my behalf, which resulted in an invitation by the late Professor Barri Jones to enrol for the degree of Master of Philosophy in the Department of Archaeology: Rosalie became my supervisor for this degree.

This chapter is presented in honour of Rosalie for her much appreciated help in developing my ancient Egyptian technology project. It summarises three areas of my research that benefited from extra evaluations using scientific methods, beginning with the experimental manufacture and test of replica copper and bronze chisels to establish what resistant materials could be cut by ancient chisels. As a matter of interest, particular scientific principles that ancient craftworkers employed in the construction and use of their tools, and in their manufacturing technologies, are discussed.

Hardness and cutting comparisons between experimental and ancient copper and bronze chisels

The experimental manufacture of twelve test copper and bronze chisels commenced by accurately weighing copper and varying quantities of other constituent metals, such as iron, tin and antimony, and then casting each individual chisel in a clean crucible. Upon becoming cold, each casting immediately received a sequential identity project number punched into it before its designated flat or crosscut taper was hammered to shape. This number referred to its metallic content, its scientifically determined hardness and its performance in cutting different wood and stone types (Stocks 1988, II: appendix C, 1–4; appendix H, 1–6).

The casting of the chisels took place in open sand moulds. Six chisels were designated as copper tools, project nos. 1–4, 6 and 26, and six chisels designated as bronze tools, project nos. 9–11, 18, 22 and 25 (see Table 35.1 for contents of both chisel types). In particular, the three bronze chisels 18, 25 and 22 contain 8 per cent, 10 per cent and 12 per tin content respectively. Some preliminary hardness testing of project bronze chisels, containing between 8 per cent and 12 per cent tin, indicated twin advantages of hardness and durability for these tools.

As an integral part in determining each chisel's capability to cut resistant materials, its edged taper received a hardness test after *cold* hammering the metal into shape, this being the only way in which to work-harden non-ferrous metals (Rickard 1932, I: 116), in contrast to ferrous alloys, such as steel, which require high temperatures. Red-hot copper and bronze become brittle because of changes to their crystal structures at elevated temperatures (Rickard 1932, I: 116). For example, a project-manufactured bronze chisel, containing 5 per cent tin, when raised to a bright red heat and hammered immediately, fractured into several pieces (Stocks 1988, I: 77). Copper and bronze tools – chisels, adzes and axes – normally require these metals to be annealed during the hammering process in order to restore malleability and to delay cracks from forming, particularly for bronze tools containing significant amounts of tin. However, metallurgical studies have revealed that ancient tools were sometimes heavily cold-worked without any annealing (Maddin *et al.* 1984: 39). Annealing is achieved by heating the metal to a dull red heat and allowing it to cool slowly in the air: quenching in cold water is inappropriate for non-ferrous metals. However, the project chisels were hammered to shape without annealing in order to obtain the highest possible hardness results.

In order to determine each numbered chisel's hardness, testing was carried out on its hammered taper using a Vickers pyramid hardness testing machine: hardness is established by the use of an inverted, pyramid-shaped diamond indenter placed under a known load for a known fixed time. Six indentations are made into a chisel's taper. The Vickers Pyramid Number (VPN), resulting from a mathematical equation, is an expression of the relationship of a known force upon a known area, and the higher the number obtained the harder the specimen. The average of the six values obtained from the six indentations gives the final VPN (see Table 35.1).

The hardness tests show that the six replica copper chisels range from VPN 132 to VPN 167, being harder than annealed (softened) mild steel of hardness VPN 131 (Rollason 1939: 3, table 1). The six bronze chisels range from VPN 161 to VPN 247, with some of them exceeding the hardness of cold-rolled (hardened) mild steel of hardness VPN 192 (Stocks 1988, II: appendix B). Bronze chisel project nos. 22 and 25 are harder than modern unworked chisel steel of hardness VPN 235 (Rollason 1939: 3, table 1), but hammered chisel

Table 35.1   Hardness results for replica copper and bronze chisels

Chisel no.	Metal type	Chisel taper	Cu %	Sn %	Fe %	Pb %	Sb %	VPN
1	copper	flat	98	0.5	1.5	–	–	132
2	copper	flat	96	1.1	2.9	–	–	134
3	copper	crosscut	96	1.5	2.5	–	–	146
4	copper	flat	96	1.8	2.2	–	–	154
6	copper	flat	96	2.0	2.0	–	–	167
26	copper	flat	98	0.6	0.5	0.7	0.2	140
9	bronze	crosscut	97	3.0	–	–	–	161
10	bronze	crosscut	95	5.0	–	–	–	180
11	bronze	flat	93	7.0	–	–	–	188
18	bronze	flat	92	8.0	–	–	–	232
25	bronze	flat	90	10.0	–	–	–	239
22	bronze	flat	88	12.0	–	–	–	247

Abbreviations: Cu = copper, Sn = tin, Fe = iron, Pb = lead, Sb = antimony

Note: The table is organised, for bronze chisels, to show increasing proportions of tin and not according to sequential project numbers.

steel's hardness is VPN 800 (Rollason 1939: 3, table 1). During the project, a test to destruction of a 10 per cent tin in bronze casting, using hammer blows of considerable force, soon caused it to fracture, the highest hardness VPN 256 being recorded.

The testing of each replica copper and bronze chisel for cutting materials, such as types of stone, could now be related to that particular chisel's known metallic content and its hardness VPN. In this study, composition analyses of some *ancient* copper and bronze chisels would provide a guide to *estimated* hardness numbers for them, and that these estimated hardness numbers would indicate ancient chisels' capabilities for cutting particular stone types when compared with the cutting tests performed by replica copper and bronze chisels of broadly similar metallic content.

Stonecutting tests commenced with the replica copper flat and crosscut tapered chisels. The stones utilised for test included two sedimentary types, red sandstone and soft limestone (both hardness Mohs 2.5), calcite (Mohs 3–4), hard sandstone and hard limestone (both Mohs 5) and rose granite and diorite (both Mohs 7). All six copper chisels cut the two sedimentary stones well, but cutting calcite, hard sandstone, hard limestone, rose granite and diorite demonstrated that all of the chisels suffered immediate blunting and jagged dents to their edges, discounting them as cutting tools for these stones.

The cutting tests with the bronze chisels on rose granite, diorite, hard sandstone and hard limestone demonstrated that all six chisels sustained serious damage. The two bronze chisels, project nos. 10 and 11, could just cut calcite, but experienced unacceptable damage. Only the bronze chisels 18, 22 and 25 cut calcite reasonably well, but required sharpening at intervals not consistent with the efficient use of the tools. Consequently, it is likely that the hardest ancient bronze chisels lost metal at a rate that was unacceptable to ancient craftworkers. The bronze chisels also cut red sandstone and soft limestone with ease, both the softer copper and bronze chisels sustaining slight wear over time. The test cutting of hard and soft woods with project copper and bronze chisels shows that all of these tools possess superior hardness to all woods, requiring only infrequent sharpening of their cutting edges.

As part of my MPhil research I studied several metal chisels found by Sir Flinders Petrie at 12th Dynasty Kahun (Petrie 1890: pl. XVII, 4; Petrie 1891: pl. XIII, 14, 16; Petrie 1917: 20, pl. XXII, C79; Stocks 1988, I: 45–6, 79, fig. 10, a–c). G. R. Gilmore's (1986: 458) composition analyses of three of the Kahun chisels, J. H. Gladstone's (1890: 227) composition analysis of a fourth Kahun chisel and composition analyses for a New Kingdom chisel (Colson 1903: 191) and for two chisels from the 12th and 18th Dynasties respectively (Sebilian 1924: 8) enabled estimates of the hardnesses of two ancient copper chisels and five ancient bronze

Table 35.2   Hardness estimates for some ancient copper and bronze chisels

Number	Metal type	Cu %	As %	Sn %	Fe %	Estimated VPN
1	copper	96.00	2.37	–	0.54	150–60
2	bronze	93.00	0.94	3.33	1.31	165–75
3	copper	97.00	1.11	0.61	–	140–50
4	bronze	96.35	0.36	2.16	–	160–70
5	bronze	84.60	–	13.30	0.30	245–55
6	bronze	92.60	–	7.40	–	210–20
7	bronze	88.00	–	12.00	–	240–50

Abbreviations: Cu = copper, As = arsenic, Sn = tin, Fe = iron

Note: Analyses 1–3 (Gilmore 1986: 458); analysis 4 (Gladstone 1890: 227); analysis 5 (Colson 1903: 191); analyses 6, 7 (Sebilian 1924: 8). Blanks indicate elements not determined.

chisels to be made. This allowed assessments of what wood and stone types these chisels could cut when compared with the project manufactured copper and bronze chisels' cutting capabilities. (See Table 35.2 for the composition analyses and for the hardness estimates).

No project replica chisel contains arsenic, although composition analyses of some ancient chisels record this metallic element (Table 35.2). J. Maréchal (1957: 132–3) conducted hardness tests on three copper and arsenic alloys. They contained 4.2 per cent, 5.94 per cent and 7.92 per cent of arsenic and reached hammered hardness VPN 195, 220 and 224 respectively. These arsenical copper alloys all exceed the hardness of cold-rolled mild steel. The third result shows reasonable hardness comparability to the writer's project no. 18 bronze chisel containing 8 per cent tin, hardness VPN 232, as opposed to Maréchal's 7.92 per cent arsenical copper of hardness VPN 224.

In conclusion, the project hardness results recorded for the experimentally manufactured copper and bronze chisels with their known metallic compositions and cutting abilities, together with Maréchal's three arsenical copper hardness results and the scientific methods for determining the composition analyses of some ancient copper and bronze chisels, allowed estimates to be made for the hardness and cutting capabilities of the group of ancient copper and bronze chisels listed in Table 35.2. Evaluation of this research suggests that no experimental copper or bronze chisel for this study, nor *any* ancient copper or bronze chisel, could effectively cut stone other than red sandstone, soft limestone, gypsum (Mohs 2) and steatite (Mohs 3). All of the experimental chisels cut hard and soft wood types easily, indicating that ancient copper and bronze chisels were practical for this purpose.

Fitting limestone blocks into the Great Pyramid of Giza

At Giza during the 4th Dynasty Khufu built his Great Pyramid (Plate 16) using large limestone core-blocks and casing-blocks for its construction. Not only did Khufu's masons make each block's top and bottom joint surfaces accurately flat, but they are also parallel to each other and truly horizontal towards the pyramid's central axis and along each of the four sides. Parallelism between each block's top and bottom joint surfaces is essential to guarantee the pyramid's structural stability. How did craftworkers achieve such remarkable accuracy in fitting millions of limestone blocks into Khufu's pyramid? There are several clues helping experimental research into this enigma.

Firstly, Flinders Petrie made careful measurements of the rising joints of several of the remaining large casing-blocks at the base of the northern side of the Great Pyramid. The measurements revealed that 'The mean thickness of the joints of the north-eastern casing-stones is 0.02 inches [0.5 mm], and therefore the mean variation of the cutting of the stone from a straight line and from a true square is but 0.01 [0.25 mm] on a length of 75 inches [1.9 m] up the face ...' (Petrie 1883: 44).

Secondly, S. Clarke and R. Engelbach (1930: 100) also examined these casing-blocks. They noticed that the tops of the blocks were dressed *after* they had been laid, and that this procedure sometimes involved part of a core-block lying immediately behind a casing-block. This observation has considerable relevance when considering the processes of producing and testing the flatness of the top surfaces of both core-blocks and casing-blocks.

Petrie's measurements of large casing-block joints, the cutting of an immense number of truly horizontal and truly vertical block surfaces, the parallelism of all blocks' top and bottom surfaces and the experiments with replica tools (Stocks 1988, II: 274–92, Stocks 2003a: 572–8; Stocks 2005: 4–9) indicate that three known surface flatness and orientation testing tools existed at the Great Pyramid site, even though these tools have never been found at 4th Dynasty Giza. A set of three wooden rods and string, used for testing surface flatness, has been found at 12th Dynasty Kahun (Petrie 1890: 27). Two model tools were found in the 19th Dynasty tomb of Senedjem (Theban tomb 1) at Deir el-Medina, each fitted with a plumb line, being the wooden frame for testing horizontal surfaces, shaped like the letter A, and the wooden frame for testing vertical surfaces, shaped like the letter F (Petrie 1917: pl. XLVII, B57, 59).

In the 18th Dynasty tomb of Rekhmire (Theban tomb 100) at Thebes, an illustration (Davies 1943, II: pl. LXII) depicts the testing of a block's vertical surface flatness between cutting and dressing operations, which is achieved by holding two short rods of wood upright on the surface, a string being tautly stretched between the tops of the rods. A mason holding a third rod of equal length against the string shows how much stone needs to be pared away at that point. Other ancient evidence (Petrie 1909: 72) suggests that, after each surface test along the string's length, a craftworker's finger dabbed red ochre on the indicated higher places, these probably being removed with flint scrapers and sandstone grinders; the rods and string would similarly test and direct adjustments to the whole surface until the third rod just touched the underneath of the string.

The 12th Dynasty set of three rods and string is displayed in the Manchester Museum (acc. no. 28). Petrie measured the rods (Petrie 1890: 27) and found that their lengths 'are 4.96 inches [12.6 cm], equal within two or three thousandths of an inch [0.075 mm]'. To make each rod of a replica set equal to a tolerance of 0.075 mm, a simple yet effective outside calliper consisting of two stones firmly set opposite each other ensures that the three rods, when each precisely fits lengthways into the gap, are indeed a *matched* set (Stocks 2003b: fig. 7.11). Measurements with a vernier calliper confirm that all three rods are equal in length within a tolerance of plus or minus 0.05 mm, supporting the probable use of an ancient outside calliper (Figure 35.1).

Tests, measurements and mathematical calculations (Timoshenko and Young 1956: 162–7) with the replica rod set used upon a known flat surface demonstrated that the taut string, over a distance of 120 cm, created a catenary curve possessing maximum sag of 0.25 mm at the string's central position. This meant that the top surfaces of core-blocks and casing-blocks, always accurately flattened and directed to be truly horizontal with the A-frame *after* blocks had been laid into position, became slightly concave. It is likely that the bottom surface of a core-block or casing-block needed to be dressed flat while in a temporarily reversed position (top surface uppermost) before being hauled up

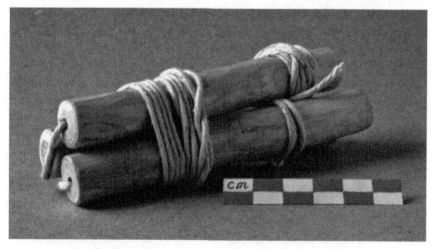

35.1 Replica rods and string set. (Photograph by the author.)

to the pyramid, turned over and laid on the blocks' prepared surfaces below it. A bottom surface of a block dressed and tested with rods and string in an upper horizontal position would also become slightly concave. However, a dressed and tested vertical surface, as seen in the tomb of Rekhmire, would remain truly straight, as a string stretched between the rods would sag not towards it, but downwards to the ground under the influence of gravity.

These procedures guaranteed that the top and bottom surfaces of any block became automatically parallel, an absolute necessity for the pyramid's construction. The gypsum mortar used for sliding a block over a lower block filled slight hollows between the blocks' surfaces, later setting hard and evenly transmitting the weight of an upper block upon supporting lower blocks' surfaces. This phenomenon prevented the blocks from cracking under load.

Henry Gorringe (1885: 83) measured one of the Luxor temple granite obelisks which is now displayed in Paris. He noted that the obelisk's north-west face, as it originally stood in the Luxor temple before its removal, is longitudinally convex, and that the opposite south-east face is longitudinally concave; the obelisk is 25 m long. Over this length, the convex north-west face has a maximum deflection of 2 cm from a straight line, while the concave south-east face has a maximum deflection of 1.27 cm from a straight line. Mathematical calculations confirm that, over a length of 25 m, a tension of 14 kg force in a 2 mm diameter string allowed it to sag 1.27 cm at its central point. The obelisk's finished surface would follow the string's catenary curve and become concave. The south-east face's concavity indicates that its surface originally occupied the quarry's floor, before extraction. The longitudinal convex surface on the opposite face may be explained by measuring from the concave face, all along it, and marking a line on each of the two opposite adjacent vertical faces and, after release of the obelisk from its bed, dressing to the lines to complete the fourth, now convex, face. Measurements and the transposition of mathematical formulae based on the scientific laws of gravity allow the calculation of the precise forces, and the catenary curve characteristics, applied to the rods and string sets used thousands of years ago by craftworkers.

Fashioned from three pieces of wood in an 'A' shape for testing horizontal surfaces (Stocks 2003b: fig. 7.2), the replica frame's plumb line hangs from a hole drilled into the apex (see Figure 35.2). In calibrating a replica tool, the frame's two free ends need just to touch the surface of still water, a vertical mark being made on the horizontal bar exactly behind the hanging plumb line. Reasoning skills are likely to have suggested to ancient craftworkers that still water equated to the flat, horizontal limestone block surface required to build the pyramid, reinforced by knowledge of irrigation techniques that highlighted one of still water's characteristics, a flat horizontal surface in all directions. Further, craftworkers probably reasoned that plumb lines always hang vertically to the flat

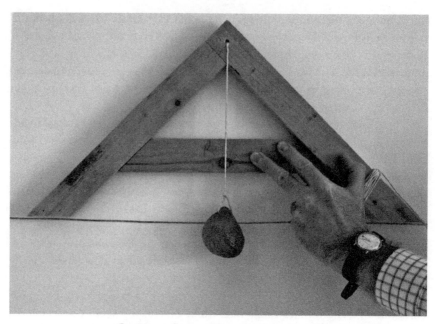

35.2 Replica A-frame. (Photograph by the author.)

surface of still water. The water calibrated replica A-frame, when employed to test two adjoining core-blocks' horizontal surfaces at the Great Pyramid (undertaken with the kind permission of the Supreme Council for Antiquities), demonstrated that the plumb line hung directly over the calibration mark, proving that the blocks are still precisely horizontal and suggesting that craftworkers used the still-water method accurately to calibrate the frame for testing horizontal surfaces in ancient times. The replica rods and string verified that these particular blocks are still accurately flat.

A replica vertical testing F-frame (Stocks 2003b: fig. 7.3) needs the two horizontal pieces to be of exactly the same length, using the outside calliper to achieve this requirement *after* firmly fastening them to the vertical length of wood (Figure 35.3). A hole drilled in the top of the vertical piece, and another hole drilled at an angle of forty-five degrees through the end of the upper horizontal piece, permitted the plumb line to be threaded through the two holes, leaving the line hanging freely against the lower horizontal piece when truly vertical. Provided that each piece of timber was accurately made and fitted together, using an outside calliper for final adjustments, ancient instruments automatically became calibrated at the end of the construction process.

A test with the replica F-frame upon the exposed joint-face of a large casing-block at the Great Pyramid showed that it had been made truly vertical, the

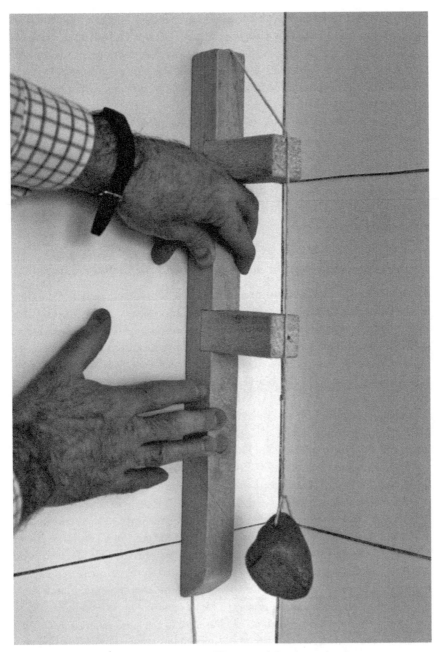

35.3 Replica F-frame. (Photograph by the author.)

plumb line just touching the upper and lower wooden pieces of the F-frame, indicating its use for building this pyramid. The replica rods and string set verified that the casing-block's joint-face is truly flat, suffering no discernible concavity. Bringing two casing-blocks together, their rising joint surfaces truly flat and truly vertical to the already prepared bottom surfaces, achieves the joint accuracy seen today.

The experimental use and evaluation of the three calibrated replica tools demonstrate that they are capable of directing stone block surface and orientation accuracy similar to observed surface and orientation accuracy for blocks in the Great Pyramid, and the verification of several Great Pyramid blocks' surface flatness and orientation with the replica tools strongly suggests that ancient calibrated rods and string sets, A-frames and F-frames existed in the early 4th Dynasty at Giza.

Sliding technology for stone blocks and for inclined ramps

Ancient Egyptian masons mitigated the effects of friction and gravity for sliding heavy limestone blocks by employing gypsum mortar as a lubricant (Edwards 1986: 284). For reducing friction between the runners of a loaded sledge on level surfaces and on shallowly inclined ascending ramp surfaces, craftworkers probably utilised a wetted, compacted clay or lime marl track (Newberry 1895, I: pl. XV; Lehner 1999: 641), but not for moving objects down steeper descending tomb corridor surfaces.

In scientific terms (Timoshenko and Young 1956: 50) the friction that must be overcome to move any block is proportional to the coefficient of friction, μ (mu), and the Normal force, N. (The coefficient of friction is a function of the type of surfaces in contact and the Normal force is the vertical force of gravity acting on the block.) The force F required to move a block is $F = \mu N$. If F is taken as the force necessary to *start* sliding, μ is called the coefficient of *static* friction. If F is taken as the somewhat smaller force necessary to maintain sliding, μ is called the coefficient of *kinetic* friction: only static friction is considered here.

The coefficient of static friction is the tangent of the angle of a ramp on which a block just starts to slide down. It can, therefore, be measured experimentally. The force required is independent of the area in contact, and, since the weight is fixed, the ease of moving a block can only be altered by changing the coefficient of friction, which is the character of the surfaces in contact. This is what the ancient Egyptians accomplished: they prepared blocks' sliding surfaces to a considerable degree of accuracy, using a lubricant between them, and wetted marl as a lubricant for level and ascending ramp track surfaces.

In order to investigate the sliding characteristics of dry and lubricated horizontal limestone blocks, together with lubricated ascending inclines and dry descending inclines, experiments began with two prepared limestone blocks and a wooden sledge runner. The *dry*, accurately flat surfaces of the prepared experimental limestone blocks were placed in contact, one block above the other, and the bottom block was slowly tilted until the top block just began to slide across its surface (Stocks 2003b: 195–6, figs. 7.17, 7.18), the angle of tilt being thirty-six degrees, and similarly for the dry sledge runner (Figure 35.4). The tangent of this angle gives a coefficient of static friction of 0.73. The test was then repeated with liquid gypsum mortar applied to the bottom block's top surface. The upper block now commenced sliding at an angle of eight degrees, giving a coefficient

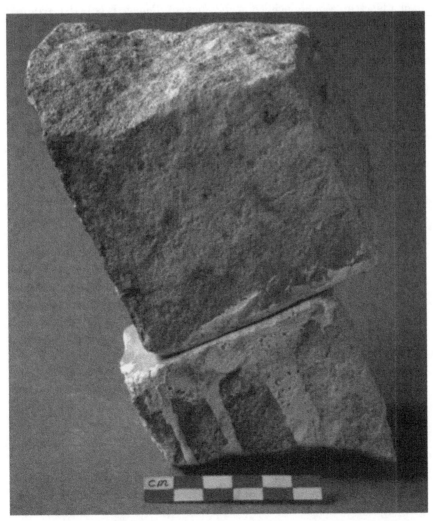

35.4 Stone blocks for sliding experiments. (Photograph by the author.)

of static friction of 0.14, and similarly for the sledge runner operating on a wet clay surface.

If the experimentally obtained dry and lubricated coefficients of static friction are respectively substituted in the formula $F = \mu N$, when applied to a base casing-block weighing 16,000 kg (Petrie 1883: 44), it can be shown that just over *five* times less force is needed to start a lubricated block moving than for a similar dry block. Under the laws of friction this reduction factor applies to all blocks, no matter what their weight and area of surface contact.

Hauling a block on a sledge up a ramp required a balance between the force required and the angle at which slippage occurred. The force needed to haul a block up a slope inclined at the angle of slippage is *twice* that required on the flat (Timoshenko and Young 1956: 162–7) lubricated or dry. This fact, and the risk of losing a block through slippage, mean that the ramp should be inclined at less than the angle of slippage. This explains why the angles of slopes for extant ancient Egyptian ascending ramps are less than eight degrees, the angle of slippage for wet marl lubricated sledge runners (Stocks 2003b: 576).

For example, the 19th Dynasty Papyrus Anastasi I in the British Museum (BM 10247) gives measurements for a hypothetical ramp inclined at an angle of five degrees. The causeway in front of Khafre's pyramid is inclined at six degrees (established by the writer for this study). The ramp angle of the unfinished 4th Dynasty mortuary temple of Menkaure is just over seven degrees (Edwards 1986: 280). Two stone-built loading ramps in Lower Nubia have a calculated gradient of seven degrees (Shaw *et al.* 2001: 33–4).

However, ramps steeper than eight degrees could have been in use by workers for *dry* sliding objects downwards, allowing friction and gravity to work in their favour (Stocks 2009: 38–43). An example is the ascending corridor of Khufu's Great Pyramid, sloping at just over twenty-six degrees, down which three granite plug blocks were probably dry-slid to the bottom, this angle of slope being confirmed by the writer for this study. Experiments and calculations demonstrate that moving a heavy object down a ramp's dry surface, even one on a wooden sledge, which inclines ten degrees less than the dry slippage angle of thirty-six degrees requires a relatively small increase of force to overcome friction, thus permitting workers carefully and safely to move a heavy object down the ramp. A safety margin of at least ten degrees of slope angle prevents a resting heavy object on a dry ramp's surface from sliding down it, because of friction continually overcoming the force of gravity.

The application of scientific studies in Egyptology develops fresh areas of research, engaging the interest and expertise of a wider body of people: this enables Egyptologists further to interpret archaeological evidence of many kinds. The value of scientific studies in Egyptology, allied to those of a technological nature, is to reveal new, exciting and important insights into many aspects of ancient Egyptian civilisation.

References

Clarke, S. and Engelbach, R. (1930), *Ancient Egyptian Masonry* (Oxford: Oxford University Press).

Colson, M. A. (1903), 'Sur la fabrication de certains outils métalliques chez les Égyptiens', *Annales du Service des antiquités de l'Égypte* 4, 190–2.

Davies, N. de G. (1943), *The Tomb of Rekh-mi-Rē' at Thebes* (New York: Metropolitan Museum of Art).

Edwards, I. E. S. (1986), *The Pyramids of Egypt* (Harmondsworth: Penguin Books).

Gilmore, G. R. (1986), 'The composition of the Kahun metals', in A. R. David (ed.), *Science in Egyptology: Proceedings of the 'Science in Egyptology' Symposia* (Manchester: Manchester University Press), 447–87.

Gladstone, J. H. (1890), 'On copper and bronze of ancient Egypt and Assyria', *Proceedings of the Society of Biblical Archaeology* 12, 227–34.

Gorringe, H. H. (1885), *Egyptian Obelisks* (London: J. C. Nimmo).

Lehner, M. (1999), 'Pyramids (Old Kingdom), construction of', in K. A. Bard (ed.), *Encyclopedia of the Archaeology of Ancient Egypt* (London and New York: Routledge), 639–46.

Maddin, R., Stech, T., Muhly, J. D. and Brovarski, E. (1984), 'Old Kingdom models from the tomb of Impy: metallurgical studies', *Journal of Egyptian Archaeology* 70, 33–41.

Maréchal, J. R. (1957), 'Les outils égyptiens en cuivre', *Métaux, corrosion, industries* 32, 132–3.

Newberry, P. E. (1895), *El-Bersheh* (London: Egypt Exploration Fund).

Petrie, W. M. F. (1883), *The Pyramids and Temples of Gizeh* (London: Field and Tuer).

Petrie, W. M. F. (1890), *Kahun, Gurob and Hawara* (London: Kegan Paul, Trench, Trübner, and Co.).

Petrie, W. M. F. (1891), *Illahun, Kahun and Gurob* (London: David Nutt).

Petrie, W. M. F. (1909), *The Arts and Crafts of Ancient Egypt* (Edinburgh and London: T. N. Foulis).

Petrie, W. M. F. (1917), *Tools and Weapons* (London: British School of Archaeology in Egypt).

Rickard, T. A. (1932), *Man and Metals*, I (2 vols; London: Arno Press).

Rollason, E. C. (1939), *Metallurgy for Engineers* (London: Butterworth–Heinemann).

Sebilian, J. (1924), 'Early copper and its alloys', *Ancient Egypt*, 6–15.

Shaw, I., Bloxam, E. G., Bunbury, J., Lee, R., Graham, A. and Darnell, D. (2001), 'Survey and excavation at the Gebel el-Asr gneiss and quartz quarries in Lower Nubia (1997–2000)', *Antiquity* 75, 33–4.

Stocks, D. A. (1988), 'Industrial Technology at Kahun and Gurob: Experimental Manufacture and Test of Replica and Reconstructed Tools with Indicated Uses and Effects upon Artefact Production' (MPhil thesis, University of Manchester).

Stocks, D. A. (2003a), 'Immutable laws of friction: preparing and fitting stone blocks into the Great Pyramid of Giza', *Antiquity* 77, 572–8.

Stocks, D. A. (2003b), *Experiments in Egyptian Archaeology: Stoneworking Technology in Ancient Egypt* (London and New York: Routledge).

Stocks, D. A. (2005), 'Auf den Spuren von Cheops' Handwerkern', *Sokar* 10, 4–9.

Stocks, D. A. (2009), 'Das Bewegen schwerer Steinobjekte im Alten Ägypten: Experimente in der Ebene und auf geneigten Flächen', *Sokar* 18, 38–43.

Timoshenko, S. and Young, D. H. (1956), *Engineering Mechanics* (Tokyo: McGraw-Hill).

36

Snake busters: experiments in fracture patterns of ritual figurines

Kasia Szpakowska and Richard Johnston

When we speak of interdisciplinary research in Egyptology, we often mean the use of a tangential approach or resource as a tool to explicate an Egyptological problem. Few Egyptologists have so effectively succeeded in actually melding disciplines as has Rosalie David. She has inspired me to explore scientific methodologies to answer Egyptological questions: to make use of experimentation, and to have the courage to team up with scientific colleagues 'across campus'. It is in this interdisciplinary spirit that we offer this discussion of initial experiments in the arts, crafts and engineering of making and breaking clay figurines.

Over 700 fragments of solid clay figurines in the shape of rearing cobras have been discovered in fifteen settlements, military and administrative centres in Egypt along the Mediterranean from Libya and into the Levant (Szpakowska 2012, 2003). The rituals and beliefs associated with the cobra must have been an important part of the self-identity and ethnicity of the Egyptians, important enough for them to take their cult with them on the road. Interpreting them is difficult as most of them are not inscribed, and there are no texts definitively associated with their use. Their fabric, manufacture, style and breakage points, as well as their context, do provide clues to the original function of the serpents as votives, avatars, components of spells, apotropaic devices or decorative elements. Because most have been found fragmented, and some with surprisingly 'clean' breaks, it could be suggested that this was the result of ritual or at least intentional breakage. However, no experiments have ever been carried out on figurines such as these to establish whether the cause of the breakage can be ascertained with any degree of certainty on the basis of the fractures themselves. Barring the existence of external supporting evidence, the only way to test this is to actually replicate the destruction in a number of different ways (accidental, 'ritual' or crushing, or a combination thereof) to determine whether they reveal any diagnostic fracture features. Since we cannot destroy the original artefacts, the idea was formed to experiment on modern versions.

Related to the problem of their breakage are questions related to their production. Did professionals create these objects, or could unskilled individuals have made them? What kind of variation might we expect if they were not produced in a specific workshop or by a skilled person?

Between 2010 and 2013, a series of experiential and experimental events were held in the hope of adding a new dimension to our understanding of these figurines. This chapter focuses on two of these events: a workshop on making figurines and a fracturing experiment performed on replica figurines. Three basic stages constituted the process to begin to answer all of these questions.

1. As part of the conference 'Experiment and Experience: Ancient Egypt in the Present',[1] a session was held called 'Making and Breaking Ritual Clay Objects'.
2. A professional potter produced and fired forty nearly identical replica clay cobras based on illustrations and photos of an excavated complete figurine.
3. The fired replicas were then subjected to breakage tests at the Materials Engineering Department of Swansea University.[2]

Conference experience

In 2010, the conference 'Experiment and Experience: Ancient Egypt in the Present' took place at Swansea University. One of the main goals of the conference was to demonstrate the usefulness of both experimental and experiential archaeology. Experimental archaeology is defined by Bahn (2001: 150) as 'the controlled replication of ancient technologies and behaviour, in order to provide hypotheses that can be tested by actual archaeological data'. As Graves-Brown (forthcoming) discusses, definitions of experiential archaeology are less well established. She notes that three characteristics of this methodology are:

- The reconstruction of aspects of life in the past;
- The explicitly sensory;
- Practice or action.

Graves-Brown concludes that 'the experimental deals with empirical hypothesis testing whereas experiential is more exploratory'.

1   Podcasts from the conference can be found online at www.egypt.swan.ac.uk/index.php/conferences/397-technology-podcasts (last accessed 12 August 2015).
2   The project was supported by a Swansea University 'Bridging the Gaps' grant.

One of the goals of the conference was to measure the usefulness and effect of both *experience* and *experiment*, as well as to demonstrate the value of cooperation between scholars, crafts and art professionals and the public. Audience participation was encouraged throughout the three days, and for the final session, all delegates, including the speakers and the audience, were invited to be involved in the experience of creating their own ritual objects.

A local coarse clay and tap water were provided, and the members of the audience were encouraged to make their own 'ancient Egyptian' clay cobras. The goal was to gain an impression of the skill set required to create such a figurine, as well as providing participants with opportunities to work with the clay themselves. The individuals in the audience included children and adults, some of them elderly, and ranged from those who had never touched clay to experienced potters. Four volunteers were selected to sit at a table on the top of the stage and create figurines for the benefit of the live streaming broadcast.[3]

Although the results may not have been as visually impressive as the 'Field Project' conceived by Antony Gormley (Gormley 2015), the event was partly inspired by it. For his projects, Gormley asked people in various countries (in Mexico it was a family of brick makers, in the UK it was volunteers and families from schools) to create humanoid figurines. They were given clay with instructions purposefully left vague: 'the pieces were to be hand-sized and easy to hold, eyes were to be deep and closed and the head was to be in proportion with the body' (Tate Liverpool 2004). In a similar vein, the participants at the Swansea University conference were asked to create their own rearing cobra. While they had seen excavated ones during the preceding presentation, the images were not shown during the experience itself, thus allowing for variation (the ancient Egyptian cobras also display a great deal of variation). The result, as with Gormley's work, was artistic and moving in its own right (Figure 36.1).

This event was of value not only for answering the questions noted at the beginning of this chapter, but in particular in relation to the experience shared by all at the conference. Clay is a medium that can be underestimated for the level of skill required to work it and for its value in the creation of ritual objects. Because it is readily available and seemingly simple to work, it may initially be assumed that it was selected as the medium of choice for these reasons alone. However, for many conference delegates it was more difficult to work than they anticipated. The production method chosen by the participants was also simpler than one used for the fabrication of a number of the artefacts. Some of the cobra fragments excavated at Beth-Shean (James, McGovern and Bonn 1993),

3   The podcast of the making can be seen beginning at about the 32:00 mark via the podcast at www.egypt.swan.ac.uk/index.php/conferences/397-technology-podcasts (last accessed 12 August 2015).

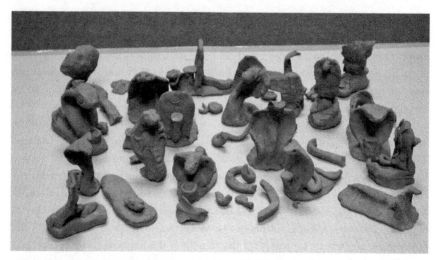

36.1 Sample of clay cobra figurines produced at Swansea University's conference
'Experiment and Experience: Ancient Egypt in the Present', 10–12 May 2010.
(Photograph by the author.)

Kom Rabi'a (Giddy 1999), Akoris (Hanasaka 2011), Tell Abqa'in (Thomas 2011),
Sais (Wilson 2011) and possibly Kom Firin (Spencer 2008) reveal that the figurine as a whole was produced by creating a socket in the base into which the
'tang' of the torso of the cobra would be inserted. This 'tang' would then be
smoothed and more clay applied to strengthen the join. The use of this method
has been confirmed through X-rays of cobras from Beth-Shean (Glanzman and
Fleming 1993: 95–6, pl. 15). However, this technique was not used by anybody
at the conference.

Following the conference, the cobras were curated. Between the year 2010
and the present, the 'decay' of the cobras has led to some interesting questions.
Because the clay was initially not consistently kneaded, and was worked by
amateurs, it was likely that many of the pieces would contain air-bubbles and
had the potential to explode if fired in a kiln. Not surprisingly, at the time of the
conference no professionals were willing to risk their kilns being damaged by
firing the pieces. The pieces were thus allowed to harden naturally. When the
photograph in Figure 36.1 was taken a year later, in May 2011, already some of
the pieces were beginning to naturally fragment and break apart. By the time
of the writing of this chapter, few of the cobras remain intact, emphasising how
remarkable it is that twenty unfired clay cobras managed to survive at Abydos.[4]

4   Factors affecting survival would include the composition of the clay and the
    surrounding burial medium as well as the general environmental conditions of Egypt
    as opposed to Wales.

This also provided us with the opportunity to compare these objects created by amateurs with those created by an individual experienced in working ceramics. While the conference experience was engaging, there were many questions that had yet to be addressed, particularly those related to breakage. These would be better answered through experimentation.

Breakage experiment

In terms of clay figurines, the previous scholarship on breakage experiments is slim at best; many scholars discuss possible ideological or metaphorical reasons for intentional fragmentation, including feelings of repugnance or fear, or ritual killing (Grinsell 1960; Chapman 2000; Becker 2007; Graves-Brown 2010; Bailey 2014). The subject matter is usually objects that have been placed in graves or anthropomorphic figurines. The intentionality of breakage in these cases is often assumed rather than questioned.

Mariko Yamagata's (1992) summary of research concerning Jomon rituals in Japan included examinations of 1116 figurine fragments found at the site of Shakado. Upon physical examination, it was noted that during the fabrication process, those figurines must have been intentionally designed to be easily broken. It was suggested 'lumps of clay were shaped into the head, torso, arms and legs, and attached to each other, often with small wooden pegs. A thin layer of clay was then applied over this basic structure before firing.' The author notes that this creates an inherent weakness in the joints, and that most of the fragments were indeed broken where expected (Yamagata 1992: 131–2). Unusual fabrication is also noted by Lauren Talalay (1987) in her work on eighteen Neolithic Greek split leg figurines. To ensure that separate clay elements will join securely, the edges of the surface of the areas to be joined are usually scored. Talalay notes that the area of the inner surface of these figurines' legs did not in fact show the scoring expected in circumstances where the potter wishes to maximise the strength of the join. She thus suggests that these figurines were created with inherent weaknesses.

Other scholars present less compelling evidence for intentional breakage. In their discussion of over 4000 figurine fragments from Chalcatzingo (Mexico), David Grove and Susan Gillespie (1984: 28) simply state that 'almost all of the figurines had been intentionally broken sometime in the past. The heads had been snapped from the bodies, apparently an important action during the final ritual function of these small artifacts.' Mark Harlan (1987) revisits the enlarged corpus of 6000 Chalcatzingo fragments. While he is mainly concerned with developing a typology, he does note that 'complete figurines are extremely rare. Our large sample clearly shows that most had been broken at the neck area, a pattern so regular that it strongly indicates purposeful breakage. Such decapitation may be akin to the decapitation of monuments' (Harlan 1987: 252). Ann Cyphers Guillén (1993) revisits the Mexican figurines, but her corpus consists of over 8000 fragments from secure archaeological contexts, including Chalcatzingo. She notes that 'despite interpretations of ritual destruction of figurines by breaking off the heads … other body parts are also broken off. Inherent structural weakness in the articulation of limbs and heads may be a more acceptable explanation in the absence of clear evidence for ritual breakage' (Guillén 1993: 213).

While he is more concerned with frameworks for arriving at meaning, Richard Lesure (2002) provides a detailed discussion of the many issues that should be accounted for in discussions of figurines in general fragmentation, but usually are not. These include find-spots, associated artefacts in the same context, statistical analyses, fabrication and use-wear. He also recognises the weakness of claims concerning intentional ritual breakage.

A growing number of scholars are carefully examining the breaks and fragment lines of clay figurines to determine intentionality related to the ancient Mediterranean world (Simandiraki-Grimshaw and Stevens 2013). Elizabeth Waraksa's (2009) work on the female figurines from the Mut precinct is one of the most balanced discussions in terms of Egyptian artefacts and formed an important foundation for this study. However, few experiments have been performed to determine whether or not intentionality can leave visible traces.

One of the goals of our project at Swansea was to see whether or not fractures caused by unintentional breakage could be differentiated from objects intentionally broken. Funding was received to pilot a project to perform more systematic tests with the aid of the Materials Research Centre at Swansea University and an artist familiar with working with clay.

Making figurines

Alicja Sobczak, an artist who studied at Swansea Metropolitan University, was commissioned to create forty replica cobra figurines. During two meetings she was provided with images of a range of cobra figurines and background information. Two videos were made to document the process of making a clay cobra.

The model we chose for replication was one of the Amarna cobras: Ägyptisches Museum und Papyrussammlung, Berlin, ÄM 21961 (Plate 17). Amarna was chosen as this was the site of the earliest known cobra figurines and the location at which were discovered most of the fully and nearly complete ones. In addition, because most of the surviving fragments lack protuberances, we selected one that did not have visible protrusions on the torso.

The clay fabric of most of the Amarna figurines was Nile Silt B2. Sobczak selected a similarly coarse fabric to use for the replicas (10 per cent sanded terracotta) but did not add temper. It should be noted that both the clay and temper thus differed from the originals. As the originals showed no sign of being mould-made, the replicas were hand-formed as well. Sobczak noted that this would create some variability in the form, as would the process itself. Clay itself shrinks during both hardening and firing. This variability and inconsistency is obvious in the archaeological record as well. While many of the ancient figures are similar, no two are identical. The variation can be as subtle as the tilt of the head or the shoulders, and that particular variability (as well as size) became apparent in the replicas.

The replication process took approximately an hour for each model. However, this was in part because the potter was carefully replicating a specific model. Sobczak estimated that it would take an experienced potter who was not attempting to be so precise in replication only approximately twenty minutes to fashion each one. She also suggested that someone with experience would have produced the originals. This was consistent with our findings from the conference.

Experimentation in forming the figurines further supports that they were hand-made. Interestingly, it was difficult for Sobczak to produce a figurine using the technique revealed through X-rays of Beth-Shean figurines. In those figurines, the base was created separately with a concave indentation into which a 'tanged' cobra figurine would be slotted (Glanzman and Fleming 1993: 95–6, pl. 15). Sobczak instead used an easier technique that was probably used for many figurines (based on the fragments): she produced all parts, including the head and tail, from a single slab of clay. The experiment also clarified that the tails were functional, helping support the weight of the torso. This helps explain why many of the Egyptian figurines have stubby bases and fat tails; some 'tails' are simple triangular lumps melded to the torso. Both archaeological remains and the modern production confirm that these figurines were not structurally designed for intentional fracturing as were those of the Jomon (Yamagata 1992), nor did they require scoring, as the elements were not created separately.

After drying but before firing the figurines were covered with slip (a mix with stoneware). Then, after being dried for five days, they were painted with red ochre (from Egypt) mixed with water. They were then allowed to dry for another five days before firing.

The fifty replicas were placed in the kiln close together and on a single level. To reach the desired temperature of 800°C, they were fired in the following stages:

1. The temperature was raised by 10°C per hour until 150°C was reached. The objects 'soaked' at this temperature for 30 minutes.
2. The temperature was increased from 150°C at a rate of 25°C per hour until 250°C was reached.
3. The temperature was increased from 250°C at a rate of 35°C per hour until 573°C was reached.

4. The temperature was increased from 573°C at a rate of 50°C per hour until a temperature of 800°C was reached. This temperature was maintained for one hour.

5. They were then left to cool.

There was little fragmentation; only one head was separated during removal from the oven. Overall, producing the replicas provided important insights into the likely manufacturing process of many of the ancient Egyptian cobra figurines that can be summarised as follows:

- They were probably made by experienced potters (or amateur talented individuals).
- The figurines were hand-made, not moulded.
- The head was easier to make at the same time.
- The tail was important for structural support.
- The 'tanged' process that was at least partially used at ancient Egyptian sites was more difficult and its utilisation requires further investigation.

Breaking figurines

In preparation for the fracturing experiments, each of the replicas was numbered, photographed from six sides, and placed in a numbered box that eventually held all the collected fragments. Rather than dropping the objects on the concrete floor, we decided to create a surface that would be closer to the material of an ancient Egyptian floor. The project assistant, undergraduate engineering student Josh McMahon, created a 'mud floor' using mud from the Swansea University field, clay from Swansea Bay and straw from harvest mouse bedding. He mixed it together in a turkey roasting tin, and because the weather was not dry enough to allow the mud to harden in the sun, it was baked in an oven in the engineering building at 60°C for two days (all the while apparently emitting a most noxious odour).[5]

To record the process, we borrowed a Photron Fastcam SA-3 monochrome high-speed camera, recording at a speed of 3000 frames per second and with a frame size of 1024 × 576 pixels, from the EPSRC loan pool. This turned out to be very important, as the impacts were more unpredictable than anticipated and some fragments bounced on the 'mud floor' to further shatter on the concrete floor. The super-slow-motion camera allowed us to identify fragments that were created by the initial impact, and only these were used for this study. A measuring rod was used to ensure that each figurine was dropped

---

5   At the 2012 annual conference of the American Research Center in Egypt Salima Ikram suggested that a floor of cardboard and sand would have more closely mimicked the floor of an ancient Egyptian dwelling.

consistently from the height of 90 cm. This height was selected as it was the maximum height of many of the emplacements in Amarna homes, and it is not too far off the height of a hand which can accidentally drop an item while carrying it.

The possible causes for object breakage after successful creation are numerous: accidental impact by being dropped while transported or falling off a shelf or niche and intentional impact by smashing, snapping, crushing or being subjected to external force, as well as a range of post-depositional processes. With our limited number of replicas and limited time we chose to perform twenty-four 'accidental' drop tests from various angles. While forty figurines were initially produced, some of them were much larger or thicker than the average, and these were excluded from the tests. Four figurines were initially held horizontally face down, four face up and eight on the side (both sides), and four were held vertically by the base and four by the top of the head. It should be noted that the point of impact was often very different from that expected on the basis of the position in which it was held at the start of the drop.[6]

Aside from the ritualistic 'breaking of the red pots' there is little detailed ancient Egyptian evidence of the specific methods that could have been used. In her discussion of ancient Egyptian female figurines, Waraksa (2009: 70) presents possible scenarios wherein a figurine could have been intentionally broken. These include being snapped at midpoint and, based on the 'breaking the red pots' descriptions, by the figurine being placed 'on a hard surface and then deliberately and precisely smashed at its mid-section with a pestle, hammer, or similar instrument, or cracked across a person's knee'. On the basis of Waraksa's discussions, our 'ritualistic' breakage was performed through two tests: one consisted of striking the object with a rock, the other of holding it horizontally with two hands and snapping it.

Discussion and conclusions

The results of the experiments were not always as expected. For example, when held horizontally by the base and the top and then intentionally snapped with equal pressure on each part, cobra no. 36 did not break into the expected two cleanly fractured parts at midpoint (Waraksa 2009: 70). Instead, our figurine snapped into *three* parts (Figure 36.2). While the two fragments held in the hands did show relatively clean breaks, a third section broke free and launched dramatically into the air. The high-speed camera allowed us to see that this 'third' section consisted of a middle section, from the front down to the front

6   So the impact of a figurine dropped vertically head first was not necessarily on its head; it might rotate in the air and fall on its side or base instead.

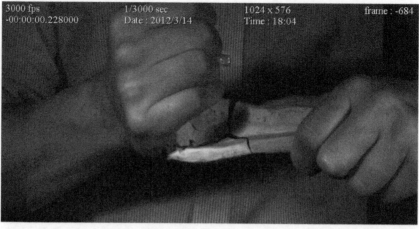

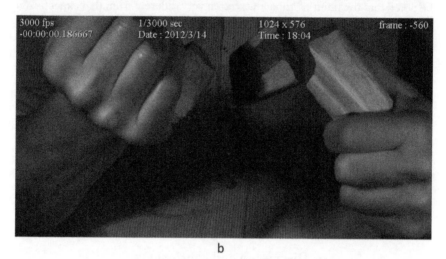

36.2 Replica cobra intentionally snapped at midpoint. (Photograph by
the author.)

of the base. The two end pieces, which included the thicker section of clay
running down the back to the base, remained firmly held in the hands. Many
of the cobra fragments show varying thicknesses caused either by adding inte-
grated 'tails' for support or by protuberances (offering bowls or snakes) added
to the front. However, it would be worthwhile to perform fracture experiments
on replicas shaped like the Mut female figurines discussed by Waraksa as well
as on replicas of cobras shaped with 'bare torsos' and no additional thickness
down the back, or at least ones where the thickness begins much closer to
the base. Our piece fractured at the join; without the added material there it

might well have broken into two equal pieces, but at this point it is impossible to tell.

Other interesting observations included the creation of 'clean breaks'. While intuitively it would seem as though accidental breakage would not cause fractures with sharp straight edges, again, the experiments proved otherwise. As an example of intentional breakage, cobra no. 33 was placed standing upright upon the replica floor. When deliberately hit with a stone upon its head, the figurine remained standing with the head and shoulders cleanly breaking off. But 'accidental' breakage also caused strikingly straight fractures across the shoulder. Sharp clean fractures occurred on cobra no. 25 (initial impact with the floor occurred on the back of the base), no. 18 (impact was on the neck and shoulder) and nos. 11 and 9 (which were impacted on their bases). The high-speed camera revealed a possible mechanism for the fracture of no. 9: spallation or internal rupture under shock loading, resulting in failure at a remote point away from the local point of impact or contact with the floor (Figure 36.3a). Again, the breaks usually occurred just above the thickness added to the torso. It could be that if the thickness had begun lower, the fracture would have occurred lower as well.

Clean fractures such as this occur on cobras from ancient Egypt as well as on various parts of cobra figurines (as is the case with the replicas). A sample of ones with clean fractures across the base of the shoulders includes fragments from the Workmen's Village in Amarna (WV.330 in Kemp 1981: 15), Memphis (EES 518 and 530 in Giddy 1999), Beth Shean (984113/9 in David 2009), Akoris (016 in Hanasaka 2011: 70, fig. 4) and Sais (S390 in Wilson 2011; Figure 36.3b). This could suggest that factors that might intuitively be thought to indicate ritual breakage, such as clean or even consistent breaks, might occur through accidental breakage as well.

As the data for all the archaeological specimens has not yet been fully input or analysed, full comparative results await future publication. The fragments were classified using the same coding as is being used for the ancient ones (for example, a fragment consisting of a head only is classified as 'b', head plus shoulders is 'bc', base only is 'f', etc.). The angles of the breaks are classified as well. This will allow patterns to be discerned. For example, is there any consistency in terms of which fragments remain based on the point of impact? Is there any pattern related to the angle of the break? Figure 36.4 demonstrates one of the simpler results based on twenty-four drop tests.

From the initial twenty-four whole objects, impact from the floor resulted in sixty-three fragments, and the secondary impact with the concrete resulted in forty-two more. Figure 36.4a graphically shows the statistics for the number of fragments occurring from the initial impact with the replica floor versus secondary impact with the concrete floor of the laboratory. For each impact point, the pie charts show the median number of fragments that each figurine breaks into

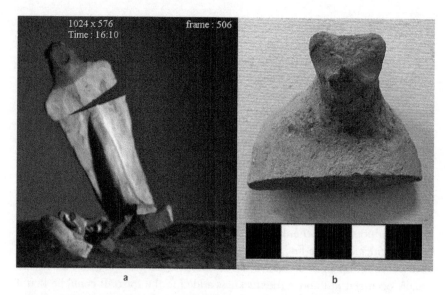

36.3 (a) Dropped replica cobra showing clean break. (Photograph by the authors.)
(b) Sais S390. (Photograph by Penny Wilson.)

(note that a value of '1' implies that the figurine did not break; a null value would suggest that no fragments remained). The overlying black bar shows the range of fragmentation for each figurine subset. In the top graph of Figure 36.4a, labelled 'Primary impact on mudbrick', the maximum number of fragments (and thus the radius axis) is five. When taking into account the secondary impact via concrete, the radius axis is ten (although fragmentation into this number of pieces is very much an outlier). The length of the black bar could indicate that the number of fragments obtained from impact on the base or the head of the figurines is less predictable with impact on other parts, since the bar spans the whole length of the radius axis.

Figure 36.4b reflects the angles at which the breaks occurred based on point of impact. The break angle was recorded according to whether it occurred on the top (i.e. the top of the head, or upper part of torso) or front (i.e. the front of the base) versus fracture of the base (i.e. the bottom of the head or torso) or the back (i.e. the back of the base). Here again there seem to be indications of some sort of consistency. Booth notes the similarity between the 'Base' and the 'Head' pie charts, perhaps indicating that impacts occurring on either of these points could cause the figurine to fragment in the same way. The 'Back Base', 'Back Neck/Shoulder' and 'Front' charts also look to share characteristic break patterns. A more nuanced analysis will take into account the fragment part classification (i.e. whether the fragment includes the head and shoulder, 'bc', or base only, 'f'), and compare it with the ancient fragments.

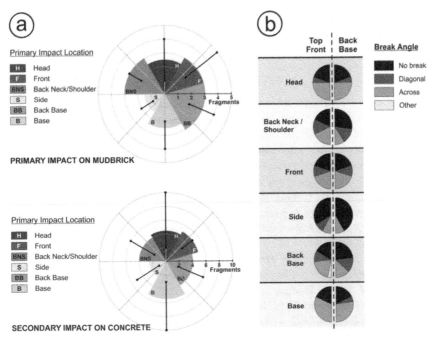

36.4 Results of twenty-four drop tests: (a) number of fragments based on impact with mud floor only, versus mud floor and cement floor combined; (b) break angle correlations with point of impact. (Graphs courtesy of Adam Booth.)

In the end, the pilot projects suggest that it would be worthwhile to perform further full-fledged experiments. Ideally, one replicating the ancient Egyptian conditions more precisely would follow this pilot project. The replicas would ideally be based on two models: one with no protuberances or supporting tail and one with an offering tray and cobras on the front of the torso. The production could take place in Egypt, using local Nile silt clay and temper, and fired in local kilns. The breakages could occur on an actual mud floor or at a site. More cobras could be 'ritually' broken as well. The results could also provide a model for determining causes of breakage of other animal figurines.

Acknowledgements

We acknowledge the use made of a Photron Fastcam SA-3 monochrome high speed camera which was borrowed from the Engineering and Physical Sciences Research Council (EPSRC) Engineering Instrument Pool. The project was supported by an EPSRC 'Bridging the Gaps' grant (EP/I00145X/1). We are grateful to Adam Booth of Imperial College London for creating these graphs in Figure 36.4 and for patiently explaining their significance and bringing these observations to our attention. We are also grateful to Adam Booth and Carolyn Graves-Brown for their helpful comments on this chapter.

References

Bahn, P. (2001), *The Penguin Archaeology Guide* (London: Penguin).

Bailey, D. (2014), 'Touch and the cheirotic apprehension of prehistoric figurines', in P. Dent (ed.), *Sculpture and Touch* (London: Ashgate), 17–43.

Becker, V. (2007), 'Early and middle Neolithic figurines – the migration of religious belief', *Documenta Praehistorica* 34, 119–27.

Chapman, J. (2000), *Fragmentation in Archaeology* (London: Routledge).

David, A. (2009), 'Clay Cobras: Ramesside household cult or apotropaic device?', in N. Panitz-Cohen and A. Mazar (eds.), *Excavations at Tel Beth-Shean 1989–1996: The 13th–11th Century BCE Strata in Areas N and S* (Jerusalem: The Hebrew University of Jerusalem), 556–60.

Giddy, L. (1999), *The Survey of Memphis II. Kom Rabi'a: The New Kingdom and Post-New Kingdom Objects* (London: Egypt Exploration Society).

Glanzman, W. D. and Fleming, S. J. (1993), 'Fabrication methods', in F. W. James, P. E. McGovern and A. G. Bonn (eds.), *The Late Bronze Egyptian Garrison at Beth Shan: A Study of Levels VII and VIII* (Philadelphia: University Museum, University of Pennsylvania), 94–102.

Gormley, Antony, 'Field' (2015), www.mymodernmet.com/profiles/blogs/antony-gormley-field (last accessed 12 August 2015).

Graves-Brown, C. A. (2010), 'The Ideological Significance of Flint in Dynastic Egypt' (PhD dissertation, University College London).

Graves-Brown, C. A. (2015), 'Building bridges: experiential and experimental', in C. Graves-Brown (ed.), *Egyptology in the Present. Experiential and Experimental Methods in Archaeology* (Swansea: Classical Press of Wales), ix–xxxviii.

Grinsell, L. V. (1960), 'The breaking of objects as a funerary rite', *Folklore* 72 (3), 475–91.

Grove, D. C. and Gillespie, S. D. (1984), 'Chalcatzingo's portrait figurines and the cult of the ruler', *Archaeology: An Official Publication of the Archaeological Institute of America* 37 (4), 27–33.

Guillén, A. C. (1993), 'Women, rituals, and social dynamics at ancient Chalcatzingo', *Latin American Antiquity* 4 (3), 209–24.

Hanasaka, T. (2011), 'Archaeological interpretation of clay cobra figurines: based on the study of objects from Akoris', *Journal of West Asian Archaeology* 12, 57–78.

Harlan, M. (1987), 'Chalcatzingo's formative figurines', in D. C. Grove (ed.), *Ancient Chalcatzingo* (Austin: University of Texas Press), 252–63.

James, F. W., McGovern, P. E. and Bonn, A. G. (1993), *The Late Bronze Age Egyptian Garrison at Beth Shan: A Study of Levels VII and VIII*, 2 vols. (Philadelphia: University Museum, University of Pennsylvania).

Kemp, B. J. (1981), 'Preliminary report on the el-'Amarna expedition, 1980', *Journal of Egyptian Archaeology* 67, 5–20.

Lesure, R. G. (2002), 'The Goddess diffracted: thinking about the figurines of early villages', *Current Anthropology* 43 (4), 587–610.

Ritner, R. K. (1993), *The Mechanics of Ancient Egyptian Magical Practice* (Chicago: The Oriental Institute of the University of Chicago).

Simandiraki-Grimshaw, A. and Stevens, F. (2013), 'Destroying the snake goddesses: a re-examination of figurine fragmentation at the temple repositories of the palace of Knossos', in J. Driessen (ed.), *Destruction: Archaeological, Philological and Historical Perspectives* (Louvain: UCL Presses Universitaires), 153–70.

Spencer, N. (2008), *Kom Firin I: The Ramesside Temple and the Site Survey* (London: British Museum Press).

Szpakowska, K. (2003), 'Playing with fire: initial observations on the religious uses of clay cobras from Amarna', *Journal of the American Research Center in Egypt* 40, 113–22.

Szpakowska, K. (2012), 'Striking cobra spitting fire', *Archiv für Religionsgeschichte* 14, 27–46.

Talalay, L. (1987), "Rethinking the function of clay figurine legs from Neolithic Greece: an argument by analogy', *American Journal of Archaeology* 91 (2), 161–9.

Tate Liverpool (2004), 'Antony Gormley: Field', www.tate.org.uk/whats-on/tate-liverpool/exhibition/antony-gormley-field (last accessed 12 August 2015).

Thomas, S. (2011), 'Chariots, cobras and Canaanites: a Ramesside miscellany from Tell Abqa'in', in M. Collier and S. Snape (eds.), *Ramesside Studies in Honour of K. A. Kitchen* (Bolton: Rutherford Press), 119–31.

Waraksa, E. A. (2009), *Female Figurines from the Mut Precinct: Context and Ritual Function* (Fribourg: Academic Press Fribourg).

Wilson, P. (2011), *Sais I: The Ramesside-Third Intermediate Period at Kom Rebwa* (London: Egypt Exploration Society).

Yamagata, M. (1992), 'The Shakado figurines and Middle Jomon ritual in the Kofu Basin', *Japanese Journal of Religious Studies* 19 (2–3), 129–38.